# ARIANE SHERINE & DAVID CONRAD

# How to Live to 100

## What Will **REALLY** Help You Lead a Longer, Healthier Life?

ROBINSON

ROBINSON

First published in Great Britain in 2020 by Robinson

1 3 5 7 9 10 8 6 4 2

A CIP catalogue record for this book
is available from the British Library.

ISBN: 978-1-47214-388-4

Typeset in Adobe Garamond by Hewer Text UK Ltd, Edinburgh
Printed and bound in Great Britain by Clays Ltd, Elcograf S.p.A.

Papers used by Robinson are from well-managed forests and other responsible sources.

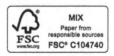

Robinson
An imprint of
Little, Brown Book Group
Carmelite House
50 Victoria Embankment
London EC4Y 0DZ

An Hachette UK Company
www.hachette.co.uk

www.littlebrown.co.uk

*For Lily, with all our love*

# Contents

# Contents

# Contents

# Introduction by Ariane Sherine

If you're reading this, you probably want to live to a hundred.

And why *wouldn't* you want to live a super-long life, if you could remain in good health? You'd get to meet your great-grandkids, try out space travel and the teleporter, and gross out all your descendants by having noisy old-person sex.

I've always been determined to live into my hundreds, but never knew how. My grandmother is ninety-five, so I might have inherited her lucky genes, but I had no idea what I could be doing proactively to help me lead a longer life. I'm a comedian, not a scientist, and there was so much conflicting and confusing health information out there, I didn't have a clue where to start.

Luckily, last year I bumped into David Conrad, a public health expert, and told him about my quest for longevity.

It turned out I'd met the one person willing and qualified to weigh up all the research and evidence and let me know exactly what I needed to do to live a long and healthy life. As someone with both 'evidence' and 'intelligence' in his job title, a Fellow of the Faculty of Public Health, and author of various academic papers and books for health professionals, I figured he ought to know what he was talking about.

I asked David endless questions about all kinds of health topics, and he went away, researched them and provided clear and helpful answers. Then we decided it wasn't entirely fair for this information to remain between us, so we agreed to write it up as a book and let everyone else live to a hundred too.

This is that book, featuring the detailed conversations between us, including all the facts, stats, inappropriate jokes and shameless puns you could ever need to make it to your eleventh decade. David has researched the evidence behind a hundred things that can affect your health – everything from green tea to gardening, fish to flying and sex to sweeteners – and provides tips to maximise your chances of making it to a century.

This book is especially helpful these days, as we often read sensational 'shock horror' health pieces in newspapers. Although great at grabbing our attention, they're often based on a single scientific study and present an oversimplified account of its findings. And, of course, the article you read this week may totally contradict the one you saw last Wednesday.

I needed someone who could look at the balance of evidence across a big list of hot topics and give an accurate picture of what the research is really telling us. Many of David's findings surprised me (who knew that vegans aren't cruising to victory in the race for longevity? Or that the fitter you get, the longer you'll live, with no upper limit?) and I now feel I know which risks are worth taking. (Riding a motorbike? Not even to impress the world's sexiest Hells Angel!)

While we were writing *How to Live to 100*, I asked some celebrity friends what they thought about the subjects discussed, so you'll find interviews with them throughout the book too.

I hope you enjoy it, laugh a lot and learn how to stay in good shape until you get featured in the newspapers as the world's oldest person.

Wishing you a hundred candles to blow out on your birthday cake,

Ariane x

# Part One: Relationships

# Marriage

*It's only chapter 1 and I'm already bracing myself. I just got divorced.*

You'd be right to brace yourself. A lot of research evidence has shown that people who are married tend to have better physical and mental health than those who are unmarried. Scientists have discovered lower rates of death and illness among married people for a range of different health threats, including cancer, heart attacks and surgery.[1]

*Yeah, that's not making me feel any better.*

Sorry, it gets worse: marriage is associated with greater life satisfaction, too. Married men and women have also been found to make better use of healthcare services and are more likely to rate their own health as 'good', 'very good' or 'excellent'.[2]

*You're really not helping. Let's move on – why does marriage extend your life?*

Broadly, two theories have been suggested to explain why married people have better health outcomes – 'selection' and 'protection'. The idea of selection is that people who are in better physical and mental health, or who lead healthier lifestyles, are simply more likely to be considered 'marriage material' and are therefore more likely to get married (and stay married).

*Is 'protection' where they use a condom?*

Protection is the idea that marriage is good for our health because it provides benefits, such as practical and emotional support and a positive influence on our lifestyles.[1] Research shows that it's common for spouses to actively try to improve each other's health behaviours.

*Like shouting 'Move AWAY from the pizza!' through a megaphone?*

Yes, this can include efforts to increase healthy eating and reduce excessive drinking and other risky behaviours, as well as encouraging trips to the doctor and regular health checks.[3] A combination of both selection and protection is likely to explain the link between marital status and health.

*Hang on: I'm sure I read somewhere that marriage is only healthier for men and that it's actually single women who live longer . . .?*

Marriage brings health benefits for both sexes, although yes, they do appear to be greater for men than women.[1] One explanation for this difference which has been proposed by researchers is that wives have a greater tendency to attempt to control their husbands' unhealthy habits than vice versa.[3]

*You mean, by nagging them?*

Let's call it 'making constructive suggestions'. Another factor which could help explain this phenomenon is that wives are less likely to be reliant on their marriage as a sole source of emotional support, with women tending to have more close confidantes with whom they share personal problems.[1]

*Not in my case – my ex-husband was also my best friend. But he and I were barely speaking by the end, so it definitely wasn't emotionally supportive.*

Being happy with the marriage is as important as the marriage itself. Research suggests that it's the satisfaction and support which people get from being in a *good* marriage which are key. Better health outcomes, such as lower stress, lower blood pressure and less depression, are associated with high marital quality.

If you're single, having a strong support network doesn't appear to deliver the same health benefits as being married – suggesting that the relationship with one's spouse may be particularly important for health, compared with other relationships.[4] A large American study using data from 1978 to 2010 found that people who described their marriage as 'very happy' or 'pretty happy' had significantly lower odds of dying over the same period of time than those who described their marriage as 'not too happy'.

*Don't people just let themselves go and put on loads of weight after they're married?*

Again, the quality of the marriage is a critical factor here. A Harvard University study looked at weight gain during marriage over ten years, analysing data from over 2600 married men and women in the US. Although the proportion of people who were obese did increase over that period, having a supportive marital relationship and a good quality marriage were both associated with less weight gain.[5] Being overweight or obese increases the risk of a range of health conditions which can limit the quality and length of our lives, so this in itself is a good reason to seek out a happy marriage.

*How about gay marriage? Do same-sex couples get the same perks?*

Research into the health impact of same-sex marriage in California uncovered a more complex picture compared to heterosexual marriage.[2] The study looked at a range of outcomes, including self-reported health, use of healthcare services and health insurance coverage. Overall, people in gay and lesbian marriages did not experience the same health benefits as people in heterosexual marriages, although there were still some advantages.

*They didn't have to shag straight men?*

Both lesbians and gay men in legally recognised same-sex partner-ships were more likely to have consistent health insurance and use healthcare services than those who were not legally partnered. While gay men in legally recognised partnerships scored better than hetero-sexual married men on some health measures, lesbians in legally recognised partnerships generally fared worse than heterosexual married women. It's not yet clear why gay marriage appears to bring fewer health benefits than heterosexual marriage, although the life-long stress of being in a minority group has been suggested as a possible explanation.[2]

*Do people in gay marriages also nag their spouses to be less fat and lazy, or is that just a straight thing?*

Research has shown that people in same-sex marriages also seek to influence their spouse's lifestyles to try and improve their health. Compared with how this typically plays out in heterosexual marriages, however, there are some differences. Gay and lesbian spouses tend to want to change their partners' exercise habits more than people in heterosexual marriages, and this reflects generally lower levels of physical activity among heterosexual spouses.

*Do they have a view on their partners shovelling doughnuts into their gobs?*

Wives and husbands of all sexual orientations have an equal desire to change their partners' eating habits.[3] We also know that women in lesbian marriages are a lot more receptive to their spouses' attempts to influence their behaviour than women married to men (men married to men also tend to be less appreciative of these efforts).

*So, wedded lesbians get healthier, plus they get to shag women, who generally smell a bit nicer. Some people have all the luck.*

6

*Reality check*

While married people are generally healthier, any marriage isn't necessarily better for you than no marriage. Research shows that being in a low-quality marriage is actually worse for your health than being unmarried.[4]

Although there's good evidence that one of the key benefits of being married is the influence that spouses have on each other's lifestyles, it's been shown that people who are less physically active or heavier than their spouses are more likely to feel irritated by or simply to ignore these efforts. Marrying a fitness fanatic may not be a magic cure for an unhealthy life-style, therefore, if you're not motivated to fix it.

*So basically, we're saying . . .*

Getting married is likely to be a good move in your quest to live to a hundred but ending up hitched to the wrong person could leave you worse off than staying single.

## Charlie Brooker on marriage

*Charlie, you regularly speculate on our possible technological futures in* Black Mirror. *In the future, do you think we'll all be married to solar-powered sex robots instead of people?*

I don't know that they'd replace people, so much as augment their marriage with the robot. Maybe that would mean everyone was in a polyamorous marriage . . .? Would the robots have to resemble people? Maybe instead the robot would be a walking thing with lots of legs and every sort of genital you could imagine. But we won't be married to them, we'll be issued them by the government.

*You're putting me off wanting to live to a hundred now!*

# Cohabitation

*Does living in sin confer the same health perks as marriage, or do you actually have to tie the knot?*

Research across five countries published in 2017 looked at differences between how those who were married and those who were cohabiting with a partner rated their own health. The results showed no differences between cohabiting and married people in Australia, Germany and Norway, while in the UK and US marriage was significantly associated with better self-rated health.[1]

*Then maybe I'll shack up with a Norwegian. The Beatles extolled the virtues of Norwegian wood.*

The researchers, however, found that much of this statistical association between marital status and health was explained by differences in the childhood experiences of married versus cohabiting people. Once childhood factors, such as the structure of people's families and the socio-economic status of their parents, were controlled for in the analysis, differences between the mental health of married people and cohabiters in the UK and US were greatly reduced (although notable differences persisted in the case of British men).[1]

*Stand down, Norwegians! I've changed my mind.*

The experiences we have as children are also important in explaining differences between the mental health of people who are married and those who cohabit with a partner. Certain childhood factors are correlated with marital status in later life.

Researchers in one study took into account how likely people were to marry based on their childhood circumstances to see if this explained any differences between the mental health of married people and cohabiters. They looked at a range of underlying factors which predict the likelihood of marrying, including people's social class at birth, whether they were living with their biological parents at age ten and their educational aspirations. Their analysis showed that in the case of those who were more likely to marry there was no mental health benefit to being married compared with cohabiting.[2]

*That's a relief. I can live in sin without worrying about a hen night full of penis straws.*

In the case of women whose childhood circumstances predicted that they were less likely to marry, however, marriage was associated with better mental health. Even in this group, though, marriage appeared to offer no benefit for cohabiters with shared children who were in a long-lasting relationship.[2]

*OK, so I need a boyfriend, at least to start with.*

Try to choose a healthy one, as there's evidence of an association between our own health and that of our partners. A Dutch study which looked at data for 12,000 married and cohabiting couples found that those whose partners described themselves as in poor health were nearly three times more likely to do the same. This phenomenon is likely to be explained by a combination of factors.[3]

*Shared late-night tiramisu?*

Not necessarily. Firstly, the data showed a connection between people's own level of education and that of their partners. We know that generally those with a higher level of education are more likely to have better health and less likely to engage in unhealthy behaviours, such as smoking.[4] In other words, to an extent, we simply tend to end up living with partners who are already similar to us in terms of their health profile.

*Yeah. You don't want your partner trying to drag you to the gym when* Bargain Hunt *is on.*

Secondly, households develop norms and values relating to health and lifestyle which can affect the health status of the individuals in them. These influences can be either beneficial or harmful – for example, it can be much harder to give up cigarettes if your partner is an ardent forty-a-day smoker than if you're living with someone who has already quit successfully.[3]

*Any other reasons why living with a partner should be good for my health?*

There's evidence that having an affectionate relationship with a supportive partner may help the way your body responds to stressful life events. Researchers tested how people reacted to the stress of a public speaking task after ten minutes of hand-holding with their partners while watching a 'romantic video', followed by a twenty-second hug.

*I hope it wasn't the researchers doing the hugging.*

They compared these participants' responses with those of a control group who had no contact and rested quietly for the same amount of time. Both men and women in the 'warm contact' group showed lower blood pressure and lower increases in heart rate. Over time, the cumulative effect of this kind of intimate contact for couples in supportive relationships may result in a lower risk of cardiovascular disease.[5]

*Noted: always bring a hugger when public speaking. What about flatmates?*

Sharing a home with someone with whom you're not in a relationship does not appear to offer the same health benefits as living with a partner. While differences in childhood circumstances appear to account for much of the variation in health outcomes between cohabiters and people who are married, living with a partner is still associated with better health once these factors are taken into account.[2]

A Finnish study which examined the relationships between people's living arrangements and their mental health found that those who lived alone or with someone other than a partner were around twice as likely to suffer from anxiety or depressive disorders.[6]

*I'm guessing inflatable partners don't count.*

Neither do same-sex partners, oddly. Danish research which looked at data from a thirty-year period found that those who were cohabiting in a heterosexual relationship were less likely to die in that time compared with people who were living alone, with their parents, in shared houses with multiple adults or in same-sex cohabitation. The researchers acknowledged, though, that lifestyle factors such as smoking, excess weight and alcohol intake may account for some of these differences.[7]

*Yeah, I think that if I lived with my mum I'd have to get paralytically drunk in order to cope. She'd probably say the same – so at least we have that in common.*

> ### Reality check
> While the evidence suggests that, for many of us, cohabitation can offer much the same health benefit as marriage, this may not be the case when it comes to keeping in shape. A study of over 20,000 German adults looked at differences in weight gain during cohabitation compared with marriage, with data covering a sixteen-year period. The results showed that, after four years or more, cohabitation led to significant weight gain in both men and women. Marriage was also associated with weight gain but only around half that associated with cohabitation.[8]

*So basically, we're saying . . .*
If you're not currently cohabiting in a warm, supportive relationship with a romantic partner, you should probably start
(but keep an eye on your waistline).

# Divorce

*OK, I just got divorced. Give it to me straight.*

Studies on the impact of marriage breakdown have shown that divorce is associated with poorer mental and physical health, and increased risk of death.[1]

*Can't live with 'em, can't live without 'em.*

A review of published research on the subject, which brought together data from eleven countries, showed that people who are separated or divorced have a significantly increased risk of early death compared with those who are married.[2] A separate review of published research studies on marital status and mortality in the elderly also found that those who were divorced or separated were at higher risk of death, although this was also the case for people who were widowed or never married.[3]

*So why is divorce linked to kicking the bucket?*

Four main theories have been proposed to explain the link between poorer health and divorce.[2] The first explanation is that less healthy people are simply more likely to get divorced. A US study showed that health-related risk-taking behaviours, such as smoking and drug use, are strongly related to a higher risk of divorce for both men and women.[4]

*But I don't smoke or take any drugs! Kinky sex is my only vice.*

Also, divorce itself could result in changes to people's lives which impact negatively on their health. One mechanism might be the loss of access to resources.

*That didn't happen in my case. I was the only earner in my marriage.*

Well, this could either manifest itself in material terms, such as greater financial hardship and living in poorer quality housing, or in relation to more intangible resources, such as emotional support and warm contact – all of which can have an impact on our health.

It's also possible that after getting divorced, people's lifestyles and behaviours change in ways which are bad for their health.

*Well I did have a rebound one-night stand, but I'm not sure it actually went in.*

Finally, if someone were to experience chronic psychological distress as a result of divorce, this could have a detrimental health impact.[2] Research into the effects of divorce and separation on mental health in the UK found that they were associated with increased anxiety and depression. This association remained after a number of other factors were ruled out in the data analysis as possible causes, including aspects of mental health in childhood, financial hardship, and a lack of social contact and support.[5]

*That bit's true in my case. I felt so miserable the Christmas I got divorced, I ate two entire boxes of Quality Street in one sitting. Except for the blue coconut ones, because who likes those?*

I do. Another study, looking at the mental health impact of divorce on women, showed that in the years immediately after divorce, they experienced significantly higher levels of psychological distress compared with married women, leading to higher levels of depressive symptoms in later life.[6] There's also evidence that the impact on mental and physical health is worse for single mothers who marry and then divorce, compared with women who were childless when they got married.[7]

*Oh whoop-de-doo – that's me. Well, there's only one thing for it: I'll just have to get married again. Time to install some dreadful dating apps.*

> *Reality check*
> Although we have good evidence that marriage is associated with better physical and mental health, we also know that the quality of the relationship is of vital importance. A US study using data collected over a twenty-year period found that high levels of marital happiness were associated with better health, while high levels of marital problems were associated with poorer health.[1] When the relationship is primarily a cause of stress rather than a buffer from it, separation followed by divorce is probably the healthiest option.

*So basically, we're saying . . .*
Marital breakdown generally isn't good news for your health but staying in a bad marriage is unlikely to help you live longer either.

# Sex

*Let's bang this one out quickly: will regular bonking make me live forever?*

Although we can't say that having more sex will necessarily mean a longer life, there is some evidence to suggest that a good sex life might have a beneficial impact on life expectancy.

*I think you need to sex up your chat a little. It's not exactly making me aroused.*

That's a relief. Now, do you want the facts or not?

*Ooh baby, I like it when you get all stern with me! It makes me want to—*

I think I'll just carry on. A twenty-five-year study which followed the lives of over 250 people found that a greater frequency of sexual intercourse predicted a lower annual death rate in men, while enjoyment of sexual intercourse predicted a lower death rate in women.[1]

*'Enjoyment'? Does that mean making like Meg Ryan in bed?*

Only if you're not faking it.

*Uh-uhh-uhhhhh! Sorry, where were we?*

I was about to say that another study, which looked at British men over ten years, found that a greater frequency of sexual intercourse was associated with lower death rates, after controlling for other factors such as age and smoking.[1]

*Lower death rates? How much lower are we talking?*

Compared with men who reported having sex at least twice a week, those who had sex less than once a month had twice the death rate. The link between more frequent sexual intercourse and reduced death rates was strongest in the case of coronary heart disease mortality – the major cause of death in most developed countries.[1]

*But hang on – can't sex actually* cause *a heart attack?*

A US study found that a small percentage of sudden cardiac arrests are related to sexual activity; however, the patients in these cases were more likely to have a history of cardiovascular disease, with a majority taking cardiovascular medication.[2] The American Heart Association suggested in 2012 that patients with cardiovascular disease who wish to engage in sexual activity go and see their doctor.[3]

*Why, are their doctors likely to have sex with them?*

Probably not. Mine's never offered.

*Mine neither. He just keeps telling me to exercise for two-and-a-half hours a week. Does sex count towards that tally?*

Exercising your heart is important for maintaining good physical health, and there's no doubt that having sex is one way to achieve this. Sexual arousal will increase your heart rate, with the number of beats per minute reaching a peak during orgasm. Just like other forms of exercise, however, the degree of benefit you'll get depends on how regularly and vigorously you're doing it.[4]

*What about a sneaky hand shandy in the loos at work? Does that count?*

Scientists have compared the exercise value for men of masturbating, being masturbated by a partner, and having sexual intercourse in two different positions ('man on top' and 'woman on top').[1] Unfortunately, they didn't look into the benefits for women.

They studied the men's oxygen uptake, blood pressure and heart rate stimulation and concluded that full sex provides the best workout at the point of orgasm compared to manual stimulation. The 'man on top' position offered men the greatest exercise value; however, 'woman on top' was still superior to either DIY masturbation or masturbation by a partner.

*You said earlier that sex makes men live longer, but what's in it for women?*

Evidence suggests that good quality sex with a partner promotes cardiovascular health for women, specifically reducing the risks of hypertension (high blood pressure).[5]

*Sounds promising. Anything else?*

Some research has shown that a greater lifetime number of sexual partners is associated with a decreased risk of breast cancer.[1]

*I should be safe then! Er, I mean, that can't be right, surely . . .?*

Well, we know that nuns have very high rates of breast cancer, although this is possibly explained by the fact that the risk of breast cancer is known to be reduced by childbearing and breastfeeding, rather than an absence of frequent sexual intercourse in itself.[1]

*Just in case, I think you should pledge personally to save all nuns from this fate.*

*Reality check*

Some of the apparent health benefits of sex have been found to only occur in penile–vaginal intercourse without the use of condoms. Having unprotected sex can bring its own health risks, however. Using a condom will help protect you and your partner against sexually transmitted infections (STIs) as well as unplanned pregnancy.[1]

Studies have shown the average peak heart rate at orgasm is the same as during light exercise, such as walking upstairs, which is not enough to keep most people fit and healthy. Adults should do at least 150 minutes of moderate-intensity aerobic activity every week. Unless you're having 150 minutes of orgasms a week, you should perform other forms of exercise to supplement your sexual activity, such as cycling or walking briskly.[4]

*So basically, we're saying . . .*
Try to have sex twice a week if possible.

## Lou Sanders on sex

*The optimum healthy frequency for having sex is twice a week. Do you have any ideas as to why this might be?*

I think I'm the wrong person to ask because I've just had to throw away a box of condoms which went out of date A YEAR AGO.

But thinking about it, it kind of makes sense because if you're not banging at all, that can't be good for the soul, or morale, or confidence. But if you're constantly banging, something is going to go. Hips, knees, groin – it's all taking an impact.

Yes, a nice twice a week sounds lovely. Still a lot of room to get some admin done.

# Having children

*Having my daughter Lily is the best decision I ever made. Could it mean I live longer, too?*

Overall, parents do live longer than people who don't have children. A nationwide study in Sweden has shown that both men and women who have at least one child experience lower death rates than their childless peers.[1]

*That's amazing. I thought the death rates would be higher due to fatal accidents from tripping over My Little Ponies. Does it matter whether you have a daughter or son?*

The results showed that it doesn't matter whether the child is male or female, although male parents experience a greater boost to their longevity than female parents.[1]

*Boooooo! How much longer?*

By the age of sixty, men with children had two more years of life expectancy than their childless counterparts. Among women, parents had an extra one and a half years than non-parents.[1]

*Not too shabby, then. But is this boost to longevity just because people who are married are more likely to have children?*

Although being in a good marriage or a supportive relationship is associated with better health, the researchers took account of this in their analysis and found that it didn't explain the link between parenthood and life expectancy. They did find, however, that the effect of having children became greater in older age and that it was stronger in people who weren't married. This suggests that the additional social support that parents get from their children, particularly in old age, might be the reason why they tend to live longer.[1]

*I see. Well, this book is dedicated to Lily, so looking after me in old age is the least she can do.*

*Reality check*
Although generally being a parent improves your chances of reaching a hundred, having a child is a major life transition which brings new pressures, and the stresses of parenthood can have a negative impact on well-being. Research shows the sense of increased pressure which comes with having children is greater for mothers than fathers.[2]

*So basically, we're saying . . .*
Generally speaking, having children is a good move in your quest for longevity but there's a chance it could take a toll on your mental health.

# Family and friends

*Don't tell me family are important for a long life. I'm estranged from most of mine.*

The importance of social support for health has been well established by a wealth of research. It's been said that the evidence for a link between social ties and health is no less compelling than that behind the landmark US government report in 1964 linking smoking with specific diseases.[1]

Our relationships with our families and friends, or the lack of them, are an important factor to consider if we want to live long lives in a good state of well-being.

*Well-being? Ha ha! You haven't met my folks.*

While the family can undoubtedly be harmful to both physical and mental health, for many people it's a primary source of social support throughout the life course.[2] For this reason, scientists have been keen to understand the impact of family ties on our well-being and how long we live.

*Hit me with the data that's bound to depress me . . .*

One study brought together data from fifty research publications, looking at the impact of perceived social support on over 100,000 people. The analysis of the data showed that having lower levels of perceived social support was associated with an increased risk of death within a particular timeframe. This applied to both men and women.[3]

*So far, so unsurprising. Anything else?*

The study also found that support from family members was more beneficial to health than support from friends, and that only a moderate degree of additional support was necessary to have an impact. Having social support appeared to become more important with age.[3]

*I guess my daughter is my family, and she's awesome. Though she also says she's my best friend.*

Having good friendship networks, with strong levels of reciprocal everyday support, also increases our chances of receiving assistance in response to specific events in our lives. This targeted support helps to buffer us against the health impact of stress when we need it most.[4]

*We can be friends too if you like?*

Quality counts when it comes to the health impact of our social ties, just as it does with intimate relationships. Irrespective of how much contact with others we have, when we feel that there's something lacking in our social lives and family relationships we can experience loneliness.

*What are you saying?! Anyhow, doesn't everyone feel lonely, especially if they live in a big city?*

We all feel lonely at times, but when loneliness becomes a more constant feature of our lives it can spell bad news for our health in the long term. Links have been found between loneliness and a range of health problems, including increased risk of coronary heart disease and stroke, increased risk of Alzheimer's and increased stress response, as well as early death.[5]

*As if lonely people didn't have enough to feel sad about.*

*Reality check*

Loneliness shouldn't be confused with solitude. It's possible to feel lonely while surrounded by people, or to have relatively little social contact without experiencing loneliness. How we feel about our social ties and the level of emotional support we get from them matters most, rather than the amount of social contact we have.[6, 5]

It's also important to remember that all relationships aren't necessarily a source of warmth and support – some may even be detrimental to our well-being. The lifestyles and beliefs of those around us matter too. Social networks can propagate unhealthy habits just as they can encourage and normalise healthy ones.[6]

*So basically, we're saying . . .*

Regular warmth and emotional support from others is important for physical health, as well as quality of life. Avoiding chronic loneliness, particularly, will help maximise your chances of a long innings.

# Social media

*Hang on, are you saying my love for Twitter could affect how long my life will be?*

Health experts have long worried about the negative impact of the media and electronic entertainment on our health – from TV ads for junk food and alcohol, to the influence of violent computer games and the impact of spending our work and leisure time staring at a screen all day.

The rise of social media and smartphone use has brought an added dimension to this field of research and triggered a new moral panic about the effects of this omnipresent technology on the well-being of our children and young people.[1]

*Yeah, but that's just pearl-clutching technophobes getting in a tizzy, isn't it? They probably think social media means reading someone else's newspaper.*

Quite a lot of studies have been done looking at the mental well-being of people who spend more time on social media platforms, such as Facebook, Twitter and Instagram.

*And they found it was perfectly fine? Great! Let's move on.*

Particularly high levels of social media use have been shown to be correlated with low self-esteem and high level of depression symptoms in adolescents.[2] Research into the experiences of lesbian, gay and bisexual minorities with social media has also shown an association between cyberbullying and depression and suicidality.

25

*Oh no. I guess I'm lucky I grew up before smartphones were a thing. It was hard to get addicted to playing Snake on your Nokia 3210.*

Addiction to social networking platforms isn't simply determined by the amount of time you spend on them or how many times a day you log in. If you experience a compulsion to spend time on social networking apps and sites in a way that is negatively affecting your psychological health or impairing other aspects of your life, such as your work or studies, sleep, or personal relationships, then this might be considered problematic.[3, 4]

*Does this affect small mixed-race women aged forty? No reason for the question, just wondering ... .*

A large Norwegian study found that a number of characteristics were associated with scoring higher on a scale for measuring social media addiction, including lower age, not being in a relationship, having lower self-esteem and narcissism. Those who were students, women, or with lower levels of education or income were also more at risk.[5] We also know that people with social anxiety are more likely to engage in problematic social media usage.[6]

*Social media usage is a problem when I find out a much-loved ex has had another baby.*

There is a substantial body of evidence showing that people who experience problematic smartphone usage are more likely to suffer from depression.[7] Excessive use of social networking sites has also been found to be associated with heavy drinking in college students.[8]

*It's not all bad though, is it? Whose life isn't enhanced by endless cat videos?*

As with most things, it's a question of balance. Constant monitoring of one's social media profile can become a source of stress.[9] Some research found that while people generally expect that using Facebook will make them feel better, in fact there's a tendency for it to dampen mood because afterwards a feeling kicks in of having wasted time.[10] Use of Facebook has also been shown to be associated with loneliness and social anxiety, although we can't infer that it's the cause of these problems.[6]

*What about using lots of social media platforms but only spending a little time on each?*

This might not be the answer. One study showed that the more social media platforms people used, the more likely they were to suffer from depression or anxiety, irrespective of the amount of time they spent on social media in total.[11]

*Fine, I'm deleting my MySpace account.*

And that's before we get to exercise. A study of Chinese international students in Korea found that those with smartphone addiction were less physically active than their non-addicted counterparts. We know that exercise is important for preventing a number of life-limiting diseases; if you're not getting enough of it because you're staring at your phone all day, over the long term that's not going to be good for your life expectancy.[12]

*So, let me get this straight: social media will make me a bloated, pale couch potato with depression and anxiety?*

Not all of the evidence around social media usage and mental well-being is negative. Evidence shows that social media can provide a mechanism for minorities to share experiences, build a sense of identity and community, and gain support.[13, 9]

*I'm a minority, though I rarely tweet about it. I mostly make jokes about sex.*

There's also evidence that the more women use Twitter, the less stressed they are. Quite why this is, we don't know. Researchers have speculated that as an instantly accessible outlet for expression the platform may serve as a coping mechanism during stressful times. In addition, there's evidence that social media users tend to perceive that they have higher levels of social support, which might play a role.[14]

*There's definitely a high level of support for my sex jokes.*

Scientists have even begun trying to utilise social media as a mechanism for encouraging and helping people to achieve positive lifestyle changes.[15] So far there has only been very modest evidence that this approach is effective, although research in this area is very much in its infancy.[16, 17]

*Well this is all very contradictory. What's your overall judgement?*

Like any other form of communication, social media is used to spread both positivity and negativity. Isolating one from the other in a free society may be impossible, but we can at least be alert to the dangers of harmful social media usage and try to limit our own exposure to negative messages.

*Very interesting. I'm off back to Twitter now. Follow me at @ArianeSherine for sex jokes. My tweets won't depress you – I promise.*

*Reality check*
Although lots of evidence shows an association between negative health outcomes and excessive social media and smartphone usage, it's much harder to untangle the relationship between them. The extent to which problematic social media use actually causes all of these health issues or is just more likely to occur in people who have them is still a question for further research. Clearly, however, things like cyberbullying can have a very real negative impact.

> *So basically, we're saying . . .*
> Spending time on social media platforms can bring benefits
> and disadvantages for your health, depending on how you use
> them and your individual experiences, but letting them take
> over your life is a bad move.

## Josie Long on social media

*What are your views on social media?*

I think for all of the wonderful positives of social media, there are so
many negatives. It sort of amplifies social contagions, for good and
for bad. So, it can help people connect, it can help people feel great
– but it can also, as we've all seen, disseminate fascism in a really
terrifying way. The mixture of these apps that are purportedly about
human connection but are then floated on the stock market, and the
way it fucks with the morality of it . . . it scares me basically.

But I do think there will be a generation that rebels against it. I
like to think that my daughter will have seen me and my boyfriend
on our phones enough – even though we don't really want to be on
our phones the whole time in front of her. I like the idea that she'll
be like, 'Oh God, that's such a boring sad thing my parents do! I'm
gonna climb a tree and whittle some sticks!' Like the way that people
whose parents are 'wild childs' are always really strait-laced. Little
kids will be like, 'My parents are online, that's so sad. I'm out in a
river!'

That's my ambitious dream, that people will be more natural. But
not me, I don't want to be. I want to be on my phone!

# Volunteering

*I can't volunteer. I'm too busy trying to look after my kid and scrape together a living.*

That's a shame, as a substantial and growing evidence base suggests that volunteering is good for people's health and that volunteers have lower death rates compared with non-volunteers.[1]

A number of studies suggest that volunteering can improve mental health, reduce death rates and increase how healthy people feel.[2] Research in the US found that volunteers were more likely to use preventive healthcare services and spend fewer nights in hospital than non-volunteers.[3] Another study concluded that volunteering brought health gains which were the equivalent of being five years younger.[4]

*All this is good news for my mum. Since retiring, she's volunteered at her local Citizens Advice pretty much full time. But why does this mean she's going to live longer?*

There's no clear consensus on the mechanism by which volunteering benefits health. One theory is that it provides access to a social support network, which we know is linked to health and well-being.[1] Another is that volunteering improves health by buffering the effects of stress in our lives.[5] It's been linked with the release of certain hormones which can help regulate stress and inflammation in the body, and a US study which used data from 1320 people found that helping others had the effect of buffering volunteers from the negative impact of stressors in their own daily lives.[4, 6]

Researchers have also suggested that volunteering may help keep people physically active and help older people to keep a sense of control over their lives, making them more likely to maintain a healthy lifestyle.[4, 7]

*Is it the volunteering itself that makes a difference, or something else?*

Researchers have tried to take account of other differences between people who volunteer and those who don't that might account for the association between volunteering and better health. The types of studies it's been possible to undertake in this field mean that it's hard to be sure that it's the volunteering itself which improves people's health rather than some other characteristic of people who do volunteer work that hasn't been factored in.[8] Proving a causal effect on health from volunteering would require studies in which people are randomly assigned to either doing or not doing volunteer work and then measuring their health over a period of time.[9, 4] There is growing (though not yet conclusive) evidence, however, to support the theory that volunteering has a direct positive impact on health and longevity.[8]

*What if you're already ill? Can volunteering make you well again?*

Data from thirteen European countries showed that simply having a chronic condition doesn't reduce the likelihood of someone volunteering, but having a worsening health condition does.[8] On the question of whether people with an existing illness experience the same health benefits from volunteer work as the rest of the population, though, the evidence doesn't paint a consistent picture.[2, 1]

*Do the benefits just apply to vicars' wives in nice English villages, or is my tiny widowed Asian mum in with a shout of living to a hundred?*

There's continuing debate over whether volunteer work primarily benefits those with certain characteristics.[10] Some research shows that those who have a generally negative attitude towards others don't experience the same health pay-off from volunteering.[5]

*My mum hates all her clients and calls them 'thundering wanksocks'. Kidding! She loves her role and tries hard to help everyone. Any more info?*

Evidence of a positive association between volunteering and health has been found in different countries (not just high-income ones) and different age groups.[4, 11]

Also, we shouldn't think of it as just something to do in retirement. Research into the effects of environmental volunteer work in midlife, for example, found that it was associated with better levels of physical activity, better mental well-being and feeling healthier.[9]

*What if you volunteer to walk a housebound lady's Dobermann and it bites you and gives you rabies?*

Volunteering opportunities vary considerably, of course, and not every experience will necessarily be a positive one. Contextual factors, such as the type of role, the level of training provided and the amount of time taken up are important in determining whether voluntary work is health-enhancing.[2]

*Ah, then maybe I'll follow in Mum's footsteps and stick to Citizens Advice when I get older. Pretty sure no one's ever got rabies there.*

Well, if they did, at least someone could tell them who to sue.

> *Reality check*
> More is not necessarily better when it comes to volunteer work. There's some evidence that the health benefits diminish once you start doing a large amount of volunteering and that too much could make your mental health worse.[5, 7, 10, 12]

*So basically, we're saying . . .*
Doing some volunteer work could help you stay healthy for longer (as long as you don't overdo it and you don't hate people).

# Community

*I live next to a weird lady who plays loud music in her garden. Is that what you mean by 'community'?*

The idea that we accrue benefits through participation in community groups and building social networks is captured by the concept of 'social capital'. Whereas we usually think of capital as being about money and tangible assets, social capital represents the benefits we get from investing ourselves in a group or network, like a sense of belonging, shared norms, mutual trust and a willingness to help others. These resources are embedded within the fabric of a neighbourhood or community, rather than a bank account or physical location. In the twenty-first century, there's been a huge amount of interest among researchers in how levels of social capital influence health and well-being.[1]

*Are you saying I should go and dance in the weird lady's garden for my own health?*

Different studies have found varying results regarding the extent to which social participation improves health.[2]

A Swedish study that looked at data over a five-year period found that low levels of social participation were linked with higher rates of total deaths and higher rates of death from cardiovascular diseases and cancer. This relationship remained after taking account of people's BMI, perception of their own state of health, unmet health-care needs and other potentially related factors.[3]

Living in a neighbourhood with higher levels of social capital is linked with lower death rates. This relationship isn't explained simply by differences in levels of poverty and deprivation (which are very closely linked to people's health: see Social class, pages 66–8).[1] Researchers in the US also found that communities with higher levels of social capital had lower levels of drug overdose, and there's evidence that social capital helps people to better manage chronic conditions, such as diabetes and chronic lung disease.[1, 4]

*Oh gosh. I'm inviting the weird lady over right now. Should I invite the rest of the neighbourhood too?*

It's not a bad idea. A high level of perceived neighbourhood social cohesion, characterised by a sense of solidarity and connectedness, has been shown to help protect against adverse health outcomes, such as high blood pressure, heart attacks and death from stroke. A low level of social cohesion, on the other hand, has been linked with higher rates of certain adverse health outcomes, such as depression and smoking.[5]

People living in neighbourhoods which they perceive to have good levels of social cohesion are also more likely to go for flu vaccinations, cholesterol tests and some types of cancer screening (but not prostate examinations). Again, socio-economic factors don't account for this link.[6]

*That's OK, I don't need my prostate examined. My cervix, on the other hand . . .*

You could be in luck. The findings of one study suggest that perceptions of neighbourhood social cohesion act as a stress buffer for women with cervical cancer.[7] Another found that South Asian women in the US living in neighbourhoods with high social cohesion had 46 per cent lower odds of having high blood pressure than those living in areas with low social cohesion.[8]

*That's great, but if I invite the neighbours over, they might nick my stuff.*

Research has shown that a high level of general trust (not just trusting people we know individually) is associated with lower death rates in both men and women. This relationship also can't be explained by differences in socio-economic factors – it's not simply the case that those who have more trust in those around them live in better-off neighbourhoods.[9]

A lower level of trust between neighbours is associated with greater cardiometabolic risk, both in the present and several years into the future. Greater levels of anxiety and lower levels of physical activity appear to partly explain this relationship.[10]

*OK, I'll stop being so suspicious. Why does all this affect health though?*

Various theories have been suggested as to why levels of social capital affect health. It's been suggested that living in high social capital neighbourhoods may have a psychological benefit which has an impact on aspects of physical health, or that it may create social norms for healthier living, such as not smoking. Another theory is that it reduces barriers to accessing healthcare. Lower levels of violent crime in areas with more social capital have also been suggested as something that might contribute to the link with health and mortality.[3]

*So, if I join a community group, I'll live longer?*

Evidence indicates that participation in community organisations leads to lower death rates, better mental health and higher brain functioning among older people. Researchers have suggested that this kind of social participation may improve health as a result of psychological benefits, such as higher self-esteem, a greater sense of purpose in life and a buffering of the impact of stressful experiences.[2]

*I wouldn't mind joining an organisation if I could be in charge.*

A study of almost 15,000 Japanese people aged sixty-five and over found that those who were in a leadership position in a community group or other form of local club or organisation had lower death rates than those who were regular members. It's possible that having a position of authority brings greater psychological benefits, including greater self-esteem, social status and sense of control over one's life.[2]

*In that case, I might start playing loud music in my own garden myself and invite everyone round.*

*Reality check*
Despite being the subject of countless research studies over the last twenty years, looking at a whole range of outcomes and different contexts, there's still no universally accepted definition of what social capital is. Combinations of a number of different but related concepts have been said to comprise social capital, including social networks, social support, a general sense of trust in other people, and participation in civic and community life.[3, 11]

As well as researchers having different definitions of social capital, there's also no consistency in how they measure it. Even among those who share the same concept of what social capital entails, there can be different methods of quantifying the amount of social capital in a community.[3] This means that it's hard to build a clear picture from the evidence of which aspects of social capital are most important for health and how best to bolster them.

*So basically, we're saying . . .*
Joining a community group and getting to know your neighbours could help you live longer. You don't have to play rave music in your garden if you don't want to.

# Religion

*I created and ran the Atheist Bus Campaign back in 2009, so I don't think this chapter is going to convert me, even if practising religion makes you live forever.*

There's definitely a possibility it could mean you live longer. A US study published in 2018 found that overall people who attend religious services at least once a week live between 1.1 and 5.1 years longer than those who attend less frequently or never.[1] Other researchers have also found evidence that weekly attendance at religious services brings health benefits and reduces mortality, even after accounting for a range of other factors which might have explained the relationship.[2,3]

*OK, but I bet most of those extra years of life are spent at church, which can be very boring, so it's swings and roundabouts. Actually, swings and roundabouts would make church more fun. I heard that religion makes you happier too though?*

Although studies have found mixed results, overall there is good evidence that religiosity and spirituality are associated with some aspects of better mental health, including lower risk of depression and suicide.[4]

Researchers in the US found that women who attended religious services most frequently had a lower risk of developing depression than those who never went.[5] Whether there's a causal link between the two is a different matter, of course.

Japanese research has suggested that the well-established link between religiosity and well-being in elderly people could be accounted for by differences in personality traits – specifically with regard to agreeableness and conscientiousness.[6]

*Could religious people being more health conscious account for greater well-being? I bet they're not snorting lines off the pulpit.*

A study of people aged fifty and over in Europe found that those who prayed at least once a day were less likely to smoke.[7] Religious beliefs don't go hand-in-hand with a healthier lifestyle across the board, however. Researchers in the US conducted a study looking at Christians' attitudes to different behaviours affecting health.

It turned out they believed drug use, smoking and excessive drinking were sinful, but the same didn't apply to lack of exercise, overeating and obesity – even though they regarded them as destructive to God's temple (the body).[8]

*What about spirituality (as opposed to religion)? I'm not completely against the odd bit of mindfulness . . .*

A study of patients with congestive heart failure found that experiencing spiritual peace resulted in a 20 per cent reduction in the risk of death over five years. Demographics, health status and health behaviours, such as smoking, were ruled out as explanations for this association.[9]

Whether being spiritual is good for your health overall remains unclear, though. Some research has shown that spirituality is linked with a higher risk of depression and anxiety.[10, 11] A study of over 5500 people in the US, China and India, on the other hand, found that a high level of spirituality halved the risk of depression.[12]

*I've also heard that turning religious could help slow the ageing process?*

Yes – surprisingly, people have been looking into this. Scientists have found evidence of a relationship between religiosity and telomere length.[13, 14]

*Telo-what?*

Telomeres are DNA–protein structures found at both ends of each chromosome. As we get older, they get shorter. This shortening of our telomeres is believed to play a key role in the ageing process.[15] More research is needed to understand what's behind the link with religion, though, and what the implications might be.

*Well, God moves in mysterious ways. Which is code for saying he doesn't exist (probably).*

**Reality check**
Although studies have shown that attending religious services is associated with lower death rates, US research published in 2015 found that the same didn't apply to other measures of religiosity, such as how often people pray, or whether they believe in a god or an afterlife.[10] Evidence suggests that the link between attending religious services and life expectancy might be due to the increased access to social support which this can bring about, rather than the religious nature of the activity itself.[16]

*So basically, we're saying . . .*
The jury is still out on whether being religious or spiritual improves your health, but regularly attending religious services could possibly help you live longer.

## Sanjeev Kohli on religion

*Why do you think people who attend religious services live longer on average?*

I have two theories.

1) Incense. Incense is very much the common denominator of services over a broad spectrum of religions. And there is no denying

its calming influence. It is very much the gaseous equivalent of the theme to *The Antiques Roadshow*. Indeed, I would theorise that if incense were more prevalent outwith places of religious worship then there would possibly be no wars or skirmishes or gangs or ANY need for Ross Kemp at ALL.**

2) Logic (or lack thereof). Most religious texts, in order to justify its utterly ridiculous tenets, will not hesitate to bend all reasonable logic back in on itself. Perhaps this Möbius strip of logic impacts materially on the space–time continuum so that when you exit a religious service you are in fact YOUNGER THAN YOU WERE WHEN YOU WENT IN. (I accept that this doesn't explain 1978, the year of seven popes.)

*Despite being non-religious, would you consider going to religious services in order to live longer?*

Only if I was guaranteed that the length of time added to my life would be as LEAST as long as the length of time spent at said religious services. And I would want value for those lost hours. For example, an hour spent in church would have to be counterbalanced by an hour of paintball/Laser Quest. Or the enjoyment of two episodes of *Cheers*. Or the consumption of five Viennettas.

Also, the food REALLY needs to be better. Although I hear that langar, the free food given out to anyone who enters a Sikh temple, now includes pizza and chips to entice the Instagram generation. Smart move. If God exists, this is what I'd tell her. 'God,' I'd say, 'you catch more devotees with pizza than vinegar.

'And garlic mayo wouldn't hurt. You know, for the crusts.'

---

* See Scented candles and air fresheners, pages 217–19, for the science on incense.

# Part Two: Well-being

# Sleep

*I need a lot of sleep and am often exhausted. Am I headed for an early grave?*

It's well-established that sleep is important for our health, although we're not always aware of the implications of too little sleep – other than the obvious one of feeling tired. Experiments have demonstrated that short-term sleep deprivation can result in a range of adverse effects, including high blood pressure, impaired glucose control and increased inflammation.[1]

*What are the long-term effects?*

Studies have shown that those who have too little or too much sleep each day have a moderately increased risk of cardiovascular disease, diabetes, stroke, obesity and death, as well as a greater risk of incurring a long-term disability at work.[1-6]

*Crikey. Are the effects universal?*

Researchers have found that these kinds of relationships between short and long sleep and long-term health effects exist in both men and women, in rural and urban settings, and in different countries.[7]

*Does sleeping too much or too little affect how healthy you feel?*

Research conducted in Italians aged fifteen and over found that subjective health (how healthy we feel) is also negatively affected by both short and long sleep. This was also the case for fragmented sleep (waking up during the night and going back to sleep), as well as people's own perceptions of getting too much or too little sleep, rather than the actual amount.[6]

Scientists have also found that sleep loss can affect our emotions and social interactions.[8]

*I know a few people who can make me nod off. So, what's the right amount of sleep?*

There is some variation in the definitions used in different research studies, but seven to eight hours of sleep a day is typically regarded as the desired amount.[7]

*My ex-husband used to snore like an obese hippo. He didn't believe me until I recorded his snoring and played it back to him. Does snoring affect life expectancy?*

A study of adults in the UK published in 2019 found that around 30 per cent of women and 38 per cent of men reported that they snore at night.[9] Snoring is caused by parts of your body vibrating as you breathe and usually isn't related to anything serious, although it's known to be more common in people who are overweight, smoke or drink too much alcohol.

Sometimes, snoring can be caused by obstructive sleep apnoea, a condition in which your airways become temporarily blocked as you sleep. Poorly controlled sleep apnoea can increase the risk of having a heart attack or developing other long-term health conditions, such as high blood pressure, stroke and type 2 diabetes.[10]

*If that's all, I'm off for a nap. Hopefully it won't kill me.*

*Reality check*

The extent to which too little or too much sleep cause the negative longer term health outcomes with which they're associated remains a subject for further research.[11] Similarly, it's not clear how much the risks can be reduced by switching to the recommended seven to eight hours from an established pattern of suboptimal sleep duration.[2, 3]

Studies on this topic have tended not to distinguish between those who choose to sleep less and those who are unable to get as much sleep as they'd like due to external factors or underlying health conditions, such as sleep apnoea, so we don't know if we'd see different outcomes in each of these groups.[7]

It's also important to bear in mind that different people need different amounts of sleep and that it's normal to need less sleep as we age.[11]

*So basically, we're saying . . .*

Not everyone requires exactly the same amount of sleep, but consistently getting too much or too little may have implications for your health. Aim for seven to eight hours a night and consider a good night's sleep to be an important element of a healthy lifestyle, rather than a luxury.[1]

## Charlie Brooker on sleep

For years, I couldn't get to sleep, and I tried everything: hypnosis, sleeping pills, staying up until I was so tired I'd collapse . . . that sort of thing.

Finally, what seems to have cured it is three things: an eye mask; a pair of flat headphones called 'SleepPhones' – they're like a headband and they go over your ears, but they're flat so you can lie on them and it doesn't hurt; and then I plug them into my phone and

I'll listen to a podcast. It has to be a podcast on a subject that I'm quite interested in, but not so riveted by that I'll have to stay awake and be on tenterhooks.

Every night, the eye mask goes on, and then the SleepPhones and the podcast. And I'm asleep within fifteen to twenty minutes, every single night, whereas I used to just stay awake. It's a bit like waving a bit of string at a cat – you know how a cat has to go and chase it?! – it's sort of like that, for the bit of my brain that would otherwise be worrying or swirling round and round. That part of my brain is listening to the podcast and forgets to worry about stuff, and the remaining 90 per cent switches off and goes to sleep. It's been genuinely revolutionary in my own everyday life.

# Happiness

*I've heard that happier people live longer. That seems a bit unfair on depressed people . . .?*

A study looking at happiness and longevity among a nationally representative sample of people in the US found that those who were not happy had a 14 per cent higher risk of death than those who were very happy, independently of socio-economic status, religious attendance and marital status.[1]

*That's adding insult to injury. Why does happiness make you live longer though?*

Little is known about the mechanisms by which happiness might impact health. One theory is that being unhappy over a substantial period of time can trigger the body's 'fight or flight' response, which is well known to have a negative impact on health if sustained over the long term.

Another theory is that happier people are more likely to have healthy lifestyles – smoking and drinking less, taking more care over what they eat and getting more exercise. It's also been suggested that happiness might be a factor in helping to grow and maintain supportive social networks, which have a beneficial effect on health.[2]

*Aren't ill people just more down in the dumps because they're ill?*

It may seem obvious that health and happiness are linked – few people reading this book will be happy about the idea of dying prematurely or living out their old age in a state of poor physical and mental health. The extent to which happiness might cause people to be healthier, rather than the other way around, has yet to be established though.

A study in the Netherlands, which looked at deaths over a fifteen-year period, found happier people were less likely to die, but once the researchers factored in people's health status and levels of physical activity this relationship wasn't statistically significant. This suggests that people who are in a better state of health and do more exercise may be happier, but their lower risk of dying is a result of those factors, rather than their state of mind.[3]

*Excuse me – I'm just off to do some star jumps.*

Similarly, a UK study of over 700,000 women showed that how well they rated their own health was strongly linked to how happy they reported feeling: 39 per cent felt happy most of the time, 44 per cent usually felt happy and 17 per cent stated that they were unhappy. Within ten years, 4 per cent of the women had died, but the researchers found that after taking into account other contextual factors, including health status and lifestyle, there was no association between happiness and mortality.[4]

*You mentioned marital status earlier. Married people are happier, aren't they?*

An analysis of data from a UK population survey showed that people who were married were happier (and that it wasn't simply the case that people who were happier to begin with were more likely to marry). Married people experienced a particular advantage in midlife, when happiness levels tend to drop before rising again as we get older, with marriage appearing to lessen the extent of this dip. The researchers also found the benefits to happiness of marriage were twice as large in those whose spouse was also their best friend.[5]

*We've established you're my friend. Vegas or Gretna Green?*

*Reality check*
When individual research studies fail to provide a clear picture, experts tend to look to scientific reviews which bring together the results from a number of studies and assess their quality before concluding what the overall evidence base can tell us at that point in time. Researchers who published a scientific review of studies on this topic in 2008 did not find evidence to support the idea that happiness has a healing quality, or that it can prolong life in people with serious illnesses. They did find evidence, though, to support the idea that happiness has a preventative effect on ill health.[2]

*So basically, we're saying . . .*
There is a well-established correlation between happiness and health – particularly people's own perceptions of their health status. The question of whether happiness can actually affect health and longevity, however, is one which researchers are still unclear about.[2]

## Derren Brown on happiness

*It's evident from your book,* Happy, *that happiness is far more nuanced, complex and elusive than most of us imagine. Say somebody's reading this book and they want to feel happier – what would you say to them?*

The book *Happy* is mainly about Stoicism, which was a major popular philosophy for 500 years before Christianity took over. They had an approach to happiness which I think is very useful and helpful, even 2000 years later. Their basic approach was to see happiness as a kind of tranquillity – an avoidance of disturbance, that was their aim; how you remove frustrations and anxieties and disturbances from your life.

Their basic approach was to say: first of all, it's not things in the world that cause our problems, it's how we respond to those things, the judgements we make about those things. So, somebody doesn't actually make us angry or upset – we at some level decide to get angry and upset in response to what they've done.

Once you've got your head around that, the second part of it is that you shouldn't try and control things that aren't under your control, and the only things that are under our control are our thoughts and our actions. So, if we limit our efforts to just those, and not try and control what other people do and think – what happens out in the world that is nothing to do with our thoughts and actions – then it's a good recipe for a more tranquil state, which I think really makes sense.

There are some areas where it needs a bit of teasing apart – like, what if you want to change things that are wrong with the world? Then you *are* trying to change stuff in the world. But you can limit yourself to doing the best job you can of changing those things and not get emotionally attached to an outcome – like success – because that is something that is out of your control.

And that is quite a useful thing, isn't it? Because we're all trying to make changes and do things in the world, somewhere, but it's about not getting too caught up in an end result that is out of our control, and just keeping focused on doing the best we can, and so on.

So, I think Stoicism holds up as a really useful approach. I think it definitely has some weak spots, and it's not going to make you 'happy' in the sense of bouncing around with joy! But it would be a bit weird if we were like that all the time. It's more about moving in an easier way alongside what life throws at you. It's going 'lots of stuff happens in life that we can't control, that isn't fun and is going to work against us' – and rather than getting angry and frustrated, we can move with those things more easily.

And I think, particularly, we're told so much today that we should 'believe in ourselves', and if we do we should set our goals and basically make anything happen the way we want it to, and I think that's quite a damaging way of approaching life. It sounds great when you first come across it, as it makes you feel 'I can do anything!' But when life throws stuff at you that puts you in a bad place that you can't do anything about, you're just going to feel that you've failed – there's nowhere to go.

So, I think the Stoic approach is a much more sensible one. It's not as overtly optimistic – in a way, it's more pessimistic! But it's a strategic form of pessimism that I think is actually really helpful.

# Sense of humour

*As a comedy writer, I'm ready for you to tell me I'm going to live forever. Laughing and joking has got to be good for you, right?*

Generally, we tend to think of humour as being good for our health and well-being, although studies looking at sense of humour and longevity have found mixed results.[1-3] Though quite a lot of evidence has suggested that there may be a link between health and humour, when you look across the results of all the research conducted on this topic there isn't a consistent pattern. Some results have even suggested that a good sense of humour might be linked with worse health in some regards.[4]

*Worse health? But having a sense of humour might help you live longer, right?*

Some evidence suggests that it might increase your chances of reaching old age. In a study published in 2014, researchers in Norway followed over 50,000 people for fifteen years to investigate links between sense of humour and mortality. Their results showed that sense of humour was associated with reduced risk of death from cardiovascular diseases among women and reduced risk of death from infections among men.[5]

*So, could you laugh your way to a hundred?*

Overall, the results of the Norwegian study showed that sense of humour was linked with a reduced risk of death up until the age of eighty-five.[5] An earlier study undertaken by some of the same researchers found that sense of humour appeared to increase the probability of survival into retirement, but it ceased to be linked with longer life beyond age sixty-five.[6]

*What about laughing in the face of death? Does that help an ill patient's prognosis?*

People may use humour as a coping mechanism when they have a long-term or life-limiting illness and there's some evidence that this may be linked with longer survival in these situations.[3] Clowns have even been used in nursing homes to improve residents' well-being.[1]

*As long as it's not Pennywise. So, the $64,000 question is: do comedians live longer? I'm crossing my fingers, toes and eyes that they do . . .*

Quite the opposite. Studies of comedians have shown that the funnier they are, the more likely they are to die prematurely.[7, 8] Also, a study of over 500 amateur improvisational comedy performers found that they suffered from infectious diseases more frequently than the general population. The results couldn't be explained by differences in age, sex, weight issues or the number of antibiotics they used.[2]

There's also the old cliché, of course, that comedians are all tortured souls, crying on the inside and drinking themselves to death. Certainly, one can find plenty of examples to support that notion, but that doesn't necessarily mean that a career in comedy is bad for your mental well-being. One theory is that people prone to mental health problems might be more likely to go into comedy in the first place.[9]

*And then they die prematurely if they're any good. Christ on a bike! I actually feel depressed now. Maybe I should cheer myself up by going to a comedy night . . .*

*Reality check*
Building a strong evidence base on the relationship between humour and health isn't straightforward because there's no standard definition of what a sense of humour entails. Is enjoying comedy the same as having an ability to perform it? Is it necessary to routinely find humour in everyday situations or just to occasionally laugh at other people's jokes? What about different types of humour? Is laughing at others' misfortune comparable to a penchant for innuendo? There are many variants of the concept of humour, so it's possible that some bring health benefits which others don't. Some types may also have negative effects on health and well-being.[2]

*So basically, we're saying . . .*
A good sense of humour might help you reach old age, but a career in comedy is probably best avoided.

# Stress

*Stress is a huge killer, isn't it?*

Yes. Stress-related disorders increase the risk of cardiovascular disease. One example is post-traumatic stress disorder (PTSD), which can occur in people who've previously experienced a stressful event in their lives – this could be a traumatic, life-threatening experience or a significant life change, such as a divorce or the death of a loved one.[1]

*Work can be really stressful too, can't it?*

It can. In one year, 12.8 million working days were lost due to work-related stress, depression or anxiety in Britain alone.[2] Stress in the workplace has also been shown to increase the risk of cardiovascular disease. A high level of job strain and a poor balance of effort-to-reward can both cause work stress and increase your chances of dying from conditions such as stroke and heart failure.

*'Job strain'? Sounds like constipation.*

Job strain results from a combination of high work demands and low control over your job. An effort-reward imbalance occurs when how hard you have to work doesn't seem to be adequately compensated for by your wages or other benefits, such as job security, career opportunities or a sense of social approval.[3]

*What kinds of jobs cause the most stress?*

In the UK, government figures show that those working in the 'professional occupations' category have the highest chance of suffering work-related stress, depression or anxiety. Tight deadlines, too much work and too much pressure or responsibility were the most frequently cited causes.[2]

Generally, research shows that types of work in which excessive or unrealistic demands are the norm, with little opportunity for staff to exercise any choice or control and a lack of support from others are the most stressful. If you routinely feel that you're not respected or recognised for your work, it may be time for a change of scenery.[4]

*Unless you're a theatre set designer. Other than changing job, what are some alternative ways of managing stress?*

You can find lots of advice online on ways to cope with stress, including exercise, breathing and relaxation techniques and learning to recognise your stress triggers.[5, 6] Evidence also shows that mindfulness can be effective in helping to reduce stress.[7] There's no quick fix though, and no single method that will work for everyone. See your doctor if stress is still causing you problems after trying self-help approaches.

*I feel like I need a massage now.*
*   Hello . . .?*

*Reality check*
When it's short-lived, stress can be positive in moderate doses – helping us to be more alert and perform better in certain situations. Trying to eliminate it from your life altogether would be an unrealistic goal, but the important thing is to avoid long-term stress.[8]

*So basically, we're saying . . .*
Stress is a normal part of life, but too much of it could shorten your lifespan.

# Employment

*I love writing for a living. It's a lot of fun.*

Keep at it, as there's a well-established link between unemployment and poorer health.

*Unless your job is mining asbestos.*

Asbestos aside (we'll come to this on pages 214–16), being involuntarily out of work is associated with an increased risk of chronic illnesses, such as cardiovascular disease and cancer, as well as an increased risk of death from various causes (including accidents and violence).[1-4] Even the anticipation of unemployment before it actually occurs has been shown to have negative effects on health.[5]

*Even if your job is cleaning the toilets in a curry house? I bet unemployment can't come fast enough for those poor buggers.*

Not necessarily. Unemployment is also associated with poor mental health and suicide, as well as physical illnesses. Evidence shows that generally the longer someone spends out of work, the worse their sense of well-being.[1]

*Does this apply to everyone not in work?*

No. It's important to draw a distinction between being unemployed and being economically inactive. People who are unemployed are actively seeking and available for work, while many others might not be in work due to studying, caring responsibilities, retirement or simply personal choice. The research we're talking about here is all looking at those who are classed as unemployed.

*So, why is there a link between unemployment and lower life expectancy?*

Research suggests that several mechanisms may contribute to the adverse health impact of unemployment. Some people develop more unhealthy lifestyles following a job loss, increasing the risk of serious illnesses, such as cardiovascular disease and cancer.[1, 6] The financial impact can lead to poverty, which itself is linked with higher death rates, while the stress of unemployment is also likely to play a role.[6]

*Does this affect some people more than others?*

This relationship is seen in both men and women, although there's evidence that men are particularly negatively affected by unemployment, possibly due to the strong cultural association between masculinity and work.[7]

*'Me man. Me provide food. Me light barbecue.'*

Evidence shows that as men get older, those who are better qualified experience the greatest increased risk of death following unemployment – this is the opposite of the pattern seen in young men. A possible explanation is that those who least expect to find themselves unemployed later in life tend to experience greater stress as a result than those whose different expectations and experiences have made them better equipped to cope.[6]

*Is the link between unemployment and poor health definitely causal? Couldn't it just be that unhealthy people are too depressed to attend job interviews?*

This possibility has long been considered a limitation of studies on illness and unemployment; however, research designed specifically to look at this issue found no evidence that this explanation accounted for the apparent overall health impact of joblessness.[8] The relationship between unemployment and poor mental health has actually been shown to be even stronger once any existing tendency towards depression has been taken into account.[7]

*That sucks. Still, whatever happens with the writing, I draw the line at cleaning toilets in a curry house. Imagine filling a balloon with korma sauce and then—*

*Reality check*
The relationship between employment and health isn't just a simple dichotomy between being out of a job and being in work. Research suggests that job insecurity also has negative health effects which in some aspects are comparable to those associated with unemployment, including an increased risk of suicide.[2, 9] Many people who wouldn't be counted in the unemployment statistics are in insecure and low-paid work. Financial struggles and the risk of losing their income can remain an everyday source of stress for people in this situation.[10]

Aside from the monetary aspects of employment, we also know that the position of a job in the workplace hierarchy has important health implications. The level of status and the degree of control which you have in your role has been shown to have biological effects related to a greater risk of ill health.[10]

*So basically, we're saying . . .*
Find a secure, stable job in which you're not at the bottom of the food chain and avoid losing it.

# Education

*I'm educated to MA level. I hated the whole of my education though and have barely used it for anything.*

I have good news for you – there's a well-established link between how well-educated people are and their risk of an early death. Generally, the higher the level of education you've received, the greater your chance of reaching a ripe old age.[1, 2] This link between education and health is seen across developed countries and it's not going away.[3] Researchers in the US report that educational attainment has become a better predictor of life expectancy than race and sex, and that the relationship has grown stronger since the 1980s.[4]

*Why is this, though?*

There are probably various reasons why the link between education and health is so strong. It's hard to pin down to what extent learning in itself leads to better health, because there are multiple aspects to the education experience. It can play a key role in shaping our beliefs and values, as well as helping develop emotional intelligence, self-esteem and social skills.

Your level of education can affect what type of work you end up doing and how much you earn – both of which are also linked to life expectancy.[1] How well off you are financially influences other things which can affect your health, such as living conditions and exposure to stress.[5]

*Any other associations?*

Education levels are also closely linked with poverty. In the UK, considerable differences in educational attainment emerge from a very young age, with children from poorer backgrounds tending to lag behind their peers.[1]

Some of the link between education and health is explained by differences in behaviours.[6] Those who drop out of high school are more likely to abuse drugs and alcohol, for example. They're also more likely to have experienced a traumatic upbringing – something which is also a predictor of poor health in later life (see also Adverse childhood experiences, pages 362–4).[7]

*Oh dear – I tick that particular box. I'm quite healthy though. Are people with lower levels of education more likely to smoke as well as doing drugs and drinking?*

Differences in smoking rates between people with different levels of education account for some of the link with life expectancy, but not all of it. Among white men and women in the US, between a quarter and a third of this life expectancy gap can be explained by smoking.[6]

*Thanks for that. I feel more educated now.*

> ### Reality check
> The extent of the relationship between education and premature death varies once you start drilling down to look at different segments of the population. A study of over 35 million Italians published in 2018, for example, found that it was stronger among people who were single rather than married. The results also showed that the strength of the association varied across different causes of death and between the sexes.[2]

*So basically, we're saying . . .*
People who are less well educated generally die younger.
Maybe look into some evening classes?

# Social class

*I've had a shit life overall but am lucky to be middle class.*

You *are* lucky. It's very well-established that the worst-off people in society typically have the worst health. Generally speaking, the lower your social class, the more likely you are to die prematurely. This pattern occurs in low-, middle- and high-income countries and shows no sign of going away.[1, 2]

*But it's not that bad in the UK, surely?*

Some countries, such as South Africa, are well-known for their extremes of wealth and poverty. Even in England, though, there's a gap in life expectancy of several years between those with the lowest and highest incomes. The gap in how many years people can expect to live free of disability is into double figures.[3]

*Is it not just that posh people eat quinoa and go to the gym more than once a year?*

No. British academic Professor Sir Michael Marmot has been at the forefront of efforts to publicise this phenomenon. His work highlights that it's not just that there's a gap in life expectancy between the people at the top and those at the bottom – there's a social gradient in health, which means that health improves with every rung of the class ladder.[3]

Marmot led an influential study of over 17,500 London civil servants which proved that the better paid and higher status people's jobs were, the lower their risk of certain diseases and the less likely they were to die over the duration of a ten-year period. Some of this inequality could be accounted for by differences in known health influences, such as smoking rates, but much of it remained unexplained.[4]

*Does this affect children?*

Social class is related to mortality at all ages. Children in the poorest households have the highest chance of dying before reaching adult-hood and the risk reduces the further up the social scale you go.[5]

*What if someone jacks in their job at the laundrette to become a lawyer?*

Research shows that your social class in childhood is related to your health in later life, even if you move into a different class in adult-hood.[6] A study of British men published in 2007 found that being in a low social class in childhood appeared to have an influence on their risk of heart disease in middle age. The effect remained after factoring in differences in smoking, alcohol, exercise and weight in adulthood, although it was a modest one. Whether people engaged in unhealthy behaviours as adults played a big role in determining the level of influence that their social class in childhood had on their heart disease risk in later life.[7]

*So, you can't fake it by buying a lordship online?*

There's good quality evidence that our own perceptions of our social status also play a role in determining our health, irrespective of which social class we're actually in. Believing that you're in a lower social class, even if you're not, is associated with an increased risk of heart disease, high blood pressure and diabetes.[8]

*If the reverse is true, Chris Eubank is going to live a very long life.*

*Reality check*
The relationship between class and how healthy we are isn't always simple and there may be variations in different cultural contexts. Research in India, for example, has shown that while people in a lower socio-economic position are more likely to have behavioural risk factors, such as smoking, those at the other end of the social spectrum are more likely to be obese, and to have high blood pressure and diabetes.[9]

It's also important to remember that while social class in itself might have some protective effect on our health, for many of us, the choices we make still play a big role in determining our chances of a long life, irrespective of our position in society.

*So basically, we're saying . . .*
Generally, the further down the social scale you are, the less likely you are to live a long healthy life, but a healthy lifestyle will maximise your chances whichever social class you're in.

# Subjective age

*What's 'subjective age' when it's at home?*

While there's no escaping the fact that we're all getting older, many of us aspire to maintaining the mindset and physical vitality of someone considerably younger as we creep into our later years.

*Yeah, duh! That's what this book's about.*

Well, how old (or young) we feel compared to our actual age is known as our 'subjective age'. It's a concept which has attracted the attention of scientists looking to understand how the way we perceive ourselves relates to our physical health.

*Do most people feel older or younger, then?*

A study of almost 1500 Danish adults aged between twenty and ninety-seven found that up until the age of twenty-five, people tend to report feeling older than they actually are. From age twenty-five onwards, people generally report feeling younger than their real age.[1]

*It's not just a Danish thing though, is it? I've felt twenty-two since I was, well, twenty-two.*

It's definitely not just the Danes. A tendency for people to report feeling younger than they actually are is found in many cultures, although it does appear to be more pronounced in those which place a high value on youthfulness, such as the USA.[2]

*Maybe that explains why I feel young: I'm half-American.*

The same study showed that generally beyond the age of forty the ratio of subjective age to chronological age stabilises. Once we get past 'the big four-zero' we typically go through the rest of our lives feeling 20 per cent younger than whatever our actual age is at the time. The research showed that this applied pretty consistently, with very little variation between men and women, or people with different levels of income or education.[1]

*Isn't this just about being in denial, though? What's it got to do with health?*

Evidence shows that how old we feel is related to a range of health outcomes. Those who have lower subjective age tend to have better physical and mental health, better cognitive functioning and lower risk of hospitalisation.[3] A smaller waist circumference and better grip strength are also associated with feeling younger.[2]

*I've got it: we should all become adult babies. You know, like those infantilists who wear nappies and—*

Anyhow, when scientists looked at the results of a number of studies which tracked people over time, they found solid evidence that those with a younger subjective age tended to go on to live longer.[4]

*Any idea why this is?*

Various theories have been proposed. One idea is that a lower subjective age helps people to maintain a positive view of themselves in a culture which generally regards ageing as negative, and that this contributes to mental well-being (which is known to be linked to physical health and longevity). Another possibility is that subjective age influences how we act, with some evidence suggesting that people who feel younger are more likely to engage in health-promoting behaviours.[4]

*I don't have any aches or pains yet. Does this have anything to do with subjective age?*

Physical health is itself a strong predictor of subjective age and the extent to which feeling younger than your actual age is a cause of good health rather than a consequence of it remains unclear.[2, 5] People who are in better health may feel younger because they experience fewer restrictions and less pain when making physical efforts in their daily lives – things which we typically associate with ageing.[2] There is some evidence, though, that our perceptions of our own health play a greater role than our actual physical status in influencing our subjective age.[6]

*I see. Well, I'll go right on pretending that I'm twenty-two. At least I won't have to pay for nappies that way, at least until I become incontinent.*

*Reality check*
Although there's quite a bit of scientific literature exploring associations between health outcomes and subjective age, we still don't know enough about the nature of the relationship, and we have to be cautious when thinking about causality.[4]

It's also not clear what kind of things might be effective at preventing people from developing older subjective age or reversing it in those who already feel older than they are. More research would also be needed to establish whether reversing older subjective age led to the same improved health outcomes experienced by those who had always felt younger in mid and later life.

Some evidence suggests that the relationship between subjective age and future health is more pronounced in some cultures than others. Feeling younger is more strongly associated with staying alive in countries with less welfare provision and has a greater effect on well-being in the US compared to Europe.[2]

*So basically, we're saying . . .*
People who feel younger than their years tend to live longer, but we don't really know to what extent it's a reason *why* they live longer, rather than just a consequence of being in better health to start with – it might be a bit of both. Either way, staying physically active and not allowing negative feelings about ageing to become a self-fulfilling prophecy are good tips to follow.

# Puzzles and memory games

*I'm scared of going doolally when I'm older. What can I do to stop it?*

A consequence of overall improvements in life expectancy has been a rise in the prevalence of age-related diseases. Many of us particularly fear developing dementia as we get older. As the proportion of the population who are in old age increases, it's becoming an increasingly common condition. It's estimated that over 135 million people worldwide will be living with dementia by 2050.[1] As more of us worry about this issue, the idea that we might be able to do something about it by exercising our brains, and not just our bodies, has started to gain attention.

*How should we exercise our brains, then?*

Numerous brain-training programmes and tools have been developed and marketed. The idea is that through intensive, targeted mental exercise we can enhance our cognitive abilities.[2] Research has shown a high level of interest in brain-training smartphone apps, particularly in young adults. Users reported that they believed this kind of app could help improve thinking, attention, memory and even mood.[3]

*I wonder if three hours a day on Twitter counts?*

Scientists have struggled to come to a consensus over the health benefits of brain-training exercises. In 2014, two large groups of scientists published open letters on the topic – one denouncing the lack of evidence that brain training, or 'brain games', are effective at preventing cognitive decline or improving brain functioning, and the other claiming that there was plenty of scientific literature demonstrating their benefits.

*That's puzzling.*

Two years later, researchers published a comprehensive review of the published research on the subject, concluding that brain-training exercises tend to only be good for improving your performance at the specific tasks they include. In other words, playing a brain game regularly will make you better at playing the game but it won't do much to improve your brain functioning beyond that.[4]

*Oh no. What else can I do to stave off senior moments, then?*

Studies looking at what might help protect against dementia have shown contradictory results.[5] Avoiding high blood pressure, diabetes, smoking and being overweight might reduce your risk of developing vascular dementia in later life, although we still don't fully understand how much it's possible to prevent the condition through lifestyle changes.[6]

A US study found that intellectual enrichment over the lifetime was associated with lower cognitive decline in old age. To what extent enrolling in a higher education course in midlife, for example, would reduce your risk of going on to develop dementia remains unclear, however.[7]

*I can't afford to go back to uni. Maybe I could take up a stimulating hobby instead? I love sudoku.*

A study of almost a thousand people published in 2010 showed that spending an hour or more a day on hobbies might help protect against dementia in later life. The time could be spent on a range of pastimes which stimulate the brain, including crossword puzzles, cards and board games (but not reading). The results also showed that engaging in a greater variety of hobbies was more beneficial, although time spent on either crossword puzzles or craft activities alone was also found to reduce the risk of dementia.[8]

*So, if I start losing my memory, should I start doing crosswords?*

There's evidence to suggest that crossword puzzles may help to delay memory loss in people with dementia, but more research is needed to assess their true potential in this area.[9]

*What about jigsaws? I do love a good thousand-piece nature scene.*

There's some evidence that completing jigsaw puzzles is good exercise for the brain and that potentially it may help to keep your mind sharp over the long term, but this isn't a quick-fix solution.[10]

*Not with a thousand pieces that are mainly sky, it isn't.*

*Reality check*
Regardless of any benefit for your brain, spending all your spare time in a chair doing jigsaws or crosswords isn't going to be the best option for your general health. Activities such as this should be treated as just one aspect of a varied lifestyle which keeps you motivated and active physically, socially and mentally.

*So basically, we're saying . . .*
Brain game apps are unlikely to reduce your risk of dementia in old age. Not enough is really known about how preventable dementia is, but maintaining a healthy lifestyle, getting plenty of intellectual stimulation and having a range of interests are probably the best things you can do.

# TV viewing and reading

*Ooh, I love watching* Black Mirror *on Netflix, and Channel 4's* First Dates . . .

I'm afraid television viewing isn't the healthiest way to spend your free time. As well as involving time sitting rather than engaging in physical activity, TV watching is linked with grazing on unhealthy foods.[1] There's good evidence that people who watch relatively little TV have lower death rates than those who take in several hours of viewing every day.[2]

*Isn't this just because they get less exercise?*

No. An Albanian study found that, in women, the more time spent watching TV every day, the greater the risk of acute coronary syndrome (a group of conditions which includes heart attacks and unstable angina). This relationship couldn't be explained by conventional coronary risk factors or variations in how much exercise people did.[3] One piece of research even showed that the more time people spend watching TV in middle age, the more likely they are to develop Alzheimer's disease – with each additional hour of daily TV viewing increasing the risk further.[4]

*At least they won't mind all the repeats.*

When researchers brought together evidence from a number of different studies, they concluded that prolonged TV viewing was linked with an increased risk of type 2 diabetes, cardiovascular

76

disease and death. Those who watched TV for three hours or more per day had a higher death rate.[1]

*They should make a documentary series about this. Can it really be that dangerous?*

The results took account of a range of other factors, although it can't be ruled out that the link between TV viewing habits and health is explained by something else which wasn't considered.[1]

*What if I watch telly while jogging on the spot?*

A US study found that even among adults who had a high level of physical activity, those who watched seven hours or more of TV per day still had a higher risk of death than those who watched less than an hour.[5]

*How about reading a book instead? Is that any better?*

There's certainly some evidence to suggest links between reading and health. Research in the US found that, among elderly people, those with limited literacy had almost twice the death rate of their peers after taking account of various other factors which affect the risk of dying.[6] Another study which looked at seventy-year-olds in Jerusalem found that over eight years – again, after taking into account various other factors – the risk of death was significantly reduced among men who read every day compared with those who didn't.[7]

*Will reading keep my brain sharp in old age?*

Possibly, although the evidence is mixed on this one. Some research suggests that reading might help protect against dementia, but not all studies have found a link.[8-10] The results of one study published in 2010 even showed that reading a newspaper was associated with a higher risk of dementia, although it's important to say that this doesn't prove a causal link between the two. The researchers suggested that the demand on your brain might vary depending on which section of the newspaper you were reading.[8]

*Maybe the people who got dementia were reading the horoscopes.*

*Reality check*
The occasional box-set binge or an hour of telly a night is very unlikely to bring about your premature death. Equally, picking up a book a couple of times a year probably isn't going to reduce your risk of dying or stop you getting dementia. It's your habits over a sustained period that really matter. No matter how you spend your leisure time, keeping your brain and body active and eating healthily throughout your life will help to reduce your risk of health problems.

*So basically, we're saying . . .*
Swapping your daily TV fix for a bit of reading might be beneficial for your health in the long term, but don't forget to get up and do some exercise as well.

## Konnie Huq on reading

*The more you read, the longer you live.*

Yeah, and you know why? Reading breeds empathy, more so than watching telly – people who read can be transported to other places, put themselves in other people's shoes, and see things from another perspective. Longevity is very much stress-related, so I think it's twofold: reading is a form of relaxation, but also the more caring people are, the more they want to give back to society rather than just help themselves. And by doing that, they're less stressed.

If people govern their lives by helping themselves, they just want the next fashionable thing. They want to keep up with the Joneses: they want a show home house like their neighbours, and trendy clothes like people around them. You're continually competing, and you always want more, as you think your happiness comes from helping yourself. Whereas if your happiness comes from helping others, I think it's a much less stressful way to be, and stress is a massive part of health.

*Have you always loved reading? Did you read a lot as a kid?*

As a kid we'd always go to the local public library and choose three books. It was the most exciting treat – making your shortlist of which three books we were going to take out. Real happiness comes from emotions, and emotions can be massively enhanced by reading books.

*What made you decide to write your children's book,* Cookie and the Most Annoying Boy in the World?

I've had young children in my extended family for a long time, so I've had this character I've made up stories about. I did the Blue Peter Book Awards for years, working with young people, and had been asked several times if I wanted to write a kids' book. The timing was right as my youngest son has just started school – but also, I didn't just want to do something for the sake of it. The book embraces being 'other' and having values of inclusivity, diversity and social awareness.

In society, we're only used to what surrounds us. I think the route to a better society is through children. Adults are fully formed, but children are a blank canvas. So, if you give them values of empathy and altruism and wanting to give back to society, you can effect real change. If you have kids with the right mindsets and values, no matter where they go – if they're the CEO of a FTSE 100 company, or if they're the President of the USA, or whatever – they'll want to make the world a better place.

# Part Three: Exercise

# Aerobic exercise

*Oh God, this takes me back to horrendous Games lessons at school . . .*

Sorry, but you should know that a large body of research has demonstrated that physical activity (whether or not in a form that we traditionally think of as 'exercise') has a range of benefits for our physical and mental health. Being more active improves quality of life and reduces our chances of dying prematurely.[1]

*I could cringe myself to death thinking about Sports Day: the other kids would all run around the track, then the girl with the gammy leg, then me.*

Running counts as aerobic exercise, even if you're slow. Aerobic exercise is any activity that you can keep up for more than just a few minutes which gets your heart, lungs and muscles working more than usual. You might also hear people refer to this type of exercise as 'cardio'.

*My only type of cardio these days is my credit cardio.*

Evidence shows that regular aerobic exercise can increase active life expectancy by helping to minimise the impact of an otherwise sedentary lifestyle and limiting the development and progression of chronic diseases.[2] It helps to protect the heart and, along with a healthy diet, provides a vital first line of defence against heart disease.[3, 4]

*Stressful flashbacks about being picked last for Games aside, will getting fitter make me live longer?*

There's a well-established relationship between levels of cardiorespiratory fitness and rates of death. Greater fitness is associated with lower mortality, independently of age, race, ethnicity and illness. It's also associated with lower rates of coronary artery disease, hypertension (high blood pressure), diabetes, stroke and cancer.[5]

*How much should I be doing, then? Does running for the bus count?*

It's recommended that adults aged nineteen to sixty-four should either do at least 150 minutes of moderate aerobic activity every week to stay healthy, or 75 minutes of vigorous aerobic activity (such as running or a game of singles tennis), or a mix of the two. Moderate aerobic activity will raise your heart rate, and make you breathe faster and feel warmer.[6]

*Warmer? I think I'll feel exhausted.*

Keep in mind that this is the minimum recommended amount, though, rather than an optimum level. Generally, the fitter you are, the greater the health benefits; for example, a study of the relationship between mortality risk and cardiorespiratory fitness among men showed that there's a gradient, with those with the lowest level of fitness of all having the highest death rate.[7]

*Oh God, that's me – except for the 'men' bit. Isn't it possible to be too fit, though? You always hear about people dying during marathons.*

A US study published in 2018 looked at data from 122,000 patients between 1991 and 2014 whose cardiorespiratory fitness had been measured using treadmills. They found that being fitter was associated with a lower risk of death and that there was no apparent upper limit at which a higher level of fitness ceased to be beneficial. Those who had extreme levels of fitness had the lowest death rate of all.[5]

*Wow. So those ultramarathon runners who bang on about energy gels have the right idea?*

Possibly. There isn't a clear scientific consensus on the question of whether there's a level of exercise which generally ought to be considered too much. If you're currently unfit, however, you should build up your level of physical activity gradually, and speak to your doctor before starting a new exercise regime if you have an underlying health condition.

*Is 'aerobic exercise' really for everyone? What about pregnant ladies and old people?*

Aerobic activity can benefit people of all ages, including pregnant women. A research trial demonstrated that a three-month supervised exercise programme during pregnancy improved women's health-related quality of life (including measures of physical function, bodily pain and general health).[8] There's also no age limit to the benefits of aerobic exercise, as the cardiovascular system is responsive to training at any age.[2] It can also improve balance and agility in old age, thereby potentially helping to reduce the risk of falls.[9]

*OK – I guess there are no excuses. I'm off to sign up at my local gym and then never go.*

*Reality check*
You don't have to be doing something primarily for the purpose of exercise in order for it to count. Aerobic exercise can take many forms, such as cycling, brisk walking, dancing or even pushing a lawnmower, as long as you're hitting the threshold for 'moderate activity'. If you find that you can still talk, but you can't sing the words to a song, then you're probably doing moderate activity.[6] There are plenty of ways to achieve and maintain fitness that don't require you to brave a gym changing room and different forms of aerobic activity might appeal more at different times of life.

> *So basically, we're saying . . .*
> Aerobic exercise is a vital tool in your quest for longevity which can benefit you throughout the course of your life.

## Charlie Brooker on exercise

*You once told me you don't trust people who exercise!*

I know, I don't. But then I got this Couch to 5k app. You put it on, you get into your running gear, miserably, and you put some music on and start the app. It says, 'start running', and it makes you run for thirty seconds, then walk for ninety seconds, then repeat. It breaks it up, so the running is never longer than thirty seconds.

It does that for half an hour, and then it tells you 'you're halfway there, so you can turn round and come home'. It says, 'thanks for that, you're going to do this again on Wednesday'. It plans it all out for you for the next nine weeks. It throws you a curveball at about four weeks in, when it suddenly makes you run for about twenty minutes – but by then, it's built you up.

By the end of nine weeks, I could run for half an hour without stopping – which, if you'd told me that nine weeks earlier, would have been the equivalent of telling me I could flap my arms and fly to the moon!

# Strength exercise

*I'm so weak, I'm like the opposite of The Rock. Maybe I should be called The Paper?*

Start strength training if you want to live to a hundred. A study which followed more than 8000 men aged between twenty and eighty years old for an average of nineteen years showed a clear relationship between their muscular strength and risk of dying over that time.

The researchers found that greater muscle strength was associated with a lower risk of death overall and a lower risk of death from cancer specifically, even after the results had been adjusted to take account of variations in the men's cardiorespiratory fitness and other factors which might have accounted for the relationship.[1]

*It's a losing battle though, isn't it – don't we shed muscle as we age?*

As we get older, we typically experience a decline in both muscle mass and strength, known as sarcopenia. This can impair our physical functioning in daily life – something which has been shown to predict disability, admission to a nursing home and death in older people. A downward spiral can occur in which loss of muscle strength is followed by a reduction in physical activity leading to a further decline in strength.[2]

*It's the beginning of the end! Why does it happen?*

Loss of muscle strength and mass as we get older is generally the result of a combination of the natural ageing process, a reduction in the amount of physical activity we do, nutritional deficiencies and chronic disease. Although we can't halt the ageing process, we can modify our levels of exercise. Reducing physical inactivity is associated with improvements in muscle strength and a lower risk of death.[2]

*Is it just about getting big muscles? Because I'm not sure they'd suit me.*

Researchers have discovered that while there's a high correlation between muscle strength and mass, it's not the size of the muscle that's important when it comes to mortality. A US study of men and women aged seventy to seventy-nine which was published in 2006 showed that grip strength and strength in the quadriceps (a group of muscles on the front of the thigh) provided a much better indicator than muscle mass of the risk of death.[3]

*Is this just something to worry about when I'm old and feeble?*

Muscle weakness, along with low body weight, is often seen in people suffering from chronic diseases. To unpick the role of muscle strength from these other factors, researchers analysed data from more than 6000 healthy men in Hawaii aged from forty-five to sixty-eight who had been followed over thirty years. The men's hand grip strength and body mass index (BMI) were measured at the start of the period and death rates were calculated at the end.

After taking account of a range of other factors which could have influenced the results (age, education, occupation, smoking, physical activity and body height), the researchers found that those with greater grip strength were less likely to have died by the end of the thirty-year period. The analysis showed that this relationship was not accounted for by variations in BMI.

The researchers concluded that muscle strength in middle age predicts an increased risk of death among men, and that increasing muscle strength in midlife may improve the chances of living longer in old age.[4]

*How do I go about getting ripped, then? And I don't mean because I'm The Paper.*

Strength exercise isn't necessarily something that involves going to a gym and pumping iron to get ripped. It can be any activity that gets your muscles working harder than usual. Heavy gardening, hill walking, cycling and even climbing stairs can count. It's recommended that you should try to do at least two sessions of muscle strengthening exercise every week, working all the major muscle groups (legs, hips, back, abdomen, chest, shoulders and arms).[5] You can find advice on the NHS website about getting started.[6]

*Any other benefits I should know about?*

Reduced bone mineral density is also something which can spell bad news as we get older, as it can increase the risk of fractures leading to physical inactivity and affecting quality of life. Weight bearing exercise can increase bone density in older adults – again, helping to prevent a downward spiral of decline.[7]

*Righto. Move over The Rock – The Paper's taking over! Please welcome me into the fold.*

*Reality check*
Although some aerobic exercises can help to strengthen your muscles, time spent doing strength exercises doesn't count towards the recommended 150 minutes per week of moderate aerobic activities. You need to be doing both in order to ensure that you're getting the full health benefits.[6]

*So basically, we're saying . . .*
You don't need to start training like a champion weightlifter but maintaining a good level of muscle strength throughout your life will improve your chances of reaching a hundred.

## Robin Ince on an unconventional type of workout

*Do you exercise?*

I've got an alibi for exercise, which is that because I go to an enormous number of bookshops and don't really use public transport, rather than go to a gym, I buy too many books from charity shops, place them in a rucksack and then walk for two to three miles. And I consider that to be exercise! Which is probably bad . . .

However, when I tour with Brian Cox, of course, because he's a millionaire astrophysicist, he has a personal trainer – and I find that interesting, as I can keep up. I'm not as fit as them, but I find the exercise of being an excessive bibliophile works.

And also, when I did stop stand-up, I found that I put on weight immediately, so that hyperkinetic two hours a night I think does count as some form of aerobicising.

# Standing

*As a writer, I don't do much standing. I do some grandstanding though.*

While scientists have long recognised the serious impact on health of insufficient physical activity, a focus on the potential health consequences of prolonged sitting in its own right is relatively new.[1]

*I'm not standing for idle speculation. Give me some facts.*

In developed countries, 80 per cent of us spend a third of the working day sitting at a desk. Many of us spend yet more time every day seated in cars or on public transport and watching TV, gaming or using the internet. Sitting for prolonged periods uninterrupted, coupled with insufficient physical activity, substantially increases your risk of death. For this reason, experts have recommended that office workers try to increase the amount of time they spend standing and walking around during work hours.[2]

*Great! A medical excuse to get up and pace aimlessly around the office. But isn't the issue just that people who spend all their time sitting down aren't getting enough exercise?*

Studies have shown that sitting down on the job is associated with higher weight and higher risk of diabetes. To what extent sitting itself, rather than lack of physical activity, causes certain health problems and increases risk of death, however, is unclear.[3] Despite this, there is good reason to think that a predominantly sedentary lifestyle may have a negative impact on our health in its own right.

*My Apple Watch seems to think so. It prompts me to get up and stand for a minute every hour. I generally just ignore it.*

Research has also shown that prolonged periods of bed rest have a rapid detrimental effect on physical health.[1]

*Don't take my lie-ins away from me too!*

Comparisons have also been drawn with evidence of the impact on the body of weightlessness in space. Studies which have attempted to unpick the impact on death rates of prolonged sitting by taking overall levels of physical activity into account have found contradictory results, however, so this is an area which requires further research.[1]

*Is there actually any evidence that standing up more is healthier?*

An Australian study of more than 200,000 mid- and older-aged adults found evidence that standing lowered the risk of death in both people who met the physical activity guidelines and those who didn't. This effect was particularly strong when standing replaced sitting, with each hour of sitting that was replaced with standing bringing a 5 per cent decrease in the risk of dying during the period of the study.[4]

*I'm sprinkling drawing pins on all my chairs so I don't forget.*

Researchers also found evidence of a 'dose-response' relationship between standing time and mortality in adults aged forty-five years and older (in other words, the more time people spent standing, the lower their risk of death). This is particularly encouraging, because it's one of the signs that scientists look for when trying to establish if two things are causally linked.[5]

Another piece of good news is that research conducted with a group of sixty-eight-year-olds showed that reducing the amount of time you spend sitting down can lengthen your telomeres.[6]

(We talked about these in Religion, pages 38–42: they're the DNA–protein structures found at both ends of each chromosome. Their shortening is believed to play a key role in the ageing process.)

*So, standing up is now officially part of a healthy lifestyle?*

It is in Australia. Government guidelines there recommend that adults should minimise the amount of time spent in prolonged sitting and break up long periods of sitting as often as possible.[7] Those with a sedentary job should break up the time they spend sitting every day with two to four hours of standing and light walking.

*Government intervention? There could be sit-in protests.*

*Reality check*
In the UK, half of all workers are office-based, spending around two thirds of the working day seated and clocking up an average total of over ten hours of sitting time per day. Although it's become more common to see special standing desks in offices, you may not have the option to avoid being seated for prolonged periods while you're at work. Even if you're not forced to sit down on the job, you might simply feel too awkward to be the first one to break with convention if there isn't already a culture of standing.

A small study of desk-based employees in the UK published in 2018 looked at their experiences of standing up during meetings in which others were seated. As well as some physical discomfort, the participants reported difficulty fully engaging in the meeting from a standing position, along with a sense of awkwardness, especially if they weren't the person leading the meeting.[8]

*So basically, we're saying . . .*
Spending too much time on your bum could reduce your chances of making it to a hundred, even if you're getting the recommended amount of exercise overall (and especially if you're not). If you work in an office, try to find ways to spend more of the day on your feet, but prepare to deal with some awkwardness if you're looming over everyone else in the team meeting.

# Part Four: Food

# Five a day

*I'm not really a veg fan, unless we're talking chips and baked beans.*

A diet high in fruit and vegetables is one of the most important components of a healthy lifestyle.[1] They're a good source of vitamins, minerals and fibre (which can help to prevent constipation and reduce your risk of bowel cancer).[2] It's the combinations of these components of fruit and vegetables and the interactions between them which are believed to give them their health improving qualities.[3] As long as you don't cook them in lots of oil they're also usually low in fat and calories.[2]

*That's the chips out of the window. So, will eating non-oily veg make me lose weight?*

Studies have shown that higher fruit and vegetable consumption is associated with less or slower weight gain over time among adults, but more research is needed to really understand this relationship.[4]

*Well that's good news, except for the fact that I actually have to eat vegetables. Will chowing down on rabbit food make me live longer, too?*

An analysis of data from a nationwide health survey in England found that higher fruit and vegetable consumption was linked to lower death rates and that this relationship couldn't be explained by a range of other factors including physical activity, smoking, social class and weight.

The results showed that the benefits didn't only apply to those who were meeting the requirements of five a day, but the more people consumed the greater the impact. Those who ate at least one full portion of fruit and vegetables per day but less than three had a significantly greater chance of survival than those who ate less than one, while those who ate seven or more portions had the highest survival rate.[5]

*How many should I eat, then? Twenty?*

Most countries have official dietary recommendations that include fruit and vegetables but there's considerable variation between them regarding how much daily intake is recommended, what constitutes a portion and what counts towards the total. In some countries, for example, potatoes can be included, but not in the UK.[6]

The UK government advises that we all consume at least five portions of fruit and vegetables a day. This message is based on the World Health Organization's recommendation that people should be eating a daily minimum of 400 grams of fruit and vegetables to lower their risk of serious health problems, including heart disease, stroke and some types of cancer.[2]

*So, what counts as a portion – 80 grams?*

Fresh, frozen, canned and dried fruit and vegetables all count. One portion is 80 grams of fresh, canned or frozen fruit and vegetables, or 30 grams of dried fruit. To get your five a day in accordance with UK guidelines you have to discount potatoes, yams and cassava. Beans and pulses are a good source of fibre, but contain fewer nutrients than other fruits and vegetables. They only count as one a day, no matter how many you have. A glass of juice also only counts once a day.[2]

*What's with the juice? Surely, it's made of fruit, right?*

The evidence is mixed around the question of whether pure fruit juice is a poor substitute for fruit and should only be consumed in limited quantity.[7] We do know, however, that blending or juicing fruit is worse for our teeth because the process releases the sugars. When fruit is left whole, the sugars remain within its structure.[8]

*I like bananas. Can I just eat five bananas a day?*

Eating five of the same thing doesn't count. The idea is to consume a variety of fruit and vegetables each day in order to get a variety of nutrients. It's recommended that you try to consume a mix of different coloured fruits and vegetables.[2]

*Do you have to eat veg, or can you just eat different coloured fruits?*

Evidence shows that vegetable consumption has a significantly greater impact on health than fruit consumption.[5] Researchers have even suggested that instead of telling people to eat more 'fruit and vegetables', official guidelines should advise people to eat more 'vegetables and fruit' to emphasise the need for them to increase their vegetable intake primarily.[9]

*Sigh. I'm off to the illiterate greengrocer, where I was once forcibly ejected for crossing the apostrophe out of 'plum's'.*

*Reality check*
Whether there's an upper limit of fruit and vegetable consumption beyond which further intake provides no additional health benefits (or leads to a reduction in benefits) is unknown.[5] We do know, however, that it's possible to turn a sort of yellow-orangey colour if you eat too many carrots (a condition called carotenemia).[10]

*So basically, we're saying . . .*
One of the best things you can do to cut your chances of an early death is to eat at least five portions of fruit and vegetables every day. Get a good mix of different types and put the emphasis on the vegetables.

# Leafy green vegetables

*Greens, greens, good for your heart*
*The more you eat, the more you fart.*

*Or maybe that's beans? The farty bit still holds true though if we're talking about Brussels sprouts.*

We're talking about all kinds of leafy green vegetables (cabbage, lettuce, kale, spinach, leeks, etc.), including cruciferous vegetables (such as cauliflower, broccoli and, yes, Brussels sprouts). Leafy green vegetables have been labelled 'anti-ageing' due to their antioxidant properties.[1] They're typically low in calories and fat and provide a rich source of nutrients and dietary fibre.[2]

*Shame they taste so rubbish then. Still, I guess I should probably eat them and nothing else if I want to live to a hundred . . .*

Not so fast. Humans require a range of different types of food in order to obtain all the protein, vitamins and minerals needed to grow, reproduce and sustain life. No single food group can provide all the nutrients that our bodies need. By eating a range of foods and avoiding over-reliance on a single food, we also minimise the chances of ingesting a toxic dose of any one component.[3]

*Toxic? How can there be toxic stuff in green veg?*

Green leafy vegetables are known to contain considerable amounts of nitrate, which is carcinogenic and toxic. This is present naturally in the vegetables and is also found in fertiliser. Research carried out in Croatia with a broad sample of leafy vegetables found that they contained significant levels of nitrate, although still at an acceptable level in terms of human health.[4]

*What about pesticides?*

A broad range of pesticides are used on leafy vegetables and their large surface area means that relatively high levels can be left on them at the point of purchase. Research has shown, however, that standard food preparation methods, such as washing, peeling, blanching and cooking, are effective in removing most of these pesticides.[2] (See also Weedkiller and pesticides, pages 231–3.)

*Anything else I need to worry about?*

Several studies have suggested that broccoli might help to reduce the risk of developing some types of cancer; however, it also contains compounds which are potentially damaging to DNA. The health benefits of modest broccoli consumption outweigh any risks, although the impact of sustaining an extraordinarily high level of broccoli intake is not known.[5]

*I can't see myself falling into that category. Any other information?*

Research has suggested that consuming green leafy vegetables and cruciferous vegetables may lower your risk of developing type 2 diabetes.[6–8]

*Ah, we're back to the sprouts.*

A similar paper published in 2018, however, concluded that the evidence for a beneficial effect of eating green leafy or cruciferous vegetables on type 2 diabetes risk wasn't convincing.[6]

*Parp.*

*Reality check*

In recent years, the concept of 'superfoods' has taken off in a big way. The idea is that certain natural foods are considered particularly beneficial for health because of their levels of certain nutrients. You might have heard leafy green vegetables as a whole, or specific leafy green vegetables, such as kale, being referred to as 'superfoods'.

Scientists have often struggled to find convincing evidence to support the idea that so-called superfoods warrant the name, however. Eating a variety of fruits and vegetables and getting a minimum of five a day is the key to ensuring that your body gets the nutrients from plants that it needs, rather than fixating on the perceived benefits of one particular variety over another.[9]

*So basically, we're saying . . .*

Try not to get hung up on which type of vegetable is labelled as life-enhancing at any one time – just try to consume a good range of vegetables and eat more of them in general. Don't consume ridiculous quantities of any single variety – remember the possibility of turning orange from eating too many carrots!

# Meat

*You do realise I'm a vegetarian?!*

It won't be for everyone, but meat is a good source of protein, as well as vitamins and minerals, and can form part of a healthy balanced diet. Red meat specifically is a source of iron and one of our main sources of vitamin B12.[1]

*Can't you get iron from dark green leafy veg and B12 from a tablet?*

You can. Although in the UK the vast majority of people do eat meat, it isn't an essential component of a balanced diet, and there are some things to consider should you choose to eat it.[1] (There are also things to consider if you choose *not* to eat it – see Vegetarianism and veganism, pages 124–7.)

*I'm sensing a list coming up . . .*

Let me start by saying some meats are high in saturated fat, which can raise the amount of cholesterol in your blood. Having high cholesterol increases your risk of heart disease. Ways to reduce the amount of saturated fat you get from eating meat include choosing lean cuts, removing the skin from poultry meat, avoiding meat products in pastry (sausage rolls, etc.), grilling rather than frying and allowing fat to drain off when roasting.[1]

*Seems easier to not eat meat than remember all that.*

Numerous studies have also demonstrated a link between the consumption of processed and red meat and the risk of developing several chronic diseases and overall risk of death.[2-7] Processed meat is meat which has been preserved by either smoking, curing, salting or adding preservatives. Sausages, corned beef, bacon, ham, salami and pâté are all examples of processed meat.

UK guidelines recommend that if you're eating more than 90 grams of red and processed meat per day (that's the weight after cooking) that you should cut down to the average UK consumption of 70 grams a day, particularly because of the link with an increased risk of bowel cancer. To put that figure in perspective, a fry-up containing two sausages and two rashers of bacon would typically contain 130 grams of processed meat.[1]

*Really unhealthy – especially for the pig.*

The additional risk isn't huge – for every 10,000 people eating 76 grams of processed or red meat a day there will be 8 extra cases of bowel cancer.[8] So, you might feel it's a risk worth taking. On the other hand, you might not if you turn out to be one of the unlucky eight.

*It's not just eight overall though, is it? It's 8 for every 10,000, so probably runs into thousands. So no, not keen!*

It's also recommended that you should avoid eating liver or liver products too often because this may cause a harmful level of vitamin A to build up in your body. Having too much vitamin A can put you at greater risk of bone fractures when you get older – something which you'll definitely want to avoid in your quest to reach a hundred. Even just eating liver or products such as liver pâté once a week may mean that you're getting more vitamin A than you need.[1]

*You're preaching to the choir. And I feel another song coming on . . .*

*Reality check*

It's not just the longer-term health consequences of eating meat that you need to think about. Avoiding food poisoning in the immediate term is also an issue. Food safety is very important when you're cooking and handling raw meat. It's very common, for example, for raw chicken sold in the UK to contain a bacterium called campylobacter, which is estimated to cause around 300,000 cases of food poisoning every year. Around 70 of these cases will be fatal.[9]

You can get comprehensive advice on food safety from the NHS website. A couple of quick tips are worth mentioning here. Firstly, don't eat burgers which haven't been well cooked all the way through. Generally, it's OK to eat a steak that's rare on the inside as long as the outside is cooked properly because that's where the bacteria will be, but with burgers the bacteria can be right the way through. Secondly, don't wash meat under a running tap before you cook it – you'll just be spraying bacteria over nearby surfaces and thereby increasing your risk of food poisoning[1]

*So basically, we're saying . . .*
Avoid eating a lot of red and processed meat because of its links to cancer and higher death rates (you may even wish to consider cutting it out of your diet completely). Always follow food safety advice when handling and cooking any type of meat to avoid food poisoning.

## Richard Osman on meat-eating

As we start this interview, Richard is tucking into a juicy steak.

*The more red and processed meat you eat, the lower your life expectancy. Will you carry on eating meat, knowing this?*

Quite apart from killing me, it's going to kill the planet. The extent to which we need to cut down on meat-eating only hit home a few years ago, so I certainly eat less than I did, and I'm very excited about this era where they make an artificial meat. I'm very comfortable with just eating that forever.

In terms of the nutritional value and whether meat will kill me, it doesn't worry me particularly. I grew up in the 1970s where there was all sorts of rubbish, and people who grew up in the 1950s and 1960s grew up smoking. We all have things we grew up with that we thought were OK; it turns out they're not, but they've become such a habit, and that's the thing that'll kill us.

Kids these days: who knows what will kill 'em? Vaping maybe, or quinoa, or avocado! By the point they find out, they'll have eaten so much quinoa or avocado they'll have to keep eating it – they won't be able to give it up.

And I'm like that with steak really, I suppose, because I guess I'm never going to give it up. I'm going to try to eat much less of it, and try to eat more responsibly sourced meat, which I know is a cop out.

I worry that it kills the planet, and I'll try and do something about that. I don't worry that it'll kill me, as *something* will kill me.

# Fish and shellfish

*Hurray! A legitimate op-perch-tuna-ty to make fish puns, for the sheer halibut. I bet, if I'm looking for fish facts, I've come to the right plaice . . .*

Fish and shellfish are good sources of a range of vitamins and minerals, and oily fish – such as sardines, mackerel, salmon and pilchards – are also high in long-chain omega-3 fatty acids, which can help to protect you from heart disease. White fish – such as cod, pollock and haddock – are a low-fat source of protein.

*So 'never mind the pollock' is inaccurate?*

Quite. It's recommended that you should eat at least two portions of fish a week as part of a healthy diet, one of which should be oily fish.[1]

*Are you saying fish and chips is good for you? Brill.*

Deep frying fish in batter isn't a healthy method of cooking because it increases the fat content. Steaming, baking and grilling are much healthier ways to cook fish on a regular basis.[1]

*I guess that's a red herring, then. Does a can of tuna in oil count as a portion of oily fish?*

No. It's the type of fish that determines whether it counts as 'oily', not whether it's been cooked or stored in oil.[1]

*Aren't fish high in mercury? And, if so, can it krill you?*

Mercury is a naturally occurring element found in the air, water and soil which is toxic to our nervous systems. Nearly all the fish we eat contain small amounts of mercury, although some contain a lot more than others. Generally, those higher up the food chain contain more because they build up accumulation from eating smaller fish, which in turn have consumed mercury from their own diet.[2]

Some groups are known to be more at risk than others – it's recommended that pregnant women and breastfeeding mothers should avoid eating fish which are known to contain higher levels of mercury. The impact of low doses of mercury exposure from a typical diet on the general adult population isn't well understood, however. So far it hasn't been possible to come up with standard guidelines on how much mercury in fish is safe to consume, partly because it will affect people differently depending on their weight, age and genetics.[3, 4]

*There's also the danger of choking on a fish bone, isn't there? Then you'd need someone to mussel in and save you.*

Getting a fish bone stuck in your oesophagus (the tube that connects the mouth and stomach) can cause potentially fatal complications, so you should definitely take care to try to avoid swallowing one.[5, 6]

It's not all bad news about bones, though. The bones of some oily fish, such as whitebait and canned sardines and pilchards, are fragile enough that they can safely be chewed or mashed up and eaten, providing a source of calcium and phosphorus which will help to keep your own bones strong.[1]

*Are shellfish as healthy as normal fish, or is that a load of carp?*

Shellfish, such as prawns, crabs, cockles, mussels, scallops and squid, are low in fat and a source of some essential minerals. You can also get omega-3 fatty acids from some types of shellfish, such as mussels, crab and oysters, although they don't contain as much as oily fish.[1]

*Aren't oysters full of sewage? They made Heston Blumenthal's profits flounder . . .*

Oysters and some other shellfish feed by filtering large volumes of water, which means that bacteria and viruses from human sewage can build up inside them.[7] In 2009, there was an outbreak of noro-virus (which causes diarrhoea and vomiting) at Heston Blumenthal's Fat Duck restaurant. The outbreak affected at least 240 people and was found to have been caused by oysters containing the virus.[8] Eating raw oysters, no matter how posh the restaurant, carries a risk of food poisoning.[7]

*OK, I've haddock with this chapter. Fin.*

> **Reality check**
> Some people take fish oil supplements as a way of getting the omega-3 fatty acids found in oily fish. Though studies had previously suggested a health benefit, a comprehensive review of the research evidence which was published in 2018 concluded that omega-3 fatty acid supplements derived from fish oils or plants have little or no impact on the risk of heart disease, stroke or on overall rates of death. This finding supported existing government guidelines in the UK advising that omega-3 should not be offered to patients as a way of preventing cardiovascular disease. While the evidence may not support the use of omega-3 supplements, however, foods which are naturally high in omega-3 (including oily fish, as well as seeds, nuts and legumes) continue to form an impor-tant part of a healthy diet.[9]

*So basically, we're saying . . .*
Overall, eating fish and shellfish, especially oily fish, is good
for your health. Avoid swallowing fish bones unless they're
delicate enough to be mashed up and be aware that eating raw
oysters might make you ill.

# Dairy products

*Ah, I love cheese. You can tell me not to eat it, but I won't give Edam.*

I'm not going to do that. As a nutrient-dense food source, dairy products, such as milk, cheese and yoghurt, have long been recommended as part of a healthy balanced diet.[1] Many of us will have childhood memories of being told by parents and schoolteachers that milk will make our bones grow strong.

*If your bones are weak, it's important to walk Caerphilly, right?*

We don't necessarily think of breaking a bone as something that could reduce our life expectancy, but fracturing a hip can have serious consequences for older people. Among elderly people who suffer a broken hip, 10 per cent will die within a month and 30 per cent will die within a year. Only half will return to their previous level of mobility.[2]

*Don't tell me sad things like that. I Camembert it.*

As we get older, we naturally lose bone density and muscle mass, although the extent of this deterioration varies. Lower bone density and reduced muscle mass both contribute to the risk of hip fracture. Adequate calcium, vitamin D and protein intake are essential for retaining muscle mass, strength and bone density, leading some scientists to hypothesise that dairy product consumption may have a role to play in preventing hip fractures.

## Dairy products

*I love to gorge myself on Cheddar, but is milk healthy?*

Milk is a natural source of calcium and protein and in some parts of the world is fortified with vitamin D. Studies have shown positive benefits from dairy product consumption on bone health, although further research is needed to gain a clear picture of the relationship between the two.[1]

*Is there any whey it could be a false correlation?*

A review of different studies looking at the relationship between dairy product consumption and the risk of breaking a hip found a mixed picture. While consuming more yoghurt and cheese was associated with a lower risk of hip fracture, greater total consumption of dairy products was not. There was insufficient evidence to establish the relationship between milk consumption and the risk of breaking a hip.[3]

*Will eating dairy make me live longer? Or is it a case of 'tough cheese'?*

A study of American adults found that those who had a higher total consumption of dairy products had a lower risk of death from all causes, as well as a lower risk of death from cerebrovascular disease specifically.

*Well, that's Gouda news.*

Those who had a higher consumption of milk, however, had a higher risk of coronary heart disease.[4]

Meanwhile, a review of research evidence looking at total dairy intake and the risk of dying from cancer found no statistically significant association. The results showed a clear relationship in men, however, between the amount of whole milk they consumed and their risk of dying from prostate cancer – the more they consumed, the greater the risk.[5]

*It's a-curd to me that this is a very mixed picture.*

Indeed. A systematic review of the latest evidence, published in 2018, concluded that the relationships between dairy products and the risk of type 2 diabetes, stroke and coronary heart disease were either neutral or beneficial.[6]

Another research review found evidence that a modest increase in dairy product consumption could help prevent type 2 diabetes, but highlighted that more robust research studies would be needed before this could be confirmed.[7]

*How about yoghurt? I think it tastes udderly awesome.*

The strongest results in the 2018 systematic review were found for the association between yoghurt and type 2 diabetes, although the authors acknowledged that this could potentially be explained by yoghurt consumption being associated with other aspects of a healthy lifestyle.[6]

Yoghurt is often sweetened to make it more palatable to the consumer and some products, including organic ones, have been found to have very high levels of sugar.[1, 8] It's important to read the nutritional information label and not to assume that a yoghurt is necessarily a healthy option.

*That's not moo-sic to my ears.*

Some final facts: a systematic review of research literature found that intake of high-fat milk was associated with a higher risk of stroke.[9] The consumption of high-fat dairy products has also been shown to be associated with poorer bone and brain health, but lower accumulation of fat around the abdominal area.[1]

Ultimately, there's more work to be done to compare health outcomes related to consumption of full-fat versus low-fat cheese and yoghurt, as well as milk and yoghurt products with and without added sugar.[6]

*Well, if it turns out dairy isn't healthy, I'll be very cheesed off.*

*Reality check*

There is evidence that consumption of milk and yoghurt is related to other behaviours which might lead to a lower risk of certain diseases. As the studies which have been undertaken in this area typically don't involve people being allocated randomly to either a group who consume dairy products or a group who don't, there remains the possibility that these other behaviours account for the observed differences in health outcomes.[6]

Although we know that calcium is important for bone health and reducing the risk of fractures particularly in older age, dairy products are not the only source.

*So basically, we're saying . . .*

Dairy products offer a convenient source of key nutrients as part of a balanced diet. Steering away from the high fat and high sugar versions should help to ensure that any health benefits outweigh the cons. Getting enough calcium, vitamin D and protein are important for staying fit and strong as we age.

# Fats and oils

*Ah, the popular 1990s dance group. Didn't one of them marry Vanessa Feltz?*

That's Phats & Small, who are unlikely to impede your progress to becoming a centenarian. We're talking food here. Two main types of fat are found in our food – saturated fats and unsaturated fats. Most fats and oils contain both types but in different proportions. There are also trans fats, which we'll come to later.[1]

*Sorry, I've got 'Turn Around' stuck in my head now and I'm struggling to concentrate.*

Saturated fat is mostly derived from animal sources, such as meat and dairy products, although it can also be found in some plant-based foods, such as palm oil. Coconut oil, which has often been touted as having health benefits, is 80 to 90 per cent saturated fat and should only be used occasionally.[2, 3] Butter contains around 50 per cent. Other foods which are high in saturated fat include meat pies, cake and cheese. Too much saturated fat can raise the level of bad cholesterol in your blood, increasing your risk of developing heart disease or having a stroke. It's recommended that men shouldn't have more than 30 grams of saturated fat a day and women shouldn't have more than 20 grams.[1]

*Right. And unsaturated fats are good?*

Unsaturated fats are found primarily in fish and plant oils. They can be either monounsaturated or polyunsaturated. Monounsaturated fats help maintain good cholesterol while reducing bad cholesterol. They can be found in olive oil, rapeseed oil, avocados and certain nuts. The two main types of polyunsaturated fats are omega-3 and omega-6. Small amounts of these are essential in our diet. Omega-3 fats are the ones we get from oily fish and omega-6 fats are found mainly in vegetable oils, such as rapeseed, corn and sunflower. Polyunsaturated fats can also help lower your level of bad cholesterol.[1]

*Trans fats are the real baddies, aren't they? If you see them, should you Turn Around?*

Trans fats can be present naturally in low amounts in dairy products and meat, but it's the artificially created trans fats used in food manufacturing which have been a cause of concern in recent years. These are produced when vegetable oils are hydrogenated to turn them into solid or semi-solid fats. Trans fats may also be created when ordinary vegetable oils are heated to very high temperatures to fry foods. They're often found in fast food, cakes and biscuits.

*Why are they so bad for you, then?*

Trans fats both raise bad cholesterol and lower good cholesterol, and are considered even worse for our health than saturated fats. For this reason, some countries have made substantial efforts to prevent trans fats getting into people's diets, both through legislation and voluntary changes within the food industry.[1, 4]

*Vanessa Feltz lost a lot of weight, didn't she? Some people say you should cut out all fat if you're dieting . . .?*

Cutting all fat out of your diet definitely wouldn't improve your chances of reaching a hundred. We all need to consume a small amount of fat because it provides essential fatty acids, which our bodies aren't able to make, as well as helping us to absorb certain vitamins. Just like excess carbohydrate and protein, though, any fat

117

we consume that the body doesn't use up will get converted into body fat.[1]

*Will reducing fat intake make me live longer?*

Research studies looking at the relationship between dietary fat intake and death have produced mixed results, but there is some evidence that consumption of unsaturated fats is associated with a lower risk of cardiovascular disease and death, while higher intake of saturated fats and trans fats is associated with a higher risk of cardiovascular disease.[5, 6]

*Is olive oil good for me?*

Olive oil is a staple of the Mediterranean diet, which has been linked with lower rates of cardiovascular disease and also shown to be an effective alternative to a simple low-fat diet for achieving weight loss.[7] Olive oil has been recommended as the best option for cooking because it produces fewer toxic compounds when heated up than many other oils, but you should still try to use as little as possible and don't reuse the oil after you've cooked with it once. Don't worry about whether it's extra virgin.[8]

*What are toxic compounds?*

When oil is heated up to a high temperature during cooking its make-up changes. Oils which are thought of as healthy at room temperature, such as sunflower oil, can be bad for us when we cook with them. This is because toxic compounds can be produced by a process called oxidation that occurs at high temperatures. These compounds have been linked with a range of negative potential implications for our health which could increase the risk of developing a serious disease.

Reusing oil for cooking after it's been heated up once can allow these toxic compounds to build up in higher concentrations. This can be a particular issue if you're regularly buying food from takeaways, where oil might be reused several times to reduce costs. [9, 10]

*My main 'takeaway' from this is to eat a little olive oil but not too much.
Also: did Vanessa marry Phats or Small?*

I have no idea.

*Reality check*
If you're trying to cut down on your intake of fat, it's important to scrutinise food labels because they can be misleading.
Foods which are labelled 'lower fat' or 'reduced fat' aren't
necessarily low in fat – they just contain less fat than a regular
version of a similar product. The lower fat version might still
be classed as high in fat. Consider anything containing more
than 17.5 grams per 100 grams as high in fat and anything
with 3 grams or less per 100 grams as low in fat.

Remember to also look at how much saturated fat specifically different foods contain. Consider anything with more
than 5 grams per 100 grams as high in saturates and 1.5
grams or less per 100 grams as low in saturates.

Bear in mind also that 'low in fat' doesn't necessarily mean
'low in calories'. Fat is often replaced with sugar in low-fat
products to keep it tasting good, so the energy content might
actually be similar. Think of managing your intake of fat as
just one aspect of achieving and maintaining a healthy diet,
rather than becoming too fixated on it in isolation.[1]

*So basically, we're saying . . .*
Try to keep your intake of saturated fats down by replacing
them with unsaturated fats, avoid trans fats, use olive oil to
cook and focus on getting a balanced diet overall rather than
just cutting out fat.

# Carbs

*I love the three Ps: pizza, pasta and potatoes. But I'm not meant to eat them, right?*

That's a misconception. The prominence of low-carbohydrate (or low-carb) diet plans for weight loss, such as the Atkins Diet and the South Beach Diet, has meant that many people assume carbohydrates to be bad news for achieving and maintaining a state of good health. The real picture is a little more complicated.

*Complex carbs? Never mind.*

Along with fat and protein, carbs are one of the three main groups of nutrients that make up our diet. Although things like pasta and potatoes often spring to mind when we think of carbs, most foods are actually made up of a combination of carbs, fats and proteins in varying amounts.[1]

*So, what are carbs?*

Sugar, starch and fibre are the three different types of carbs in the food we eat.[1] As we'll see in the chapter on sugar, pages 132–4, excess sugar has a negative impact on our health and many of us are consuming too much without realising. Starchy foods are things like pasta, rice, bread, potatoes and cereals. It's recommended that these make up around a third of our diet.

*That sounds very generous. I thought they were meant to be bad for us?*

Starchy foods are often regarded as something to avoid by people who are trying to live more healthily, but they're actually a good source of energy as well as being the main source of a range of nutrients in our diet. Wholegrain options, such as wholemeal bread and brown rice, are better for us. Leaving the skin on potatoes also helps to provide more dietary fibre.[1]

*And saves you having to peel them! I've heard that we need more fibre in our diets, but what exactly is it?*

The indigestible parts of plant-based foods are known as dietary fibre. Fibre plays an important part in a healthy, balanced diet and evidence shows that having a diet which is high in fibre reduces the risk of bowel cancer, cardiovascular disease and type 2 diabetes. Vegetables with the skins on, beans and lentils, and wholegrain foods are all good sources of fibre. Most adults in the UK are only consuming about two thirds of the recommended 30 grams a day of dietary fibre.[1]

*Don't carbs give you too many calories, though?*

Carbs should be the main source of energy in a healthy, balanced diet. They get broken down into glucose and used by your body for fuelling every activity – whether it's running a marathon or just breathing. Unused glucose can be converted by the body into a substance called glycogen. The problem comes when our bodies end up with more glucose than they're able to store as glycogen – when this happens, the extra glucose gets converted into fat.[1]

*So, if I go on a low-carb diet, where will my energy come from?*

If your body isn't able to get enough energy from carbs in your diet it will convert protein into glucose instead or derive energy from fat. Simply cutting out one food group from your diet doesn't mean that you will inevitably lose weight – it's the total calorie intake that counts. If you consume more calories than you burn, you will gain weight. This applies no matter what type of food the calories come from.[1]

*Is a low-carb diet a good idea?*

Substantially reducing your intake of carbs over the long term might stop you from getting enough of certain nutrients. Unless you find healthy substitutes to make up for the shortfall, this could lead to health problems. It's also important to bear in mind that replacing carbs with fats may end up raising your cholesterol and, in turn, increasing your risk of developing heart disease.[1]

While some people will achieve weight loss through low-carb diets, the evidence does not support the idea that they offer a better approach to weight loss compared with the more traditional approach of a balanced, restricted-calorie healthy eating plan combined with exercise.[2–4]

*How about low-GI foods – should we all be eating them?*

GI stands for glycaemic index – a system for rating how quickly foods which contain carbs affect glucose levels in the blood when eaten alone. Low-GI foods are those which cause blood sugar levels to rise and fall slowly (potentially increasing the length of time before you feel hungry again).

The limitation of focusing on GI to determine what you eat is that being low-GI doesn't necessarily mean that something is healthy. Fruit, vegetables and wholegrain foods, for example, are healthy and typically low-GI; however, chocolate cake has a lower GI rating than parsnips. The GI rating of your food will also be affected by how it's cooked.[1]

*OK, well I'm off to eat a pizza and a jacket potato.*

*Reality check*

Over time, a range of different weight-loss diet plans have gained popularity, sometimes capturing a good deal of media attention. Their requirements often contradict government guidelines on healthy eating or are likely to be difficult to adhere to in the longer term. Weight-loss diets tend to come with different pros and cons, and what suits one person may not suit another.

No matter what approach you decide to take, one fundamental rule applies – to lose weight you need to burn more calories than you take in. You should aim to achieve this through a combination of restricted calorie healthy eating and increased physical activity, ensuring that your body still gets the nutrition it needs while reducing your calorie intake. You should also choose an approach which is realistically sustainable and will enable you to maintain a healthy weight in the longer term.[4]

*So basically, we're saying . . .*

Carbs form a key part of a healthy and balanced diet, but some high-carb foods are better for our health than others. Low-carb and low-GI based diets don't offer a magic solution to weight loss.

# Vegetarianism and veganism

*I'm a veggie and eat lots of vegan foods. Does that mean I get to be smug and judgemental?*

You do according to some in the press. The potential health benefits of a vegetarian diet have been the subject of much research and attention in the media. Studying the impact of vegetarian and vegan diets on health is always challenging because those who adopt them tend not to be representative of the general population – for example, they're typically more health conscious generally than omnivores (people who have a plant *and* animal-based diet).

*Comedians always make jokes about vegetarians being weak and ill.*

It's clear from the research to date that vegetarians overall are no less healthy than their omnivorous counterparts.[1]

*I'll tell them to stop making the jokes, if I can muster up the strength. Seriously, though: are there any health benefits to being a veggie?*

The evidence has been contradictory, with some studies showing health benefits of vegetarianism and others finding no meaningful differences in outcomes between vegetarians and non-vegetarians.[1]

A systematic review of almost a hundred studies on this topic which was published in 2017 concluded that a vegetarian diet significantly reduced the risk of developing and dying from ischemic heart disease. Vegans and vegetarians had lower levels of bad cholesterol and a significantly reduced risk of developing cancer.[2]

*That sounds promising.*

A very large study of Seventh-Day Adventists in the US found that low-meat consumers, pescatarians, vegans and vegetarians all grouped together, had a lower rate of death than regular meat eaters; however, when broken down into separate categories the results were only statistically significant in the case of pescatarians.

This research provided evidence that eating less meat than regular consumers reduces your risk of death over a period of time, but didn't prove that vegans or vegetarians will experience a greater benefit than pescatarians or people who still eat smaller amounts of meat. (The data actually makes a stronger case for pescatarianism than vegetarianism.)[3] Other research studies have also provided evidence that those who consume less meat and get more of their protein from plant sources (such as nuts and pulses) have lower rates of death.[4–6]

*So, I should incorporate fish into my diet? Is this one of the reasons why the Japanese and people in Mediterranean countries live so long – they all eat lots of fish?*

Possibly – but, in contrast, a study of people in the UK found that vegetarians, pescatarians and people who eat little meat did not have significantly lower overall death rates compared with regular meat eaters.[7] One possible reason for this might be differences between the diets of vegetarians in the UK and those in the US.[3]

The researchers did find benefits, however, when looking at different specific causes of death. Vegetarians and vegans had around half the death rate from certain cancers compared with regular meat eaters, while pescatarians and low meat eaters also had lower rates of death from some causes. When they looked at the data for vegans as a group on their own, they found no statistically significant difference in death rates compared with regular meat eaters.[7]

*So, there's no point in turning vegan, then? That simplifies life.*

Overall, the evidence so far suggests that a vegan diet is unlikely to have any significant health advantages over a vegetarian diet, although of course there are also non-health reasons why you might opt to avoid animal products.[3, 8]

*Yes, ethical and environmental reasons – plus you get to have comedians make fun of you.*

*Reality check*
If you choose to become vegetarian, vegan or pescatarian it's still important to eat healthily and make sure that you're getting an adequate balance of nutrients. It's possible to have a meat-free diet which is still a very unhealthy one. Eating lots of vegetables doesn't negate the need to watch your intake of fat and sugar, for example.

In you opt for a vegan diet, there's a particular risk of not getting enough vitamin B12, vitamin D, calcium and omega-3 fatty acids, so it's important to ensure that you meet recommended intake levels through consuming fortified foods or appropriate supplements.[8]

*So basically, we're saying . . .*
Minimising the amount of meat in your diet will reduce your risk of some diseases and increase your chances of a long life, although you don't necessarily have to become a full vegetarian or vegan to experience health benefits. There are no disadvantages to giving up meat, as long as you still get a balanced diet with the right nutrients.

## Robin Ince on vegetarianism

I don't eat meat. I'm a vegetarian and I think I should be a vegan. I've tried being a vegan, I'm just not very good at it when I'm on tour. I can feel myself moving further and further towards veganism – I find animal products less and less alluring. Sometimes you look at your face and think, 'Everything's really podged up', because everything is artificial. There's too much confectionery, too many crisps, too many things that are readily available when you're touring – and I am touring all the time.

I always go and buy the 'two for £4' salads from Marks & Spencer. Normally I get the nutty wholefoods one, sometimes I get the pasta one, and sometimes I get the quinoa one. But I'm careful with the quinoa, because you do get bits in your teeth and then you're talking at a gig and a bit of quinoa flies out into the front row!

I don't eat healthily enough. I don't drink sugary drinks, but I probably drink too much alcohol – although not nearly as much as years ago, because I'm older and not as much of an idiot.

# Herbs, spices and salt

*Ooh, this takes me back. I'm dreaming of the smell of my Zoroastrian grandparents' house.*

Herbs and spices have been used to improve the flavour of food since ancient times, as well as being used as preservatives and medicines.[1]

A range of studies have highlighted the therapeutic potential of different spices for their antioxidant, anti-inflammatory and anti-carcinogenic properties among others.[2, 3]

*My nan always used to use loads of turmeric, coriander and cumin.*

Studies have been done looking at a number of herbs and spices, including, among others, garlic, mint, fenugreek, black pepper, parsley, ginger and turmeric, and reported therapeutic effects pertaining to a broad spectrum of health problems, including heart disease, alcohol abuse, high blood pressure and gum disease.[1]

*Did they show that they make you live forever? My nan's ninety-five and still going.*

Frequent consumption of spicy food has been linked to a lower risk of death from cancer, heart disease and respiratory disease, although exactly what role spices and herbs play in protecting against the development of such conditions remains unclear.[3]

*Could it be something to do with antioxidants?*

Yes, herbs and spices could be a useful source of natural antioxidants in the diet, in addition to fruits and vegetables. Natural antioxidants help to reduce oxidative stress, which is involved in a range of serious health problems, including cancer, stroke and rheumatoid arthritis, as well as the ageing process.[1, 4]

Ultimately, more evidence is still needed in order to establish any impact on cardiovascular health that can be attributed to herb and spice antioxidants.[5]

*What about cancer? Do herbs and spices help ward it off?*

Several studies have suggested that they may have a preventive effect against the early stages of cancer; however, there is a lack of research conducted in humans looking at normal levels of consumption. Without placebo-controlled clinical trials in humans it is not possible to determine the true effectiveness of herbs and spices in preventing cancers or the safe and optimal dosage required.[5]

*I don't pay much attention to dosage right now. I just chuck a load of herbs, spices and garlic into everything I cook.*

There is some evidence that consuming between half and one clove of garlic every day may lower your cholesterol by up to 9 per cent.[5] Also, a study looking at a population in China suggested that a high intake of raw garlic may reduce the risk of oesophageal cancer.[6]

*And decrease your social circle as a result of your bad breath. Anyhow: I'm sure I heard that herbs are good for your brain, too . . .?*

Although studies show that some herbal supplements can have an effect on brain health, there is little evidence that typical consumption of herbs and spices in our food directly affects cognition (the mental process involved in knowing, learning and understanding things). Our total intake of antioxidants, however, may help to protect us from cognitive decline as we age, and the inclusion of herbs and spices in our diet makes a contribution to this.[5]

*What about that Asian favourite, turmeric? It stains your fingers yellow like you smoke a pack a day, but it's good for us, right?*

As well as having anti-inflammatory properties, there is evidence that turmeric may have benefit as a treatment for people with Alzheimer's disease and symptoms of dementia.[3, 7]

A large number of studies, using a range of methods, have looked at the potential health effects of curcumin, the source of the spice turmeric, which is frequently used in curries and other spicy food from India, Asia and the Middle East. India has a much lower prevalence of Alzheimer's disease among people aged seventy to seventy-nine than the US. One study, which looked at over 1000 older people, found that those who consumed curry occasionally or often had better cognitive function than those who ate it rarely or never.[8]

*Should we all ditch our diets and get down the curry house, then?*

Although the consumption of herbs and spices has increased in recent years, and research into the potential health benefits of herbs continues to grow, there's little authoritative guidance on how much of them we should be getting in our diet. Greek dietary guidelines have highlighted that certain herbs are a good source of antioxidants; however, it's more common for the use of herbs and spices to be recommended as a way of adding flavour to food in order to help with reducing salt intake.[5]

*Salt's a killer, isn't it?*

There's a well-established association between excess consumption of salt (sodium) and adverse health effects, including high blood pressure and death from cardiovascular disease. The World Health Organization recommends a daily sodium intake for adults of less than 2 grams (equivalent to 5 grams of salt) in adults, with lower amounts for children.[9]

*Right then. You'll find me in the spice aisle, imagining a gorgeous-smelling house in Leicester with a hideous floral carpet.*

*Reality check*

Although a lot of studies have been conducted in this area, the evidence base currently has some important limitations. Much of the research has been conducted on animals or used other methods which don't test the effects of the culinary use of herbs and spices in humans.[1] Also, measuring the impact of antioxidants in the diet on people's levels of oxidative stress and health status is not straightforward.[10]

More research is needed to establish what level of exposure to different herbs and spices is required to bring about specific health benefits without any ill effects.[11]

*So basically, we're saying . . .*

Herbs and spices have a role to play in reducing your risk of certain diseases through a healthy balanced diet. Introducing more of them into your cooking can help keep your salt intake within recommended amounts and increase your intake of antioxidants. Excessive consumption of anything can be harmful, though, so ingesting unusually large quantities of herbs and spices is not the route to a longer life.

# Sugar

*I'm a chocoholic, and think sugar makes life sweeter. Should I be shutting my cakehole?*

Possibly. We used to think the only real problem with sugar in our diet was its link with tooth decay, but over time we've come to understand more about the effect of sugar on our health. Many of us consume a lot of extra calories from the sugar in our diets. This can lead to obesity and increase the risk of related conditions, such as diabetes.[1, 2] It can also increase blood pressure and chronic inflammation, and raise the risk of dying from cardiovascular disease.[3]

*If you look at food packaging though, everything contains sugar . . .*

The problem is with what are known as 'free sugars' – sugar which is added to food and drinks in the manufacturing or cooking process, as well as sugar which is naturally present in fruit juices, honey and syrups. Guidelines recommend that anyone over the age of eleven should consume no more than 30 grams of free sugars a day. A typical standard-sized chocolate bar contains around 25 grams of free sugar, while a normal can of cola contains around 35 grams, more than the recommended limit just on its own.[1, 2, 4]

*What about fruit? That's full of sugar, isn't it?*

Yes, but there's a difference. The sugar contained in pieces of fruit isn't counted as 'free' because it's trapped within the cell walls, unless it's released by juicing or blending to make juice and smoothie drinks.

132

## Sugar

*Do I need to avoid fructose, then? What about honey?*

Different types of sugar have different names, which can be confusing and make it harder to tell when sugar has been added to the food and drinks that we buy. If you see any of the following in the ingredients list, then you know that the product contains free sugar:[1, 5]

glucose
sucrose
fructose
maltose
corn syrup
honey
hydrolysed starch
invert sugar
molasses
brown sugar
agave syrup
maple syrup
cane sugar
high-fructose corn syrup
fruit juice concentrate/purée
treacle

*Well, someone just killed all the fun. I'm guessing that's the end of any desserts . . .*

Although images of sweets, cakes and chocolate tend to spring to mind when we picture sugar in our diet, it's also often added into processed foods which we would normally think of as savoury, such as soups, baked beans and ready meals. Foods which we might tend to think of as healthy, such as wholegrain breakfast cereals and yoghurt, often contain high levels of added sugar as well.

*Right, I'm off to chuck half the fridge in the bin.*

*Reality check*

As we've come to understand more about the link between excessive sugar consumption and obesity, the concept of a sugar-free diet has risen in popularity. Diet plans based on going 'sugar-free' tend to involve cutting out all or most forms of sugar, especially free sugars. While it's a good idea to try to minimise your intake of free sugars, going completely sugar-free is not considered a viable healthy approach, given that sugar occurs naturally in fruit and vegetables.[6]

*So basically, we're saying . . .*

Most of us consume too much sugar. Trying to go strictly sugar-free isn't realistic, but you should aim to minimise your intake of added sugar in its various forms and keep to the recommended limit for fruit juice and smoothies.

# Artificial sweeteners

*Zero calories! These things are a miracle, right?*

Well, artificial sweeteners have certainly become increasingly common in processed food and drinks as concern over the health effects of having too much sugar in our diets has grown. There are a number of different types, such as aspartame, saccharin, sorbitol, stevia and xylitol. They can be found in a huge range of products, including toothpaste and sugar-free chewing gum.[1] Chewing sugar-free gum has well-established benefits for dental health.[2, 3]

*So, why don't they just ban sugar and replace it with this stuff?*

A lot of consumers are wary of artificial sweeteners and distrust the claims that they are safe.[4] The question of whether artificial sweeteners are linked to cancer has been the focus of many scientific research reports. Overall, the research studies conducted in this area have not proven a link between artificial sweeteners and cancer in humans and the consensus is that they're safe to consume.[1, 5]

*Safe? Great! Hold my diet lemonade; I'm off to lobby the government and end the obesity crisis . . .*

Slow down. Studies looking at the relationship between low-calorie sweeteners and body weight have shown mixed results.[6] Though some have suggested replacing sugar with other sweeteners helps control weight and blood glucose levels in adults, these findings are not scientifically robust.[7]

Randomised controlled trials, which provide the best quality evidence, have not shown a beneficial impact on weight.[8] Other research has also cast doubt on the idea that artificial sweeteners have a role to play in helping to control diabetes.[9] Some evidence even suggests that routine consumption of artificial sweeteners is associated with increased weight and risk of high blood pressure and type 2 diabetes.[8] The inconsistencies between the findings of different studies on this topic mean that more research is needed before we can fully understand the potential long-term risks and benefits of low-calorie sweeteners.[6, 7, 10]

*Hey, I was just trying to save the world. You're quite the party pooper, you know that?*

*Reality check*
Diet soda drinks containing artificial sweeteners in place of sugar might deliver fewer calories, but they're generally still bad news for your dental health. This is because it's not just the sugar in normal soda which damages your teeth. Cola and other soft drinks can be highly acidic, causing dental erosion. Unfortunately, this applies just as much to diet sodas as it does to their sugary equivalents.[11]

*So basically, we're saying . . .*
Sweeteners are safe to consume but switching to them from sugar might not be as beneficial for your health as you might think. You're probably better off reducing your intake of sweet things altogether and replacing sugary soft drinks with water.[7]

# Probiotics

*Ah, these are the yoghurt thingies you down like tequila shots, right?*

Right. Probiotics are live bacteria and yeasts which are marketed as having a variety of health benefits. Yoghurts described as containing 'friendly' or 'good' bacteria are probably the most obvious example. They can also be purchased in the form of food supplements.

*'Friendly'! I'm not sure I could deal with that many friends. Think of the birthdays. But they're good for your health, aren't they?*

Well, the *idea* that consuming probiotics is good for your health is based on the belief that they help to improve the balance of bacteria in your gut.[1] All of us play host to hundreds of different types of microorganisms which live in the gut (collectively known as the 'microbiome') in combinations which are as unique as our fingerprints.

*What does the microbiome do?*

As well as being crucial for our digestive health, the microbiome helps to develop and shape the immune system. Emerging evidence suggests that issues with the balance of gut bacteria might play a role in the development of certain health conditions, such as obesity and high blood pressure.[2] Scientists are even exploring links between mental health and the organisms which live in our guts.[3]

*So, if everyone's microbiome is different, how can probiotics claim to restore balance?*

Probiotics are classed as food rather than medicine, so they don't go through the same kind of rigorous testing with regard to their effectiveness.[1] Although research shows that probiotics might be beneficial in some very specific circumstances, aside from this there's not much evidence to support the idea that regularly consuming them will bring health benefits for most people.[1, 4, 5]

The make-up of your microbiome is strongly influenced by your everyday eating habits. Maintaining a healthy diet overall is likely to bring much more benefit than simply consuming a probiotic.[6]

*So, they're not so 'good' after all . . . but could they be bad?*

Although it's been argued that their safety hasn't yet been fully established, based on what we know so far, as long as you have a healthy immune system, probiotics shouldn't do you any harm.[1, 4]

*I'm going to go with my gut and say you shouldn't eat your friends anyway – it yog-hurts their feelings.*

> *Reality check*
> When probiotics are used in research, scientists will typically focus on very specific organisms and carefully measure the dose that's received. This is quite different from consuming a food product with probiotics added, when you don't know exactly what you're getting or in what dose. Even when the results of a scientific study suggest that probiotics can be beneficial in some circumstances, this doesn't necessarily mean that you can replicate the effect by consuming a probiotic yoghurt from your local supermarket.[5]

*So basically, we're saying . . .*
If you're in good health, foods and supplements containing probiotics are unlikely to do you any harm, but they're also unlikely to do you much good.

# Nutritional supplements

*I take vitamin D because I'm brown and don't get enough sunlight. Should I be taking other vitamins as well?*

Getting the right balance of vitamins and minerals is essential to maintain good health. Although micronutrient deficiency is generally much more common in developing countries, it can affect people all over the globe.[1, 2] Nutritional supplements are big business and the market for them continues to grow (it's reported that three quarters of adults in the US regularly use dietary supplements), but there's limited evidence of their impact on health.[3, 4]

It's definitely not the case that 'more is more' when it comes to vitamins and mineral intake. Excessive consumption of some micronutrients can be harmful; for example, too much magnesium can cause diarrhoea and too much iron can cause constipation.[5]

*So, nutritional supplements won't make me live longer?*

Research published in 2019 looked at data from over 30,000 adults in the US to find out whether there was any relationship between death rates and intake of dietary supplements. The results showed that whether people had ever used nutritional supplements was unrelated to their risk of dying during the life of the study. Adequate intake of some vitamins and minerals was associated with lower death rates but this only applied to nutrient intake from food and not supplements.[6] It's possible that some benefits may not have shown up in the data analysis, but for now there's no evidence that taking supplements improves longevity for the general population.[7] In the UK, the advice is that a healthy, balanced diet should provide all the nutrients you need, apart from vitamin D.[7]

*I knew it! D3 for the vita-win. (Or D2 if you're a vegan.)*

It's recommended that all adults and children over one in the UK should consider taking a daily supplement containing 10 micrograms of vitamin D during autumn and winter. Vitamin D is essential for healthy bones, but our food actually provides very little of it. The main source is from exposure to sunlight but in the UK, there isn't enough of it in the winter months to allow our bodies to produce all the vitamin D we need. Almost 40 per cent of UK adults have low levels of vitamin D in winter compared with just 8 per cent in the summer. It's important to note, however, that in medical terms a low level isn't the same as a deficiency. Low vitamin D has been associated with osteoporosis and some cancers, while severe vitamin D deficiency can result in soft bones.[8]

*I had an ex-boyfriend whose bone was soft.*

I'm not sure vitamin D can fix that kind of bone.

*Reality check*
Although many people take nutritional supplements which their bodies don't need, the decision to take them or not to take them should be based on individual circumstances. There are plenty of situations in which someone may be advised to take a supplement. Vegans, for example, need to get their vitamin B12 through fortified foods or supplements, as these are the only reliable animal-free sources. Being deficient in vitamin B12 can cause anaemia and nervous system damage.[9]

*So basically, we're saying . . .*
If you're already getting a balanced diet, popping lots of nutritional supplements that your body doesn't need won't make you live longer and could do more harm than good. Check out advice around vitamin D if you're living in a country with gloomy winters.

# Obesity

*This is a sore point, as I'm having my own personal obesity crisis. So far, I've broken two toilet seats.*

It's not just you, trust me. Obesity has tripled globally since 1975: 13 per cent of the world's adult population were obese (meaning very overweight) in 2016, while 39 per cent were overweight.[1]

*Oh, to merely be overweight . . .*

There are different ways of measuring how healthy someone's weight is, but the most commonly used approach is called 'body mass index' (or BMI) which looks at your weight in relation to your height. Most adults with a BMI of 25 to 29.9 are overweight, while those with a BMI of 30 or more are obese.

*Yup, and my BMI is 37.5 right now.*

This measure isn't perfect, because people who are very muscular may have a relatively high weight for their height without this being due to excess fat.

*Ahahaha. If only.*

For most of us, however, this approach provides a pretty good indication of whether we need to lose some weight.[2] If your BMI indicates that you're overweight or obese, your waist measurement is also a useful way to tell if you're carrying excess fat. As a general rule, you're more likely to develop health problems related to obesity if you're a man with a waist circumference of 94 centimetres or more or if you're a woman with a waist circumference of 80 centimetres or more.[2]

*Try 117 centimetres. Am I going to die?*

Hopefully not, but you should know that obesity is a leading cause of poor health and death. Being obese can lead to serious conditions, including high blood pressure, type 2 diabetes, coronary heart disease and some types of cancer. It can also have a negative impact on your quality of life, and your mental health and well-being.[2]

In 2017, high BMI was the fourth biggest risk factor for death in the US (after high blood pressure, smoking and high blood sugar) and the biggest risk factor for the amount of people's lives spent with a disabling condition. The data showed a similar picture in the UK.[3]

*Why has it become such a big problem?*

In most cases, obesity is simply the result of consuming more calories from food and drink than you burn off through physical activity. The body stores this extra energy as fat.

A range of factors contribute to this overconsumption of calories, however. Obesity is becoming more and more common as a result of our sedentary lifestyles and the availability of low-cost, high-calorie food – especially things which are high in fat and sugar.[2]

*Cookie dough is my main weakness. It's so soft and hot and delicious, it's like I'm powerless to resist it.*

Well, quite. Exercise is another factor. Our dependency on motor vehicles has grown and technology has changed how we spend our leisure time.[4] It's easy to lose sight of just how little physical activity you might be getting if you drive to a desk job and spend most of your time outside work sitting down. (See Part Three, pages 81–94, for more on exercise.)

*Should I join a boot camp and get shouted at to lose the weight?*

Although physical activity plays a really important role in achieving and maintaining a healthy weight, a good weight-loss programme shouldn't be based on exercise alone.[5]

*OK, how about I try Weight Watchers or Slimming World?*

There's plenty of good evidence that some commercial weight-loss programmes, including Weight Watchers and Slimming World, can be effective, although group-based sessions will suit some people more than others.[6, 7] One alternative is a free online twelve-week weight-loss programme provided by the National Health Service in the UK.[8]

*I wonder if these programmes are drastic enough to shift my huge bulk though? Perhaps I need to live on soup and salad for a few months.*

Fad diets are unlikely to be sustainable in the long term, even if they help you to lose weight successfully in the first instance. It's advisable to choose a weight-loss plan which is based on a healthy, balanced diet and regular exercise. It's also a good idea to talk to a health professional, such as your doctor, before starting any weight-loss programme.[8]

*Hello doctor, please can you help me stop breaking toilet seats?*

*Reality check*

Although the solutions to obesity sound simple – eat less and move more – there can be underlying psychological factors to obesity which, if unaddressed, can make it very challenging to achieve and sustain a healthy weight for some people.

Once you become obese, a vicious cycle can develop which some people find very difficult to break. Being obese can make physical activity more difficult and uncomfortable, because of the strain it puts on your joints, increased sweating and breathlessness.[2] Rather than doing more physical activity to lose weight, it can be tempting to avoid it even more for these reasons – switching to always taking the lift instead of the stairs, for example. Obesity can also lower your mood or even lead to depression, possibly further reducing your motivation to exercise and increasing the temptation to take comfort in food.

*So basically, we're saying . . .*

Being overweight or obese is bad for your health and increases your chances of an early death. Regular physical activity and a healthy, balanced diet will help you maintain a healthy weight. If your BMI is too high, see your doctor to get advice on effective, safe ways to slim down which will be suitable for you.

# Part Five: Drink

# Green tea

*So, is a fragrant, delicate cup of green tea really the elixir of life?*

A very lyrical question. There's certainly been a lot of focus on whether properties of green tea can prevent cardiovascular disease and cancer, the two leading causes of death worldwide.

A large research study in Japan which began in 1994 looked at whether green tea can help stave off heart problems and cancer. The researchers tracked more than 40,000 Japanese adults aged forty to seventy-nine for eleven years, to find out whether there was a relationship between how much green tea participants drank and how likely they were to die.

When they analysed the data, the researchers took account of a number of other things that could affect someone's chances of dying in any particular year, such as age and various lifestyle factors.[1]

*And? I'm dying to know what happened.*

The study showed that green tea consumption was associated with reduced deaths overall and with reduced deaths due to cardiovascular disease – but not with reduced deaths due to cancer. Those who drank five or more cups of green tea every day were significantly less likely to have a stroke, and women who consumed that amount had a 31 per cent lower risk of dying from cardiovascular disease during the period of the study.[1]

*But I'm sure I've read tonnes of studies that say green tea cures cancer.*

Other studies looking at the impact of green tea on cancer have shown mixed results. A Chinese study of more than 18,000 men found that those who drank green tea were about half as likely to develop cancer of the stomach or oesophagus as those who drank little tea.[2]

*Result! What about bowel cancer or breast cancer?*

Research published in 2006 which combined the results of a number of studies found that high green tea consumption was associated with an 18 per cent reduction in the risk of developing bowel cancer. The same researchers also found that high consumption of green tea was associated with a 20 per cent reduction in the risk of developing breast cancer, although large Japanese studies have not shown a link between the two.[2]

*And prostate cancer?*

There have been similarly mixed results from research looking at the effect of drinking green tea on prostate cancer. A Japanese study of nearly 50,000 men found that those who drank more green tea had a lower risk of advanced prostate cancer, while a small clinical trial which studied the effectiveness of green tea extract as a treatment for prostate cancer found no benefit.[3]

Meanwhile, several studies have looked at whether green tea can help with weight loss and weight management, but the results have been mixed. Some clinical trials have shown a beneficial impact of drinking tea on weight loss, while others have not, and none of the studies has shown a persistent effect.[2, 4]

*All these studies are so wishy-washy – a bit like green tea itself, which tastes like dishwater and urine, but I might just drink it to be on the safe side. After all, it can't do any harm, can it?*

Most adults won't experience any harmful effects from drinking green tea in moderate quantities but, as with anything, excessive consumption is not advisable. The most common negative effects of consuming green tea are stomach upsets and central nervous system stimulation from its caffeine content; however, other potential risks have been identified. Green tea extract should only be taken in accordance with the recommended dosage.[2]

*You sound like one of those leaflets that comes with the contraceptive pill. Any concrete health benefits before we finish?*

Yes, green tea has been shown to be effective in treating genital warts.[4] The US Food and Drug Administration (FDA) has approved a topical ointment for the treatment of external genital and perianal warts caused by human papillomavirus (HPV), the active ingredient of which is extracted from green tea.[2]

*I wonder how you stumbled across this information . . . don't worry though, I love you warts and all.*

*Reality check*
There is a lot of conflicting evidence about the impact of green tea on various health conditions and continuing debate about the potential positive and negative effects of green tea consumption on our health.

Moderate consumption of green tea as part of a healthy, balanced diet may help reduce your risk of cancer, cardiovascular disease and stroke, but excessive consumption is unlikely to do you any favours.[4]

*So basically, we're saying that . . .*
Drinking green tea may increase longevity, but don't go overboard.

# Black tea

*Black tea's just what people call 'normal tea', right?*

Right. And though the health benefits of green tea have generated lots of media coverage, in Western countries black tea (made by fermenting the leaves of the tea plant) is drunk far more widely.[1] Scientists are interested in the biological effects of black tea, though green tea has taken over the research studies.[2]

*Green is the new black. So, what do the studies on black tea say?*

They've drawn mixed conclusions on how black tea affects longevity. Different research methods and failure to take account of other factors which influence death rates might explain some of this variation, but more studies on the health effects of black tea are needed before we have the full picture.[3–5]

*How do scientists make sense of all these different results?*

When there are lots of studies with conflicting or inconclusive findings on the same topic, researchers sometimes try to combine their results in a process called meta-analysis. This method usually produces more robust findings than the individual studies which have been fed in. In 2015, researchers published an analysis of the data from eighteen different studies looking at the relationship between black tea and mortality. They found that black tea consumption was linked with lower overall rates of death and lower rates of death from cancer. The results also showed, however, that there was no link between drinking black tea and deaths from cardiovascular disease.[1]

*Still, lower overall death sounds good to me. So, the more tea I drink, the longer I'll live . . .?*

Sadly not. The results showed that the maximum reduction in death rates was seen in those who were drinking two or three cups of tea a day. Heavy tea drinking may even have negative health impacts, although more research is needed to understand this fully.[1]

*You're ignoring the most important question: milk – first or second? I want to see the research on that . . .*

### Reality check
Studies on the potential health effects of green tea have tended to be in Asian populations, while those looking at black tea have mostly been in Western populations. Without further research, it's hard to make accurate comparisons between the health benefits of black and green tea, or to assume that these will be experienced in a similar way by different groups of people.[1]

### So basically, we're saying . . .
Less research has been done on the health effects of black tea than green tea, but the available evidence suggests that drinking two or three cups a day (but no more) may help you live longer.

# Coffee

*There's nothing like a frothy cappuccino or two to start the day. But am I being a mug and drinking it at the Costa my health?*

Studies looking at whether there's a relationship between coffee consumption and death rates have found mixed results. This may be partly explained by the different research methods used and inconsistencies in how the researchers took account of other factors which affect death rates, such as smoking and levels of exercise.

*Sounds like grounds for more research . . .?*

A study published in 2012, with the aim of reaching a clearer answer to this question, examined the association between coffee drinking and mortality among more than 400,000 people in the US aged between fifty and seventy-one. After accounting for differences in age, smoking status and other factors, the results showed that drinking one or more cups per day for men and two or more cups per day for women was associated with lower overall death rates.[1]

Coffee consumption was also found to be linked with lower rates of death from certain specific causes, including heart disease, stroke, diabetes, infections, and injuries and accidents. No link was found between coffee consumption and rates of death from cancer; however, some other studies have suggested a beneficial link between the two.[2] Although the analysis showed that drinking coffee was associated with a reduced risk of death, the researchers weren't able to conclude that this was a causal relationship.[1]

*I've bean wondering: what about its effect on the heart?*

There's good evidence that moderate coffee drinkers have a lower risk of cardiovascular disease. Those who drink three to five cups a day have been found to have the lowest risk. The evidence does not show an increased risk of cardiovascular disease among heavy coffee drinkers compared with people who drink no or very little coffee.[3]

*Won't caffeine get you in hot water, health wise?*

A good deal of research has been undertaken into the impact of caffeine on human health. The evidence to date indicates that moderate caffeine intake typical of regular coffee drinkers does not cause increased risk of cardiovascular disease, high blood pressure, arrhythmia or heart failure.[4, 5]

Although it's not easy to establish a clear threshold, research suggests that in most cases caffeine consumption of up to 400 milligrams a day in healthy adults does not lead to adverse health effects (although pregnant women are advised to consume less). Above this level, a range of negative health effects may occur, including rapid heart rate, nausea and seizures. Death from caffeine overdose is possible and tends to be associated with the accidental or deliberate intake of harmful quantities in the form of caffeine supplements or powder. For adults, around 10 grams of caffeine is generally considered a lethal dose.[5, 6]

*So, my couple of cappuccinos makes a latte sense?*

It won't do you any harm. A US study published in 2014 found that, across all age groups combined, the average caffeine intake from drinks was 165 milligrams a day. People aged fifty to sixty-four had the highest intake, with an average of 226 milligrams a day.[7] One cup of coffee only has about 94 milligrams of caffeine. So, you're free to enjoy your single cup.

*It's good to have your espress(o) permission. (OK, now I'm just milking it.)*

*Reality check*
Although coffee tends to spring most readily to mind when we think about our caffeine intake, it can also be found in other products, including tea, caffeinated energy drinks, cola, chocolate, painkillers with added caffeine and even some breakfast cereals. Even decaffeinated coffee still contains some caffeine. This can make it difficult to tell exactly how much caffeine you're getting in a day.[5] Despite this, it's very unlikely that you would unwittingly consume enough caffeine from food and drink alone to cause your own death.

Research does support the widely held belief that coffee consumption interferes with sleep quantity and quality, however. If you suffer from sleep abnormalities, it's best to avoid caffeinated drinks in the evening hours.[8]

*So basically, we're saying . . .*
Moderate coffee drinkers have lower death rates, but we don't know for sure if this is due to the coffee. As long as you stick within the safe limit for caffeine intake, though, drinking coffee is unlikely to do you any harm.

## Bec Hill on coffee

*Do you drink coffee?*

So much! I'm actively trying to cut down. I mainly drink filter coffee. We have a filter coffee machine, one of those big old ones, and it has a timer on it as well. We set it for when my husband and I are getting up, and that means when we wake up there's a full pot of coffee wait-ing for us – four cups' worth. Because I work from home during the day, I tend to brew another pot and drink all that as well.

*Apparently, it does extend your lifespan, so . . .*

I'm gonna live FOREVER!

# Fruit juice and smoothies

*I love smoothies. I even bought a £300 blender especially so I could make them.*

Juice bars have become a relatively common sight in affluent urban areas, and many of us feel we're making a healthy choice when we opt for a smoothie over a sugar-laden milkshake or can of soda. Plenty of books and articles have been written extolling the virtues of juicing and smoothie making, often authored by people with superhero-like nicknames such as Juiceman and the Juice Master.

*Can you imagine calling out their names in bed? 'Ohhh, Juice Master! You're so hot, you're making my juices run down my thigh!'*

Moving on. Some scientists have demonstrated specific potential health benefits of particular types of fruit juice.[1, 2] It's also been found that 100 per cent fruit juice retains many of the beneficial components of whole fruit.[3]

Despite this, in recent years juicing has come to be seen as a poor substitute for eating fruits and vegetables in their solid form, and it's been argued that we should limit its consumption, particularly among children.[3-5]

*So, Juice Master shouldn't be worshipped after all? We should instead bow down to Whole Fruit Master?*

Exactly. Although these drinks are a source of valuable vitamins and minerals, it's recommended that you only consume 150 millilitres of pure fruit juice, vegetable juice and smoothies per day. This is because juice doesn't contain the fibre found in whole fruit and veg, and the sugars that get released in the blending or juicing process can damage your teeth.[6]

*I wish I could take the £300 blender back now. Could fruit juice even give me diabetes if I keep knocking it back?*

There's contradictory evidence around the question of whether drinking pure fruit juice increases the risk of developing diabetes. Some studies showed no increased risk while others have suggested a possible link.[7–9]

*'Ohhh, Juice Master – it's so hot to think I might be getting diabetes!' doesn't have quite the same ring to it.*

*Reality check*
The current evidence on this topic isn't particularly robust and more research is needed for us to fully understand the relationship between juice and smoothie consumption and our health.[3]

*So basically, we're saying . . .*
While juices and smoothies have some benefits, they also deliver a lot of sugar in one quick hit. Stick to one glass a day and get the rest of your fruit and veg in whole form.

# Soft drinks and energy drinks

*I love a tall glass of iced lemonade on a hot summer day.*

I should warn you that sugar-sweetened drinks are typically damaging to teeth, calorific, nutrient poor and fill you up less than solid food.[1]

*You'll never get that job as ambassador for Pepsi.*

Research has also shown that regular consumption of sugary soft drinks is associated with a bigger waistline.[2]

*That'll be why Santa Claus advertised Coca-Cola.*

As well as weight gain, drinking sugary drinks has been identified as a risk factor for type 2 diabetes.[3] People who have one or two sugar-sweetened drinks every day have been found to have a 26 per cent higher risk of developing type 2 diabetes than those who drink no more than one a month. Research has suggested that almost 9 per cent of type 2 diabetes cases in the US can be attributed to consumption of sugary drinks.[4]

*Do energy drinks count as sugary?*

Energy drinks *can* be very high in sugar and typically deliver a large dose of caffeine. As we've already discussed in relation to coffee, a caffeine overdose can cause short-term health problems and, in extreme cases, even death. In one example, an individual attempted suicide while having a manic episode suspected to have been caused by sleep deprivation after consuming fourteen cans of energy drink over two nights.[5]

*Soft drinks and energy drinks*

*Yikes. That's energy you could do without.*

A study published in 2014 found that less than 10 per cent of people in the US consumed energy drinks, although it's been estimated that 30 per cent of adults and 68 per cent of adolescents in the EU drink them.[6, 7]

*Plenty of people drink Red Bull and vodka, don't they?*

The common practice of mixing energy drinks with alcohol can result in a kind of non-drowsy drunkenness which is believed to increase the risk of dangerous behaviour while under the influence, such as unsafe sex or getting into fights.[7]

*So drowsy drunkenness is better? Gotcha.*

Another side-effect of caffeinated drinks that I haven't yet mentioned is that they can speed up your urine production. Susceptibility to this varies from person to person, but if you find yourself having problems with urinary incontinence, it's possible that your caffeine intake may be a factor.[8]

*I do let out a bit of wee when I sneeze, but I think that has more to do with childbirth.*

*Reality check*
Evidence suggests that sugar-sweetened drinks play a fairly minimal role in the current obesity epidemic faced by some countries, although scientists have predicted that reduced consumption of sugary soft drinks would lead to a small reduction in the prevalence of obesity.[1, 9] Cutting out sugary drinks alone won't be enough for the majority of overweight and obese people to return to a healthy weight, although it's certainly a helpful step in the right direction.

161

*So basically, we're saying . . .*
Sugary soft drinks and energy drinks aren't a healthy choice, and excessive consumption can lead to potentially serious health problems which might shorten your lifespan.

# Water

*Bog-standard water's pretty dull really, isn't it?*

Plain water is the ultimate healthy drink: it has no calories and doesn't damage your teeth.[1] If you get it from the tap, it's also very cheap.

*The water in my area tastes like a dog's drinking bowl after it's dipped its balls in. Give me a lemonade any day.*

If you find water boring, you could try fizzy water instead; however, there's been some debate about whether sparkling water is damaging to your teeth on account of it being more acidic than plain still water. Some evidence has even suggested a possible link between sparkling water and obesity, although more research would be needed before reaching any conclusions around that.[2] Fizzy water is still a much healthier choice than sugary soft drinks though.

*What about flavoured water? That jazzes it up, doesn't it?*

Evidence has shown that flavoured sparkling water drinks can be erosive to teeth, as these often contain sugar and can have a higher level of acidity.[3]

*Well that puts a dampener on things. I guess you're going to tell me I don't drink enough water, too . . .*

It's recommended that we should drink around six to eight glasses of fluids a day to avoid dehydration – about 1.2 litres – although, of course, this will vary depending on the climate you're in.[4] In fact, a number of factors will determine how much water you need, including your body size and composition, how much you sweat or urinate, your diet, your health and whether you're pregnant or breastfeeding.

*How can I tell how much I need?*

The colour of your urine provides a rough guide to your level of hydration. A light-yellow colour is normal, while dark yellow or orange indicates that you need to drink more. If your urine looks like water you're getting more fluid than your body needs.[5]

It's particularly important to make sure that you're getting enough fluid as you get older because our thirst response becomes less effective with age and it becomes harder for the body to maintain its fluid balance. Getting enough fluid in older age is associated with a lower risk of both falls and constipation.[6]

*Don't people say you need 2.5 litres of water daily?*

It's a myth that you need to drink 2.5 litres of water every day or that doing so will bring health benefits for most people. It arises from a recommendation made in 1945 by the US Food and Nutrition Board that people consume this amount of water per day, but this included the water we get from our food as well as our intake of fluids.

*It's a shame I don't drink alcohol. People who do must meet their fluid requirements easily.*

Although you don't have to drink plain water to stay well hydrated, alcoholic drinks don't count towards your daily water intake. This is because alcohol is a diuretic, meaning it will make you lose more fluid in trips to the toilet than you take in.

*That really is bog-standard.*

*Reality check*
While in developed countries the pressing health issue with regard to drinking water might be the choice between getting it from a tap or a bottle and whether to choose still or fizzy, plain or flavoured, many struggle to access safe drinking water at all. The World Health Organization estimates that around the world at least 2 billion people use a drinking water source contaminated with faeces.[7]

*So basically, we're saying . . .*
Drinking good old tap water is the best way to stay hydrated throughout the day. Keep an eye on the colour of your urine and take particular care to avoid dehydration as you get older.

# Part Six: Vices

# Alcohol

*If I drink alcohol, I end up with my knickers on my head – so I don't.*

That's good. Around 800 people in Europe die every day from alcohol-attributable causes.[1] In England alone, it's estimated that there were 24,000 alcohol-related deaths in 2017.[2]

*How do people die from drinking?*

Alcohol consumption increases the risk of a number of diseases, including various types of cancer, heart disease and liver disease. On top of that, there's the risk of alcohol-related violence and accidents.[3] In Great Britain, over 200 people a year are killed in road accidents in which at least one driver is over the legal alcohol limit.[4] Drinking excessively in a single sitting can also lead to coma, brain damage and death as a result of alcohol poisoning in the most severe cases. There's also the risk of choking on your own vomit while unconscious.

*Nice. How much is it safe to drink, then?*

Until recently, it was thought that there was a safe level of alcohol consumption. Evidence now shows that any amount of drinking brings health risks. The less you drink, the lower the risks of developing a life-limiting illness as a result.[5]

In the UK, it's recommended that men and women avoid regularly drinking more than fourteen units of alcohol a week in order to keep the health risks at a low level. If you do drink this amount, you should try to spread your drinking out evenly over at least three days of the week rather than consuming it in one or two binge sessions.[6]

*Hang on – what happened to all those articles saying 'moderate drinking and red wine are good for your health'?*

Though studies have shown benefits of moderate drinking for the health of your heart, we now know that these benefits aren't as great as was previously thought, and don't apply to all adults. The latest research shows that any health benefits of alcohol consumption are easily outweighed by its harmful effects.[5, 6]

*Why does the advice keep changing?*

Our understanding of the health effects of alcohol improves as more research is undertaken. Until recently, the cancer risks associated with drinking weren't fully recognised. Now that we have better knowledge, it's become clear that any level of alcohol consumption carries some level of health risk, even if that's only a small extra risk for very occasional light drinkers.[6]

*Can I still eat sherry trifle and tiramisu?*

Maybe a small portion.

*OK. And if I end up with my knickers on my head, I'll blame you.*

*Reality check*
Alcohol is consumed by half the world's population, with Europe having the highest levels of drinking and alcohol-related harm.[5] Much has been written about Britain's culture of binge drinking, but the stereotype of young problem drinkers in the night-time economy only represents part of the picture.

Research has shown that excessive regular home drinking among relatively well-off older adults is a hidden public health problem. People in this group of middle-class drinkers who regularly consume alcohol in excess of the recommended limit may not recognise their drinking as problematic though, because of their choice of alcoholic beverage and the fact that they're not getting drunk and throwing up in a taxi at 2 a.m.[7]

*So basically, we're saying . . .*
The only way to completely eliminate the risk of shortening your lifespan as a result of drinking alcohol is not to drink it at all.[5] If you do choose to drink, familiarise yourself with what constitutes a unit of alcohol and stick within government recommended limits.

## Stewart Lee on alcohol

*Do you drink alcohol?*

I do drink alcohol. I associate it with freedom and pleasure. But I am aware I also use it as a decompression tool after shows, and as a confidence boost when I am afraid of going on stage.

I wish I could eliminate it from my life.

# Smoking

*This one's a bit obvious. Surely, it's just supermodels and builders who smoke these days?*

The health impact of smoking is now so well-established that there probably won't be many people puffing away while reading a book on how to live longer. Up to half of tobacco users will be killed by it, with over 6 million dying as a result each year globally. Despite the enormous health risks, though, there are still roughly 1.1 billion smokers in the world.[1]

*That's crazy. You know that's more than 20 per cent of all adults? Who are these people?*

Around 80 per cent of smokers live in low- and middle-income countries.[1] Smoking remains one of the biggest causes of death and debilitating illness in the UK, however, killing around 78,000 people each year.[2]

*They die from lung cancer, right? I've seen the ads.*

Many of us associate smoking primarily with lung cancer, for which it's responsible for around 70 per cent of cases; however, the list of smoking-related diseases is long. As well as causing cancer and harming the lungs, tobacco smoking damages the heart and blood circulation. It's known to increase the risk of developing over fifty serious conditions, including cancer in various parts of the body (such as the mouth, throat, bowel, cervix and stomach), coronary heart disease, stroke, heart attack, bronchitis, emphysema and pneumonia.[2]

*Crikey, you'd be safer as a crocodile's dentist.*

Yes. And just being around people who are smoking can affect your health and longevity. Breathing in second-hand smoke increases your risk of developing smoking-related health conditions, even if you've never smoked yourself.[2] Every year, globally, around 890,000 non-smokers die as a result of being exposed to second-hand smoke.[1]

*I'm staying away from smokers in the future, then. Apparently, it can also cause problems in the bedroom . . . ?*

Smoking can reduce fertility in both sexes and cause impotence in men by limiting the blood supply to the penis.[2] Women who quit smoking may become aroused more easily and experience an improvement in their orgasms.[3]

*No wonder those supermodels always look miserable. What about people who smoke e-cigarettes? Is vaping OK?*

Many ex-smokers have successfully used e-cigarettes to help them quit. Although they can't be considered entirely risk-free, they are tightly regulated for safety and quality in the UK and any risk is far outweighed by the health benefits of giving up smoking. An independent review of the latest evidence conducted in 2015 concluded that the use of e-cigarettes (or vaping) is roughly 95 per cent less harmful than smoking.[4]

*How much longer can someone expect to live if they stop smoking?*

Generally, it depends how long you've been smoking before you quit; however, it's never too late to get a health benefit from stopping at any age. We know that, on average, men who quit by the age of thirty will gain an extra ten years of life, while people who stop at sixty will gain an extra three years.[3] Those who quit smoking before their fortieth birthday will reduce their risk of dying from a smoking-related disease by around 90 per cent.[5]

*So, life really can begin at forty! What about shisha pipes? They're a Middle Eastern staple.*

Tobacco can be used in many different forms (including cigars, rolling tobacco, snuff, chewing tobacco and shisha) but all are linked to cancer.[6]

*OK, I'll steer clear and stop dating smokers, too, even if they're smoking hot.*

*Reality check*
Most of us have heard or read about people who have lived into their nineties or even to a hundred having been regular smokers almost their entire lives. You may have heard someone using these kinds of examples as a reason not to quit smoking or to argue that the science linking smoking with premature death is flawed.

Your risk of developing certain conditions and dying prematurely are greatly increased by smoking, but it isn't a certainty that each individual smoker will develop a smoking-related disease. Out of a very large global population of smokers there will inevitably be some who live to a hundred, but people who smoke are much less likely to live a long and healthy life overall.

*So basically, we're saying . . .*
Tobacco is seriously bad news for your health in any form. If you smoke, quitting is the single best thing you can do to increase your chances of living a long and healthy life. If you don't smoke, don't start.

# Drugs

*I wish I didn't have to take my antipsychotics and antidepressants, but I go loopy without them. I can't risk thinking MI5 are trying to kill me again.*

This chapter is about *misusing* drugs, whether illegal drugs or medicines. This can cause short-term and long-term health problems and possibly death.[1]

*You're Mr Cheery today, aren't you? It sounds like you need antidepressants too.*

Many studies have shown a link between drug misuse and increased rates of death, especially among those who take drugs by injecting them. People who inject drugs put themselves at risk of contracting blood-borne diseases, as well as overdose.[2, 3]

*How many readers do you think will be shooting up while browsing this chapter? 'Whoops, I've got blood all over the page! I hope I still live to a hundred.'*

Hopefully, not many. A lot of illegal drugs can also have adverse effects on the cardiovascular system, ranging from abnormal heart rate to heart attack.[4] In addition, drug misuse can cause health problems and death indirectly, for example, by affecting sleep and increasing impulsivity leading to dangerous behaviours, such as unprotected sex and violence.[5]

*I always prefer my violence to be protected.*

Although drugs such as heroin and cocaine might spring to mind most readily when we think of drug addiction, others, including ecstasy and speed, can also be addictive.[1]

People who take opioids in the form of prescription pain medications, such as codeine and fentanyl, are at risk of addiction too.[6] In 2016, more than 42,000 people died from overdoses of prescription and non-prescription opioids in the US alone.[7]

*And what about these new drugs newspaper columnists are always worrying about?*

New psychoactive substances (NPS), such as meow meow (mephedrone) and spice (a synthetic cannabinoid) can cause paranoia, coma, seizures and death.[1]

*I was going to make a pun about meow meow, but I wasn't feline up to it.*

*Reality check*
Drug misuse is responsible for a large number of premature deaths around the world every year, but alcohol kills many more people because it's used (and abused) on a much greater scale.[8]

*So basically, we're saying . . .*
Stay away from illegal drugs and use medicines only as prescribed.

# Part Seven: Healthcare

# Going to the doctor

*I can't believe there are people who don't like going to the doctor. I practically live at my GP's surgery. I swear his heart sinks every time I walk in.*

It might seem like a no-brainer to see your GP when you're ill, but many people avoid seeking professional medical help when they develop a health problem. Although minor ailments are often best dealt with by a trip to the pharmacist and bit of self-care, holding off on seeing a doctor can have bad consequences for more serious conditions. For example, some patients have been known to wait five years after noticing symptoms before seeking a diagnosis for a rectal tumour.[1]

*Perhaps they thought they could sit it out.*

The UK has a national programme of five-yearly health checks for everybody aged forty to seventy-four. Data from these checks demonstrate the benefit of regularly going to the doctor, having a health professional review your lifestyle and getting symptoms checked out early. For every 80 to 200 checks carried out, 1 person is diagnosed with type 2 diabetes; 1 person is found to have high blood pressure for every 30 to 40 checks; and every 6 to 10 checks someone is found to be at high risk of developing cardiovascular disease.[2]

*Ooh, I've just turned forty so haven't had a health check yet. Do they stick their finger up your arse?*

No, don't get too excited. They'll ask you some questions, do a blood test, take your blood pressure, and measure your height and weight.

*I'm not sure there's a tape measure in the world big enough for my girth.*

It's better to weather any embarrassment. Getting diagnosed quickly, rather than waiting until you've been experiencing symptoms for a long time, can in some cases be a critical factor in how well you recover. Early diagnosis of HIV and cancer, for example, can make a big difference to long-term survival rates.[3, 4]

*So why don't people go to the doctor? I find it baffling.*

Research has shown that there are three main types of reason people have for avoiding medical care. Firstly, they may have a negative perception of help-seeking in relation to health, based on their views about doctors or certain organisations, for instance.[1]

*Ah, the much-maligned 'Big Pharma'.*

Secondly, they may simply think that they don't really need medical attention, for example, because they expect their symptoms to clear up without professional help.[1]

*Otherwise known as The Ostrich Approach. What's the third reason?*

Finally, they might face practical barriers to accessing healthcare, such as cost, lack of health insurance or time constraints.[1]

The combination of different factors which reduce the likelihood of seeking medical help can vary between different sections of the population. Religious beliefs, differences between cultures in attitudes to help-seeking, the influence of friends, family and work colleagues, and our own perceptions of how we ought to respond to illness can all determine how likely we are to go to the doctor when we need to.[5]

*My ex-husband actually prided himself on not being registered with a doctor. Every time I told him he should seek medical attention for his depression, he'd say obstinately, 'I don't have a GP!'*

A lot of researchers and campaigners have focused on how traditional ideas of masculinity can stop men from using health services, particularly when it comes to getting help for mental health problems. Notions that men can only legitimately go to the doctor when they have a limb hanging off or once they've suffered heroically in silence until their symptoms have become unbearable are believed to be one of the factors that contribute to men's lower life expectancy compared to women.[6–10]

*When my ex was finally seen for depression, he stopped taking his anti-depressants without consulting his new GP.*

Well, going to the doctor in the first place is only part of the picture. Once you've been diagnosed with a health condition, it's just as important to make sure that you attend any follow-up appointments and stick to the treatment plan you've been given. Again, there can be reasons why people may find this challenging.[11]

How well patients stick to advice about managing their own condition can be just as important as the care they receive from health professionals. In the case of diabetes, for example, good self-management and attending check-ups play a crucial role in preventing complications, such as vision impairment and amputations.[12]

*And in the case of my hypochondria, maybe I need to stop going to the doctor? If only for his sanity. As long as I don't have a rectal tumour . . .*

*Reality check*
For many people, adequate medical help simply isn't available, no matter how motivated they are to receive it. There are big differences in people's access to healthcare both between countries and within them. Half of the world's population lack access to essential health services and 100 million people are living in extreme poverty as a result of healthcare expenses.[13]

> *So basically, we're saying . . .*
> Consult a qualified health professional if you develop a physical or mental health problem, and comply with treatment instructions.

## Yomi Adegoke on visiting the doctor

*Do you enjoy going to the doctor, or is it something you dread?*

I don't enjoy it, but it's something I do a lot – I'm probably a bit of a hypochondriac. I go to the doctor over the smallest thing, because I'm always nervous about 'web diagnosing'. It's something I used to do a lot when I was younger – I'd be sat in front of the computer typing in things like 'Am I currently having a heart attack?' or 'Do I have breast cancer?' I was being so dramatic.

And the problem with online stuff is that you can type in your symptoms for the common cold and then come away thinking that you've got the bubonic plague! So, I've realised it's better to go to the doctor for everything. I don't have that thing of, 'Oh, I'll just be stoic about it and I'll get really sick and then I'll go.' I go at the slightest sign of anything being wrong.

# Going to the dentist

*'Open wide and say ahhh' are the words I dread most. And I don't like the dentist much either.*

Many of us tend not to think of dental problems as serious health conditions, so it's easy to underestimate the importance of taking care of your teeth and having regular dental check-ups.

*I think it's more that most people are scared of going to the dentist. They put it off, thinking it won't affect them much.*

Well, there's actually good evidence that oral health conditions are linked with mortality. People with missing teeth, gum disease and caries, for example, have higher death rates than people with good dental health. Those with multiple oral health conditions have even higher mortality.[1, 2]

*Isn't that just because people with terrible lifestyle habits are also likely to have terrible teeth?*

This is one of those questions to which the science can't yet give us a clear-cut answer. Generally, research studies have tended to indicate that the link between dental disease and longevity is explained by other factors, such as age, other health issues and how well-off people are.[1, 2]

A possible causal link between gum disease and cardiovascular disease hasn't been ruled out, however.[3-5] Gum disease is a potential source of chronic inflammation, which is believed to play an important role in the development of coronary heart disease and other conditions affecting the heart and blood vessels.[3] Evidence shows that people with gum disease are at greater risk of having a stroke.[6] We also know that gum disease has a negative effect on blood sugar control and may increase your risk of developing diabetes.[7]

*I probably need to brush up on this some more.*

> *Reality check*
> Dental treatment itself isn't risk-free. Occasionally, dentists fail to adhere to the required infection control procedures, putting patients at risk of exposure to blood-borne viruses.[8] There's also a very small risk of having an allergic reaction to a local anaesthetic.[9] Although it's extremely rare, people have even been known to die as a result of dental treatment.[10]

*So basically, we're saying . . .*
Look after your teeth and gums and get regular dental checks. The research isn't conclusive, but this might help prevent you from developing a more life-limiting condition.

## Bec Hill on the Tooth Fairy

I'm obsessed with teeth, but I don't brush my teeth in the mornings. I just don't see the point, because as soon as I wake up, I'm eating food, so I don't want to brush them beforehand. And once I've eaten the food, I'm like, 'Well, I'm just going to be eating again in a few hours!' Which is so bad.

But I find teeth really fascinating, despite the fact that I don't look after my own as well as I should. I just think they're funny. Like, the Tooth Fairy as a concept – someone who collects teeth and pays for them. We tell children that and that's fine: 'Yeah, put your tooth under your pillow and you'll get money.' We teach them about body part harvesting at such a young age. If you change it and you're like 'Yeah, if you put your kidney under your pillow', suddenly that's not OK!

# Screening

*I take it we're not talking about screening films?*

No, but we are talking about testing for undiagnosed diseases. Medical screening is often used to detect conditions that have previously gone undetected, such as cervical, bowel and breast cancers. The specific screening programmes offered and the eligibility criteria vary between countries, however.[1]

*Much like cinema listings. What would happen if we didn't have screening?*

Some people with a potentially life-threatening condition wouldn't get diagnosed until it had developed further. We know that for some diseases early diagnosis leading to earlier treatment can improve survival rates.[2] Of course, most people who get screened won't have the condition, but if you do then it's much better to get it picked up early so that treatment can start before it gets worse.

*My mum sometimes gets asked to spread her poo on a card and post it. It's like an acceptable dirty protest. Who decides what screening is available?*

Although it might seem like a no-brainer, there are pros and cons with all screening programmes because the nature of the beast means that they can never be perfect. No screening test is 100 per cent accurate all of the time, so when a large population is screened

186

there will always be some false positive and some false negative results.

This means that some people who don't have the disease will have to undergo further tests and experience anxiety unnecessarily, while some who do actually have the disease will receive false reassurance. There are standard criteria which health experts use to judge whether the benefits of bringing in a national screening programme for a particular condition outweigh any potential harms.[1, 3]

*Will going for screening reduce my risk of dying early? I wouldn't want the credits to roll halfway through the film.*

Screening programmes do prevent deaths, but that's typically in a very small number of cases relative to the large volume of people screened.[4] In the case of bowel cancer, for example, one life will be saved for every 300 people screened.[5] At an individual level, the only way to know if the screening will find anything is to have the test. Familiarising yourself with the various pros and cons will help you make an informed decision before deciding whether to accept an invitation for screening.

*I guess it won't kill me and have me screaming like Jamie Lee Curtis in* Halloween . . .?

In bowel cancer screening, a thin flexible tube may be used to look inside the bowel. Although very rare, this can result in the bowel being perforated – a serious condition which could even cause death.[6] Of course, you have to weigh up the extremely small risk of this happening with the risk of developing bowel cancer (about 1 in every 18 people will get bowel cancer in their lifetime).[5]

*That's even scarier than the price of a bag of Maltesers down the multiplex.*

*Reality check*

Just because you're not eligible for routine screening for a particular condition doesn't necessarily mean that there's no risk currently of you developing it. In the UK, for example, cervical cancer screening isn't routinely offered to women under the age of twenty-five. This is because the disease is very rare in this age group, so the balance of pros and cons of including them in the screening programme has been deemed to be not right. Experts make these judgements with the welfare of large populations in mind, but at an individual level it's still important to be aware of the signs of the disease and seek medical advice if you become concerned at any time.

*So basically, we're saying . . .*

No screening test is perfect, but early diagnosis is key to survival for some diseases and screening programmes do save lives. Becoming knowledgeable about signs of potentially life-limiting illnesses, such as cancers, whether or not routine screening is available, will also help you to avoid delays in diagnosis and treatment.

## Yomi Adegoke on screening

*A lot of women find STI screening embarrassing and don't do it when they should because they're worried about how they look or smell. Do you have any qualms about it?*

Absolutely none, honestly. I think the more embarrassing thing is when they ask you 'How many sexual partners have you had within this period of time?' I used to be super-cringe about that, like 'Oh God!', particularly one year! But in terms of being in stirrups and people checking out my bits, I've always thought to myself, 'I'm not that important. They see millions of these in their career.' I'm very aware that I'm not showing them anything they haven't seen before.

I really wish people had more of that mentality. I know I'm quite different in that respect, but because I'm so cautious about my health the idea of being a little bit embarrassed because I haven't shaved and somebody's going to see my vagina . . . I'm not going to literally die of embarrassment. I'd much rather get it sorted.

In terms of cervical screening, I was the first person out of my friends to go. Generally, women have issues with it, but especially minority women. I was messaging every one of my friends, because I remember when I first went, the nurse checking me said it has to be every three years because if you don't have abnormal cells at your last check-up, it doesn't mean that they couldn't develop in the next few years.

Cervical cancer's one of those diseases where timing really makes a difference to whether you're OK or not – and if someone has to look at my vagina to make sure I don't die of cancer, or someone has to feel my boobs a bit for me to not die of breast cancer, or someone has to stick a swab up me for STI screening . . . if they have to do that so I don't die then that's fine. I mean, I know everyone's got their hang-ups, but death's a pretty big price to pay for being conservative!

# Vaccination and immunisation

*Vaccination's having a needle stuck in your arm. What's immunisation though – aren't they the same thing?*

Vaccination is the process of getting a vaccine into your body and immunisation is what happens once it's in there. The vaccine stimulates your immune system, enabling it to recognise the bacterium or virus that causes the disease and fight it off in future.

*What about all these ridiculous rumours that vaccines contain mercury, cause autism and play havoc with your immune system?*

There's a lot of misinformation online relating to vaccinations. They don't overload or weaken the immune system and the suggestion of a causal link between the MMR vaccine and autism has been solidly discredited by scientific evidence.[1]

A mercury-based chemical called thiomersal has been used in some vaccines but is no longer found in most standard vaccines in the UK. It has a different chemical structure from the mercury that can contaminate fish and build up in your body, and there's no evidence that it causes harm in the tiny amounts which have been used in vaccines.[2]

*Shame some gullible people believe Jenny McCarthy instead of doctors. By the way, I got chickenpox at the venerable age of thirty-four, courtesy of my then three-year-old. Why isn't there a free chickenpox vaccine?*

Vaccines haven't been developed for all infectious diseases but there's a pretty long list available. Some tend to be given in childhood and

190

others in adulthood, although the specific details of what vaccinations are offered to whom and when will vary from country to country. It's likely that the bulk of the vaccinations you'll receive over your lifetime will be administered when you're a baby or a child, but those which are offered in later life, such as the flu vaccination, and travel vaccinations to protect you from diseases which are prevalent in other countries, are also important.[3-5]

If a new infectious disease emerges which poses a widespread risk to health, such as COVID-19 (caused by the SARS-CoV-2 virus), work to try to develop a vaccine might begin rapidly.

*Why can't I have a free vaccination for flu, like old people get? The last time I had flu, I started hallucinating that I had a massive penis.*

Flu is unpleasant but for most healthy people it will clear up on its own without causing any serious problems. For older people and those in other vulnerable groups, however, there's a greater risk of developing potentially serious complications, such as pneumonia.[6]

*What about bird flu? They said that was going to be a disaster, but it never really took flight.*

There's no bird flu vaccine currently available to the public. It's rare for bird flu to be passed to humans, but if you're going to be in a part of the world where a bird flu outbreak has occurred you should look up and adhere to official advice about steps you can take to minimise your risk of infection.[7]

*I think you're immune to my humour. So, vaccines are pretty important, then?*

The World Health Organization estimated that between 2010 and 2015, vaccinations prevented at least 10 million deaths around the world. Countless more cases of sickness and disability from diseases such as pneumonia, whooping cough, measles and polio will also have been prevented.[3]

*That's great, but I'm still sad about the lack of a bird flu vaccine. I might tweet about it.*

*Reality check*
Vaccines aren't 100 per cent effective, so not everybody who is vaccinated against a particular disease will become immunised as a result.

The effectiveness of the flu vaccination is also limited by the ever-evolving nature of the flu virus and the way different strains will become more or less prevalent at different points in time.

It's not possible for the flu vaccine to cover you against every strain of flu, so each year the World Health Organization tries to work out which strains of the virus are most likely to be going around in the northern hemisphere next winter. A decision is then made about which strains to include in that year's vaccine. It takes several months to produce enough vaccine, however, so the decision has to be made in February for the winter starting at the end of the year.

The extent to which this forecast turns out to be accurate varies from year to year. You could get the flu vaccination and still end up catching a strain of flu which wasn't included in the vaccine.[8]

*So basically, we're saying . . .*
Vaccinations save millions of lives every year. Take up any offered as part of government programmes and check out which vaccinations you might need if you're travelling abroad.

# Access to quality healthcare

*What do you consider 'quality healthcare'? I'm not sure the frostiness of most GP receptionists is high quality.*

Good quality healthcare is based on scientific evidence. It is safe, minimises harmful delays, is responsive to the individual patient's needs, and is delivered fairly and efficiently.[1] Lack of access to good healthcare kills people.[2]

*And those receptionists scare me to death, too. But anyhow: are we talking about the UK here? Surely our healthcare is among the best in the world?*

Instances of poor-quality healthcare can occur anywhere. Inaccurate diagnoses, inappropriate or unnecessary treatment, surgical errors and unsafe clinical practices happen in all countries. However, those in low- and middle-income countries are at greater risk. Evidence from seven low- and middle-income African countries showed that healthcare workers followed clinical guidelines for common conditions less than half the time on average.[3]

*My mum grew up in Tanzania and I'd quite like to visit one day, but I might put that plan on hold.*

The availability of suitably qualified health staff can also be a problem. Over 90 per cent of low-income countries have fewer than 4 nursing and midwifery professionals for every 1000 people. In these countries, 1 in every 41 women dies as a result of pregnancy or childbirth, compared to 1 in 3300 in high-income countries.[2] Research in eight Caribbean and African countries found that just 28 per cent of antenatal care qualified as 'effective'.[3]

*Wow – when women here are fretting about having the perfect water birth complete with hypnobirthing soundtrack. What other healthcare issues are involved in lower-income countries?*

In these countries, 10 per cent of hospital patients will acquire an infection during their stay. In high-income countries, it's 7 per cent.[3]

*That still seems pretty high . . .*

Yes. It's estimated that healthcare-associated infections account for almost 100,000 deaths annually in the US and around 37,000 in Europe.[4] Lots of other things can also go wrong when you're in hospital, from mistakes with administering medication to operating on the wrong part of the body. Again, this phenomenon isn't confined to poorer countries. Around 5000 people die in the US every year due to adverse effects of medical treatment (just over 1 death for every 100,000 people in the population).[5]

*Makes me realise how important preventive care with diet and exercise is. We need to do everything we can not to end up in hospital.*

How true that is can depend on your exact location. We're all familiar with the fact that different countries have different health systems with varying degrees of accessibility and quality, but there can also be important variations in care between different areas of the same country.

In the UK, for example, there are substantial variations between different local doctors in how effectively they manage the care of patients with diabetes, affecting their risk of developing serious complications.[6] We also see differences across the country in what treatments are offered to patients in the same circumstances and how long people have to wait to receive them. This is because the UK's health system comprises lots of organisations covering different parts of the country, all making their own policies regarding the provision of services.[7]

*Ah yes – I've heard mental health provision in certain rural communities is poor.*

Living in the countryside can also restrict your access to healthcare. A quarter of people in the US, for example, live in rural areas, but around 90 per cent of doctors work in urban areas. Examples of higher rates of health problems in remote places can be found in high- and low-income countries. As well as less access to preventive care and routine treatment, being away from an urban area can also mean that it takes longer to get help in the event of an accident, leading to higher death rates.[8]

*Can cost also be a barrier to high quality healthcare, like in the US?*

Yes. Even if good quality healthcare services exist, a person's access to them is often restricted by the financial cost. Some places, such as the UK, have universal healthcare provision which is free or very low cost at the point of access, but this isn't the case everywhere. In countries where health insurance is a prerequisite to accessing good quality care, the financial cost can be a major barrier for poorer people and there are often inequalities in health insurance coverage between ethnic groups.[1] Every year, tens of millions of people around the world fall below the poverty line because of healthcare bills. This phenomenon isn't restricted to low-income countries.[2]

*Understood. I'm never going to complain about GP receptionists again – at least, not until my next appointment.*

*Reality check*

Access to healthcare isn't just about what services are provided and whether you can afford them. Simply lacking knowledge of when it's appropriate to see a doctor is also a big barrier to accessing healthcare. Even when people know that they should seek medical attention, they may not be willing to do so. Cultural factors, language barriers and social norms can make some people reluctant to use services when they really need them.[9] It's particularly common for men to delay getting help for medical problems compared with women.[10] In countries with HIV epidemics, for example, we know that men are less likely than women to take an HIV test, less likely to access antiretroviral therapy and more likely to die of AIDS-related illnesses.[2]

*So basically, we're saying . . .*

Even in a high-income country with a free universal health service, you could still end up dying as a result of poor-quality care.

# Part Eight: Home

# Where you live

*I live in Leytonstone, home of fly tippers and shops with bad fonts. Where does that leave me?*

There are vast differences in life expectancy between countries. According to 2017 data, someone born in Monaco can typically expect to live to almost ninety. In Chad, life expectancy is little more than fifty years.[1]

*Hold on, just booking a flight to Monte Carlo . . .*

Within countries there are also huge health differences between geographical areas. In England, people living in the poorest neighbourhoods will typically die several years younger than those in the richest neighbourhoods and spend longer living in poor health.[2] Particularly notable is the persistent health divide between the north and south of the country, with people in the south generally living several years longer and huge differences in the amount of time lived in good health between individual districts.[3]

*It's not just that poorer neighbourhoods have poorer people living in them and poorer people have worse health?*

Results of a large US study published in 2019 showed that the negative impact of living in a disadvantaged neighbourhood wasn't accounted for simply by individuals' socio-economic circumstances. Living in a disadvantaged neighbourhood was bad for people's health and increased their risk of dying irrespective of their income and occupational status.[4]

*So, you're telling me that if I live on vegetables, fish and green tea and run a marathon a day, I'll still die early because I live in Leytonstone? Or have I got the wrong end of the fly-tipped stick?*

A broad range of factors contribute to the difference in life expectancy between neighbourhoods. Levels of community cohesion, fear of crime and deprivation, for example, can be markedly different between areas with generally better and worse health.[2] The physical features of neighbourhoods can also impact the health of the people who live in them, by influencing things such as air pollution, levels of exercise and how easily people can get to healthcare services or reach places of education or work.[5] The density of fast food outlets in an area has even been linked to levels of obesity.[6]

*I'll say. You can't move for fried chicken shops round here. It's like they're trying to scare all the chickens away from the area.*

Some places are very obviously bad for your health. A war zone is a good example. It's estimated that around 50,000 people are killed every year directly as a result of armed conflicts.[7] Even if you're not killed directly by the violence, living in a war zone can affect your health as a result of stress and trauma and the impact on things such as access to food, clean water, healthcare and education. Wars are responsible for the deaths of many others as well as those who die directly as a result of the violence.[8]

*Leytonstone was bombed in the Second World War, but I'm not sure that counts . . .*

Clearly, your risk of dying in a war varies dramatically depending on where you live. At any one time there'll be armed conflicts going on in some parts of the world, as well as places which aren't experiencing wars where rates of lethal violence are unusually high. Almost a quarter of all violent deaths in the world happen in countries which together account for just 4 per cent of the global population.[9]

*Monaco's definitely not one of them. Now, where did I put my passport?*

*Reality check*

For some people, which neighbourhood – or even which country – they live in is something they can easily change. Many poorer people, though, become trapped in areas which are bad for their health because they simply can't afford to move anywhere else. Politics, conflict, economic decline, lack of quality affordable housing, debt, low wages, a lack of skills and education, and poor health itself can all contribute to people becoming stuck in unhealthy neighbourhoods.[10, 11]

*So basically, we're saying . . .*

Irrespective of your own individual circumstances, where you live can either enhance or diminish your health and well-being.

# Pet ownership

*Is this my cue to get a dog?*

Some research has suggested that owning a pet could bring health benefits, although it's hard to reach firm conclusions from the evidence available because different studies have shown conflicting results. Scientists have previously linked pet ownership with a range of health outcomes, including a better chance of surviving a heart attack, lower risk of cardiovascular disease, and better physical and mental health in old age.

*Sounds like I'd be barking not to get a dog.*

Subsequent studies have contradicted some of these findings, however.[1] The quality of evidence on this topic overall is generally quite limited.[2] There's enough to suggest that owning a pet might bring tangible health benefits, but this is one of those topics where further, more robust research studies are needed before we can really be sure what's going on.[3]

*What about getting more exercise by taking Rover for walkies?*

Getting a dog might encourage you to get more exercise by taking it for walks.[4, 5] That said, there's no evidence that people who own other types of pets are any more physically active overall than non-pet owners.[5]

*Well a tortoise won't give you much of a workout. So why might pet owners be healthier, then?*

There are three possible explanations. The first is that people who own pets are simply more likely to have other characteristics which make them healthier, and that owning a pet in itself doesn't cause better health. Researchers usually try to take account of these kinds of things and, so far, there's no clear indication that this explains why a number of studies have shown an apparent health benefit to pet ownership.

Another theory is that owning a pet enhances people's levels of social interaction. An example of this might be getting to know other local dog walkers and the rest of your community. We know that good quality social contact has a positive impact on health and well-being.

*And that tortoise isn't likely to bring you out of your shell.*

The third explanation is that the relationship between the owner and the pet brings benefits directly by reducing stress and being a source of companionship in itself. Again, we already know that these things have important health implications. While pets can't provide social support in the way that a person can, there is some evidence that relationships with pets can mirror certain beneficial aspects of human contact.[1]

*You've been yapping on furever, but should I get a dog or not?*

It might not simply be a black and white question of whether or not having a pet is good for you. Instead, it could be that pet ownership brings health benefits in particular circumstances and not in others.[1] Evidence suggests that the relationship between pet ownership and mental well-being, for example, appears to be more complex than we might imagine.[6]

*I guess this is only a ruff guide, then.*

*Reality check*

There are potential downsides to owning a pet when it comes to our health and well-being. Older people, for example, can sometimes be reluctant to seek medical advice if they fear it will lead to being admitted to hospital or a care home where they'll be separated from a pet. Other negatives include the stress of bereavement when a beloved pet dies.[1] There's also the potential for picking up an infectious disease from your pet, such as salmonella (from reptiles) or toxoplasmosis (from cats), not to mention the risk of being attacked and injured.[4, 7, 8] You don't have to search for long to find examples of people who were killed by their own exotic pets.[9, 10]

*So basically, we're saying . . .*

In some circumstances, getting a pet may help you in your quest to maintain good physical and mental well-being, but they can present risks to your physical and mental well-being too (and some of them might eat you).

# Home accidents and falls

*I fell all the way down the stairs at a friend's house. It was terrifying, not least because I was carrying my three-week-old daughter. Luckily, we were both OK.*

Yes, we often underestimate the threat to life posed by homes and imagine that we're more likely to meet our death on the road or at work.[1] The truth is that more accidents happen in the home than anywhere else.[2] In the UK, almost 6000 people die every year, and around 2.7 million turn up at accident and emergency departments as a result of home accidents.[3]

*Who is most at risk in these accidents, then?*

Older people are much more at risk of dying in an accident. Almost half of accidental deaths in the UK are in people over eighty-five. Women in this age group are more likely to be hospitalised as a result of an accident than men, while at every other time of life it's the other way around.[4]

*What kind of accidents are these? Falls?*

Falls are the biggest cause of death from accidents – Scottish figures show that they accounted for over 40 per cent in 2014–15.[2]
　You're more at risk of a fall once you get into old age.[2] Around a third of people aged over sixty-five who live at home will have at least one fall every year. Muscle weakness, sight problems and long-term health conditions, such as low blood pressure (which may cause

205

dizziness) and dementia, can contribute to your risk of a fall. Slip and trip hazards around the home are another causal factor, and older men especially are at risk of falling off ladders while doing DIY.[5]

*How dangerous are falls?*

Although most don't result in serious injury, falls can have serious consequences which can limit your quality of life and shorten your life.[6] Breaking a hip is one of the most serious injuries that can occur if you fall over in your old age. As we've outlined in Dairy products, pages 112–15, one month after sustaining the injury, 10 per cent of people will die and almost a third will be dead within a year.

Only half of elderly people who break a hip will return to the level of mobility they had before the accident, and many will be unable to return to living in their own homes. Up to a fifth of patients will develop complications after their operations, which increases the odds of dying in less than a year even further.[7]

*So, what can we do to prevent falls? Except for getting an Apple Watch Series 4 or later – they can sense a hard fall and send an SOS.*

There are some steps you can take to reduce your chances of a fall, including decluttering your home, using non-slip mats in the bathroom, getting your sight checked, having your doctor assess your risk of falls and doing regular exercise to maintain good balance and muscle strength as you age.[5]

*Exercise? I don't see many eighty-year-olds down the gym . . .*

There are simple exercises which can be found online to help you keep physically active and maintain muscle strength in later life, without having to be a geriatric gym-goer.[8]

*Reality check*
Although falls are a particular concern for the elderly, you should avoid unnecessary risks at any time of life if you want to maximise your chances of reaching a hundred. Dying in a fall while posing for a selfie, for example, is something that's much more likely to happen in your younger years.

In a study published in 2017, researchers found that the average age of people who died in the act of taking a selfie was twenty-three (and over 80 per cent of the victims were male). Falling from height was in the top three causes of selfie-related deaths, along with drowning and rail accidents.[9]

*So basically, we're saying . . .*
Don't underestimate the risk of dying in an accident in your own home. Take steps to prevent falls and don't pose for a selfie on the edge of a cliff.

# Fire risks

*Is this chapter about sexy firemen and their massive hoses?*

Not really. But it does contain the fact that, over a twelve-month period in 2017–18, the fire service in England attended over 30,000 fires in people's homes, as well as over 15,000 in other buildings, such as workplaces, and over 22,000 vehicle fires and over 5000 outdoor fires.[1]

*Holy smoke – that's a lot of hosepipe. How do fires begin in homes though?*

For a fire to start, three things need to be present: a source of ignition, a source of fuel and a source of oxygen. Oxygen is in the air we breathe and most of us live in homes which are filled with sources of fuel in the form of wood, paper, plastic, fabric, etc.

Anything that can get very hot or cause sparks could be a source of ignition, but common ones in the home include heaters, faulty electrical equipment, and lit candles and cigarettes.[2] In England, faulty electrics (including overloaded sockets) are responsible for around 6000 domestic fires every year. Two fires are started every day by candles and someone will die every six days from a fire caused by smoking.[3]

*Wow. Who's most at risk of dying in a fire?*

The statistics show that men are more likely to die in a fire than women, and the risk increases as we get older.[1]

*Which kinds of fire are most likely to be fatal?*

*Fire risks*

The most common types of fires aren't those which cause the most fatalities. Cooking appliances caused 48 per cent of accidental fires in dwellings in England in 2017–18, but these accounted for only 7 per cent of fire-related deaths. Smokers' materials (such as pipes, cigarettes, lighters), however, caused only 7 per cent of accidental fires in homes, but these accounted for 20 per cent of fatalities.[1]

*Aside from using common sense, how can I protect my home against fire?*

You can reduce the risk of a fire in your home by following official fire safety advice which you can easily find online. Also, local fire services will often provide people with advice and fire safety checks in the home and help with installing smoke alarms. Strong evidence shows that having a working smoke alarm will cut your chances of dying in a house fire by half.[4]

*Oh, an excuse to contact the local fire station. Nice.*

Making sure that you have working smoke alarms in your home and testing them every month is one of the most important tips to follow to reduce your risk of dying in a fire.[3] Over 90 per cent of homes in the US have a smoke alarm; however, a sizeable proportion aren't actually in working order at any one time.[5] In 2016–17, almost a quarter of households in England had never tested their smoke alarm.[1]

*I've got three high-tech Nest Protect smoke alarms which test themselves every month. Still fancy shacking up with a hunky fireman, mind.*

*Reality check*
Only a very small proportion of fires in England result in fatalities. Rates of fire deaths have declined considerably since the 1980s as smoke detectors have become more common and smoking rates have reduced.[6]

Men over the age of eighty have the highest rate of fire fatalities, although even among this group the figures are relatively very low compared with other causes of death, such as cancer and cardiovascular disease. In this age group, in England, 24.9 fire deaths per million people occurred in 2017–18.[1]

*So basically, we're saying . . .*
You're not very likely to die in a fire but having working smoke alarms in your house will substantially cut your risk further. Taking the batteries out because you keep burning your toast could be a fatal move.

# Damp, cold and mould

*'Damp, cold and mould' sounds like a description of my friend John's house.*

Sadly, it's all too common. According to the World Health Organization, in some European countries up to half of the indoor spaces in which people spend their time are damp.[1]

*What's the problem with that?*

Having damp and mould in your home means you're at greater risk of respiratory infections, allergies and asthma. It can also affect your immune system.[2] If you live in a well-ventilated and insulated home, you're less likely to be admitted to hospital with a respiratory condition than if your home is damp.[1]

*Who is particularly at risk? Apart from John, of course.*

Some people are at greater risk of suffering ill effects from living in a damp, mouldy home. Babies and children, the elderly, people with existing skin or respiratory problems, and those with a weakened immune system are particularly vulnerable.[2] Even if you're not conscious of being affected, though, you should take steps to tackle damp and mould in your home if they occur.

*What should I tell John to do?*

The first thing to do is find the cause of the damp and fix it. Excess moisture can be caused by various things, including leaking pipes, condensation, rising damp, rain seeping in or wet plaster drying. You might be able to stop condensation problems fairly easily by ventilating and heating your home more, whereas other causes of damp may require professional help.

Once you've solved the damp problem you can tackle the mould, but it's important to wear protective clothing, including a mask to stop you from breathing in the spores. Advice on removing mould can be found online. Call in a mould removal expert if it covers an area greater than 1 metre by 1 metre or is caused by contaminated water or sewage.[3]

*John's home is mainly cold because he's elderly and skint.*

Figures consistently show that proportionally more people die in winter than at other times of the year.[4] Although the winter flu season is partly responsible for this phenomenon, cold accounts for most of these excess winter deaths.[5] The difference between death rates in winter and at other times of the year is much greater in the coldest 25 per cent of homes.[4]

One research study showed that whether or not your home is warm enough in winter is actually a better predictor of health outcomes than whether your home is damp, although the two are obviously very closely linked and neither a cold nor a damp home is good for your health.[6]

*I'd better tell John he can come and live with me, then. Though he does insist on calling me his 'dusky maiden'. It fails to get me damp.*

> *Reality check*
> Many people find themselves unable to afford to heat their homes properly. 'Fuel poverty', as it's known, is driven by a combination of poor energy efficiency (often caused by inadequate insulation), relatively high fuel prices and low incomes.

It's not only the price of fuel itself that can be problematic for people living in poverty – if their heating system breaks down, the cost of repairs can be beyond some people's means, leaving them in a home without heat and potentially without hot water.[7]

The implications of fuel poverty for people's health are now well-recognised. Some countries have government schemes in place to help people who are in this situation.

*So basically, we're saying . . .*
Living in a cold, damp, mouldy home will reduce your chances of hitting a hundred. If you're struggling to heat your home adequately, contact your local government office to find out if there's anything they can do to help.

# Asbestos

*I know asbestos is dangerous, but what is it?*

It's a term for a group of naturally occurring heat-resistant minerals made up of microscopic fibres. As they deteriorate over time, these fibres can easily break away if disturbed and end up being inhaled, causing serious health problems. Before the dangers of asbestos were known, it was widely used in the construction of buildings, for things like insulation, flooring and roofing. Although it's been banned in the UK, buildings which were constructed before 2000 could still have asbestos in them.[1]

*Oh no – my house falls into this category. How risky is asbestos?*

Inhaling asbestos fibres can cause a number of serious health conditions including lung cancer and asbestosis (a serious long-term lung condition caused by prolonged exposure to asbestos).

Currently, over 5000 deaths from asbestos-related diseases occur in Britain every year. After smoking, it's one of the most common causes of lung cancer.[2] Typically, asbestos-related diseases take many years to develop, meaning that deaths happening now are the result of exposure to asbestos decades earlier when it was still widely used in the building industry. Eventually, deaths from asbestos-related diseases will become much less common in the UK as the generations who suffered widespread exposure begin to disappear.[3]

*Who is most at risk? Tradesmen?*

Yes. In the UK, the people with the highest rates of premature death from asbestos-related diseases are carpenters and joiners, electrical engineers, plumbers, and heating and ventilating engineers. This reflects the fact that they were more likely to be exposed to asbestos due to the nature of their jobs.[4] Globally, around 125 million people are still exposed to asbestos in the workplace, with tens of thousands dying each year from asbestos-related diseases.[5]

*What about my house? Is it safe?*

Between 1930 and around 1980, asbestos was widely used in house-building in the UK, particularly after 1960. If your home was built during this period it may contain asbestos, but it's not always easy to identify. A wide range of products were produced containing asbestos, including plastic floor tiles, roofing felt, lagging, drainpipes, bath panels, oven gloves and ceiling tiles. Modern asbestos-free versions often appear very similar, meaning that it can be impossible for the untrained eye to spot the risk unless the product has been labelled as containing asbestos.[6, 7]

If you have reason to suspect that your home may contain asbestos and you're planning to do any kind of refurbishment or DIY, it's advisable to have it surveyed by a trained and accredited asbestos professional before undertaking any work. Damaged or deteriorating asbestos materials should only be removed by a licensed asbestos removal contractor, and the same goes for certain types of products, including sprayed asbestos.[6, 7]

*My house was built in 1900. Does that mean I can relax?*

You still need to be vigilant – asbestos may have been introduced during building work carried out in the meantime.

*There's no escape! (Apart from the front door.)*

*Reality check*

Don't panic if you think that there may be asbestos in your home. As long as materials which contain asbestos aren't damaged or disturbed, it's unlikely that they'll do you any harm. If asbestos is in good condition, the best thing is usually to leave it alone. The worst thing you can do is embark on a hasty DIY removal of asbestos materials, releasing fibres into the air.[7]

*So basically, we're saying . . .*

If you suspect that your home might contain asbestos, get a qualified professional to do an assessment before doing any refurbishment, and never try to remove it yourself.

# Scented candles and air fresheners

*There's nothing like the scent of vanilla to disguise the smell of a poo.*

Many of us find the calming and odour-masking properties of scented candles to be good for our sense of well-being. Sadly, though, when they burn they can release a number of different substances into the air, including fine particles and chemicals, such as formaldehyde, which are known to cause health problems.[1] Air fresheners, including ones labelled as organic or green, can also emit potentially hazardous chemicals.[2]

*My poos are pretty hazardous too, though they're not often green. Should we be watching out for particular ingredients in these air fresheners?*

Consumers often have very little information about what chemicals are used to make the fragrances that these kinds of products contain because manufacturers aren't obliged to provide a full list of components on the label and often regard fragrance formulas as a trade secret.[3] Typically, over 90 per cent of the ingredients in an air freshener aren't disclosed on the packaging.[2]

*What are the negative effects they could have on our health?*

There's evidence that fragrances can be a trigger for people with certain health conditions, such as asthma, allergies and migraines.[3] In the US, over 20 per cent of the population report negative health effects from exposure to air fresheners, including breathing difficulties and skin problems.[2]

217

*What about in the rest of the world?*

Determining whether scented candles and air fresheners present a general health risk is more complicated than simply determining that they release harmful substances. We need to establish whether the level of exposure that people would receive from typical use is enough to do harm. Some researchers have concluded the emissions from scented candles don't pose a health risk when used under normal conditions, while others have been more cautious.[1]

Scientists who tested exposure to emissions from scented candles, incense and air fresheners found that under a reasonable 'worst case scenario' it was possible to exceed recommended limits for exposure to particulate matter and chemicals, including benzene and formaldehyde, within one hour. They concluded that avoiding excessive use of these products, trying not to directly inhale any smoke and ventilating the room afterwards could be necessary to avoid harm.[4]

*I got a £25 vanilla candle for Christmas. Is it safe to burn it or not?*

More research is needed to fully understand the impact of air fresheners and scented candles on our health under different types of circumstances and determine with any clarity what constitute safe levels of exposure for different groups of people.[2]

*That's a shame, it's a lovely candle. I could wax lyrical about it.*

Research published in 2000 showed that candles with metal-core wicks being sold in the US were exposing people to lead when burned. Lead helps to keep the wick upright as the candle burns; however, it's highly toxic and there is no known level of lead exposure which is considered safe. In 2003, the US brought in a ban on manufacturing, importing and selling candles with lead wicks.[3]

*Well, at least if we cut out candles there's less chance of burning the house down.*

*Reality check*

While emissions from scented candles and air fresheners may seem like very 'first world problems', air pollution within the home is a leading cause of poor health in some parts of the globe. In developing countries, a major source of household air pollution is fuel used for cooking and heating.[5] According to the World Health Organization, nearly 3 billion of the poorest people on the planet rely on burning solid fuels, such as wood, coal and animal dung, for cooking and heating. The resulting air pollution in their homes is responsible for millions of premature deaths every year, mainly from stroke, ischaemic heart disease and chronic obstructive pulmonary disease (COPD). Women and children, who typically spend more time in the home, are particularly vulnerable. Globally, more than half of deaths among children under five from pneumonia are linked to indoor air pollution.[6]

*So basically, we're saying . . .*

Use scented candles, incense and air freshener sparingly and open a window afterwards.

# Cleaning products

*Are you going to give me an excuse for not cleaning my house?*

Possibly. Typically, when we clean we expose ourselves to chemical agents which have potential harmful effects on our lungs. A number of studies have found that both professional cleaners and people who regularly clean their own homes have a greater risk of respiratory problems, including asthma.[1, 2]

*No more wet wipes for me!*

A large European study which looked at data over a twenty-year period found that women who cleaned at home or worked as cleaners experienced a more rapid decline in lung function compared with those who didn't take part in cleaning. The researchers found that use of both cleaning sprays and other cleaning agents were associated with this increase in lung function decline and concluded that cleaning may constitute a risk to respiratory health over the long term.[1]

*Should I wear a COVID-19-style mask?*

You might want to open a window at least. More research is needed to properly understand how cleaning products affect us when we inhale them, but we know that most cleaning agents can irritate the mucous membranes of our airways, and scientists have suggested that long-term exposure might cause changes in the lung tissue which could lead to a decline in function.[1]

*Blimey! I think I'll stick to cleaning with natural products like salt and vinegar. If I work up an appetite, I can always eat them.*

*Reality check*
Cleaning products are likely to pose a more immediate threat to your chances of reaching a hundred when you're right at the start of your life. In the US, thousands of children up to the age of five end up at hospital emergency departments each year as a result of injuries attributable to household cleaning products. In two thirds of cases the injury results from the child swallowing the product. Over a third of injuries are caused by bleach. Although only a very small proportion of children die as a result of poisoning from cleaning products, hundreds come to hospital each year with symptoms that are life-threatening or result in some level of disability.[3]

*So basically, we're saying . . .*
The need to clean our homes is an unavoidable fact of life, but it's wise to minimise the amount of time you spend breathing in toxic cleaning products.

# DIY

*DIY? Is this code for 'flicking the bean' or 'doing the five-knuckle shuffle'?*

No, it's about home improvement – which is a frequent cause of injuries and deaths. Almost 3400 people were admitted to hospital in England in 2016–17 as a result of accidents involving non-powered hand tools, while powered hand tools and household machinery caused over 4600 further hospital admissions.

*I've had a number of hands and tools in my lady garden, along with the odd vibrating machine. No hospitalisations yet, thankfully.*

Many more injuries which don't require hospital treatment will go undocumented.[1] Sadly the government stopped collecting data on home injuries in 2003, but the most recent figures showed that around seventy people die each year as a result of DIY accidents in the UK. Ladders, knives and even paint pots were common causes of injury.[2]

*Rather than vibrators.*

Hospitals tend to see a spike in DIY injuries during public holidays.[1] A study looking at data over a ten-year period at people who were hospitalised as a result of falling off a ladder found that the sixty-plus age group accounted for almost half of the 41,092 cases. Only 20 per cent of cases were work-related.[3]

222

*I bet that was a gory subject to research. At least one person must have chopped their head off with an electric saw?*

Deaths caused by circular saws are believed to be extremely rare, although it has been known for people to use them to commit suicide.[4]

An Australian study which looked at accidental injuries from power tools at hospital emergency departments found that almost half of all injuries were located on an upper limb, with the head and neck accounting for a further 30 per cent. Over 50 per cent of injuries were caused by power saws and grinders.[5]

*Back to tools and grinding. I'm getting worried.*

You shouldn't be – women are minority sufferers of DIY injuries. In the study I just mentioned, over 95 per cent of patients were male, and those aged over sixty were most likely to be admitted to hospital. It was common for recovery to take over three months.[5]

*What do I do to prevent a DIY injury, then?*

A lot of accidents can be prevented with some basic safety precautions, including wearing appropriate protective equipment such as gloves and goggles, not operating machinery after drinking alcohol or when drowsy from the effects of medication, and never trying to investigate or fix problems with electrical equipment while it's still plugged in.[6]

*Roger that. I'll be sure not to fix my mains-powered vibrator while it's on.*

*Reality check*
Although DIY is responsible for a lot of injuries and some deaths each year, almost all activities come with some risk. It's important to reduce those risks by taking appropriate safety precautions, but it would be simplistic to say that DIY is bad for your health. Research among middle-aged white-collar workers has suggested that spending more time doing DIY might even reduce the risk of death.[7]

*So basically, we're saying . . .*
DIY deaths are relatively rare, but thousands end up hospitalised by home improvement every year. Rather than avoiding it completely, you can reduce your risk by following basic safety guidance and instructions, as well as being realistic about your own limitations.

# Gardening

*Gardening's just for OAPs, isn't it?*

Actually, no. In the UK, around 87 per cent of households have a garden, and half of adults report that gardening is something they do in their free time. This figure rises to around 70 per cent for those aged between sixty-five and seventy-four, before falling to around 60 per cent in people aged seventy-five and over. Roughly equal numbers of men and women say that they garden.[1]

*I'm still not sure I'm old enough, but I'll do it if it'll help me live longer . . .?*

A Swedish study published in 2013 found that people aged sixty and over who frequently did some kind of 'non-exercise' physical activity, such as gardening, had better health outcomes than those who were sedentary. Over a twelve-and-a-half-year period of follow up, their risk of having a heart attack, stroke or angina was 27 per cent lower and their risk of death was 30 per cent lower.[2] There is also some evidence that gardening may have a role to play in preventing falls in older people by helping to maintain good gait and balance.[1]

*Couldn't you accidentally hit yourself in the face with a rake, though?*

Just like many other pastimes, gardening can result in freak accidents or very unusual causes of death. In 2014, it was reported that a thirty-three-year-old gardener in England died of multiple organ failure as a result of brushing past a highly poisonous plant in the garden of a millionaire client.[3]

*That sentence sounds like the plot of a horror film.*

Gardeners are also at risk of contracting tetanus – a rare condition that can be fatal if left untreated. The bacteria that cause tetanus are often found in soil and manure and can enter the body through a wound in the skin.[4] In the UK, tetanus vaccination is included in the national childhood vaccination programme, but it's possible to get fully vaccinated in later childhood or adulthood.[5]

*So, I'm at risk of being killed by a poisonous plant or getting lockjaw. Anything else I should know before I hoe?*

The piece of garden equipment which most commonly sends people to hospital is the lawnmower, with most accidents happening as a result of people trying to clean the blades. In 2016–17, 522 people in England were admitted to hospital as a result of being hurt by lawnmowers.[6] An analysis of data from two hospitals in Australia found that 40 per cent of power tool injuries among females arriving at the emergency department were caused by lawnmowers.[7]

*Yikes! Maybe I should get some of that artificial grass.*

Research in Australia showed that the most common type of lawn-mower injury in 2013–14 was a fracture to the tip of a finger, followed by the amputation of a thumb or one or more fingers.[8]

*So much for green fingers and thumbs. You're more likely to get them lopped off.*

Gardening can also result in eye injuries which require hospital treatment, especially when using power tools without appropriate eye protection.[9] Not wearing gardening gloves can also have unfortunate consequences for your health. A seemingly minor injury, such as pricking yourself on a rose thorn, can require medical treatment if an infection develops.[10]

*You know, I've gone off this gardening idea.*

*Reality check*
We don't know for certain how much impact regular gardening as a factor on its own has on longevity or the risk of developing long-term health problems. Gardening is clearly a valuable means of achieving physical activity and maintaining muscle strength, although we can't say that it has as much beneficial impact on health as more strenuous forms of exercise.[2]

While many people find that gardening is good for their sense of well-being, gardeners commonly experience some degree of lower back pain and the practicalities of looking after a garden, particularly for older people, can become something of a psychological burden.[1]

(Find out more about the health benefits of the great outdoors in Nature, pages 234–9.)

*So basically, we're saying . . .*
Regular gardening is a valid means of improving your levels of physical activity and, compared to sitting around, will boost your chances of living to a hundred. To reduce some of the risks that come with gardening, make sure that you take appropriate safety precautions, wear gloves and ensure that you're vaccinated against tetanus.

# Part Nine: Environment

# Weedkiller and pesticides

*Pesticides are sprayed on fruit and veg, right?*

Although pesticides are primarily associated with chemicals used to kill insects, the term covers toxic substances used to kill plants as well as animals. Herbicides, fungicides and rat poison are all forms of pesticide. Agriculture is the biggest consumer of pesticides, but they're also used to control infestations in homes, gardens and workplaces. In addition, pesticides are used in some countries to kill mosquitoes as part of public health efforts to reduce the spread of diseases like malaria.[1]

*They don't sound very healthy . . .*

Pesticides are poisons, so they have the potential to be harmful to human health. Exposure to pesticides has been linked with a variety of conditions, including allergies, asthma and cancer, as well as birth defects, low birth weight and the death of unborn babies.[1]

*Just how dangerous are they?*

The level of risk depends on the degree of pesticide exposure and the toxicity of the specific ingredients. Some groups, such as pregnant women and older people, may also be more sensitive to pesticides than the general population. Various studies looking at people whose work involves applying certain pesticides have found that they have an increased risk of certain cancers, including brain tumours, as well

as asthma. Possible links with Parkinson's disease and male repro-
ductive problems have also been identified.[1]

*And there was that case in the US of a professional gardener who blamed
his lymphatic cancer on glyphosate and was awarded millions of dollars
in compensation.*

Yes, glyphosate is the most widely used herbicide in the world. Over
the past twenty-five years its use has increased dramatically, with the
introduction of genetically modified crops which are resistant to it.
Most of us ingest very small amounts of glyphosate in food or water,
but people who handle it as part of their job can be exposed to much
higher levels.[2]

In recent years, a number of agencies have conducted reviews of
the current scientific research to try to establish whether or not
glyphosate poses a cancer risk to humans. Unfortunately, the
conclusions they've reached haven't painted a clear picture; for
example, the International Agency for Research on Cancer
concluded in 2015 that glyphosate is a likely carcinogen, while the
European Food Safety Authority concluded just a few months later
that it's unlikely to present a hazard. The United States
Environmental Protection Agency has embarked on further work
to look into this issue.[2, 3]

*In everyday life, should I be worried about pesticides on the fruit and veg
I'm eating? Organic food is so expensive.*

In 2016, a joint body of the United Nations and World Health
Organization concluded that exposure to glyphosate in the diet is
unlikely to pose a cancer risk to humans.[2]

It's always advisable to wash fresh fruit and vegetables before you
consume them, although that's mainly to remove bacteria which can
cause food poisoning.[4] In the UK, there are laws which set out the
maximum levels of pesticide residues which are allowed to be present
on the food we eat. These are typically set well below the level at
which there is any concern about potential ill effects. Imported foods

are tested for pesticide residues on entering the country to ensure that they don't exceed these limits.[5]

*Thanks, I'll stop pest-ering you for information now.*

*Reality check*
There's still a lot we don't know about the exact effects of different pesticides on human health. Much of the research evidence has come from studies in developed countries; however, their use has tended to be heavier and less controlled in developing countries where the resulting impact on the health of the population could well be greater.[6]

*So basically, we're saying . . .*
Wash fresh fruit and veg to get rid of bacteria and don't get a job working with pesticides.

# Nature

*Is this chapter about running around naked with your dangly bits out?*

No, it's about flowers and wildlife and green spaces – because, at the most basic level, we depend on the photosynthesis of plants and trees to provide us with the oxygen we breathe.

*Some people waste the oxygen though – like the people who panic-bought toilet roll in response to coronavirus.*

Natural resources have given us food, shelter, clothing and medicines for thousands of years. All of us, to varying degrees, live at nature's mercy – globally, around 90,000 people die every year as a result of natural disasters, such as flooding and droughts.[1]

*I flooded the bathroom once when I forgot to turn the bath taps off. When I went to apologise to the man who lived in the flat below, he quipped, drily, 'So you're the girl who's been watering my plants for free.'*

At least he had plants. Despite the massive role nature plays in our lives, it's often argued that we're more disconnected from the natural world than ever before.[2, 3] Surveys in the US have shown that on average people spend over 90 per cent of their time indoors,[4] while our daily 'screen time' has reached alarming levels.[5]

*That's all very well, but you try prising my nine-year-old away from her iPad and telling her to go for a walk instead.*

She might not be persuadable, but the negative implications of this 'nature deprivation' and the potential benefits for our health and well-being of exposure to nature have become hot topics for researchers.[2, 4]

*What are their findings?*

Studies have shown that exposure to nature has a positive impact on physical health outcomes, ranging from better sleep, improved immune function and better eyesight to lower blood pressure and reduced mortality.

*What do they say about the mentally ill? Asking for a friend.*

Mental health benefits have been found to include lower stress, reduced anxiety and depression, greater happiness and increased life satisfaction.[4]

*I need some satisfaction. I'm hitting up the garden centre as soon as this chapter's over. Why does nature improve your health, though?*

We don't have a definitive answer to that, and it's possible that more than one mechanism is at work here.

A lot of emphasis has been placed on the benefits of the natural environment as a setting for physical activity. While we might feel more like going for a walk in a pleasant bit of countryside than we would in a crime-ridden inner-city area, however, the question of whether 'green exercise' provides significant health benefits over exercise in an urban or indoor setting remains a subject for further research.[3, 6]

*I live in Leytonstone. It's a bit stabby, but it does have Epping Forest a few miles away.*

A couple of theories underpin the idea that there may be something inherently beneficial to our health and well-being about nature itself. Stress recovery theory places the emphasis on the role of nature in relieving physiological stress, while attention restoration theory emphasises nature's role in relieving mental fatigue.

*You've lost me. All I want to know is: how much nature do I need to get all these health benefits?*

Unfortunately, there's no simple answer to this question either.

*This is all a bit vague and woolly, isn't it?*

It's partly because no standard definition of 'nature' or 'the natural environment' has been applied universally in the research. There's also no agreed way of measuring someone's level of exposure to the natural environment.[7]

*Some people will argue about anything.*

Many of the research studies in this area have looked specifically at exposure to 'green spaces', although this is quite a limited concept when we consider the range of experiences that we might count as contact with nature.[4]

*My back garden's mostly decking, but it does contain ten bay trees in pots. Is that enough to have a positive impact?*

Hard to say. Some scientists have tried to work out the density of vegetation that's required to improve mental health, while others have looked at the duration of exposure that would be needed.[8] One study concluded that if we all visited green spaces for thirty minutes or more each week it could reduce the prevalence of depression in the population by 7 per cent, as well as reducing the prevalence of high blood pressure by 9 per cent.[9]

*Sounds great, but I live miles from the nearest green space. Can I just look out of the window instead?*

It's true that you don't necessarily need to be outside to get beneficial exposure to nature. Studies in hospitals, prisons and workplaces have demonstrated a range of health benefits from simply being near a window with a view of green space, including fewer illnesses and greater enthusiasm for work.[10]

*What about when it's winter and everything dies and goes crispy and brown?*

There's some evidence to suggest that simply being exposed to pictures of nature and greenery can be beneficial. One study explored the impact on recovery of viewing different images prior to experiencing acute mental stress. The results showed that those who viewed scenes with trees, grass and fields did better than those who looked at man-made, urban scenes lacking natural characteristics.[11]

Another study showed benefits to bronchoscopy patients in having a landscape photograph at their bedsides before they went into surgery.[10]

*That's sorted then: you should expose yourself to the natural environment – if only in the form of a picture – but you shouldn't expose yourself in the natural environment. Gotcha.*

*Reality check*
Although a lot of research has been published looking at the links between nature and human health, the evidence has some notable limitations. The lack of a common approach to defining 'nature', or how to measure exposure to it, has meant that scientists have often been studying slightly different things, rather than building a strong evidence base to answer the same specific questions. Researchers have often found different results depending on the methods and definitions they've applied.

Also, this is an area of research in which it's sometimes hard to prove cause and effect. People who get a lot of exposure to the natural environment, for example, may differ from those who get very little exposure in other important ways which affect their health.

> *So basically, we're saying . . .*
> Regularly getting out and about in nature might be good for
> your physical and mental health. If you're more of an indoors
> person, try sitting by a window with a nice view of some
> greenery, or at least sticking a picture of some up on the wall.
> No need to take off your pants.

## Clive Anderson on nature

Trees may not be the answer to all of the world's problems, but they can certainly help with many of them.

More or less every year, the A83, a major route through Argyll, is closed for days on end when mudslides bring huge boulders down onto the stretch of the road leading to a famous turning known as Rest and Be Thankful.

In recent years, millions of pounds have been spent putting in massive fences, metal nets and other structures in an attempt to keep the road open and safe to use – so far with only limited success. Every year, a rainstorm eventually breaks through the defences.

So the various government agencies are going to turn to tree-planting in a search for a solution. Compared to a bare hillside closely cropped by sheep, slopes held together by the roots of bushes, shrubs and trees have a better chance of withstanding the forces of water and gravity. Lots of areas of the country prone to flooding are looking to trees to help in much the same way.

In parts of the world which are less wet than Argyll, trees are being planted to try to hold back the expansion of deserts or to reverse the effects of previous deforestation. These are specific examples of how useful trees can be.

What about climate change generally? To mitigate the effects of global warming it is sometimes argued we need to invent a machine which could turn $CO_2$ into oxygen and store carbon. But you've got one or two of them growing in your back garden.

Well perhaps you haven't got a back garden with trees in it, but I daresay you pass a few trees on your way to work even if you live in the inner city. And whether growing in the town or country, extracting $CO_2$ and storing carbon is what they do – as well as looking beautiful and providing a home for wildlife.

I became president of the Woodland Trust several years ago. To give you an idea of how long ago, I remember claiming I was to be President Tree while America had President Bush.

I had always been a tree enthusiast – a tree-hugger, if you like – but it was only when I spoke about it on television that the Woodland Trust signed me to be its very non-executive figurehead. I am not actually in charge, but I do support the Woodland Trust's central aims, which are to preserve the limited amount of ancient woodland which has survived the centuries of human domination of the British countryside, and to plant millions of new trees to create new areas of woodland and forests.

While the Woodland Trust concentrates on the United Kingdom, there is an international aspect to this. Many environmentalists, quite rightly, throw up their hands in horror at the prospect of deforestation in countries such as Brazil and Indonesia. But it does mean we should put our own house in order as well.

Evidence suggests trees can be good for our health. They help filter pollution out of the atmosphere and make us feel better physically, mentally and spiritually.

Sorry to go on. All I am saying is give trees a chance.

# Air pollution

*My ex-husband says I cause air pollution. It's his term for farting.*

Although, like your marriage, the billowing factory chimneys of the industrial revolution may be a thing of the past, outdoor air pollution remains a major risk to our health in the twenty-first century. It's linked to a number of diseases, including stroke and heart disease, as well as respiratory diseases such as asthma.[1]

*Does it actually kill people though?*

Absolutely. Outdoor air pollution accounts for millions of deaths globally every year. It's estimated to cause 16 per cent of deaths from lung cancer and 17 per cent of deaths from ischaemic heart disease worldwide.[1]

*Christ, I thought lung cancer was just from smoking. Is this happening in the UK?*

In 2016, 91 per cent of the world's population were living in places where the World Health Organization's recommended air quality levels were not met.[1] Air pollution is a global problem, but over 90 per cent of premature deaths caused by outdoor air pollution occur in low- and middle-income countries.[1] In the UK, it's estimated that air pollution is responsible for between 28,000 and 36,000 deaths every year.[2]

*OK, so 0.06 per cent of the population, tops. What causes air pollution – cars?*

Outdoor air pollution in countries such as the US and UK is mainly caused these days by emissions from road traffic. Vehicles with petrol or diesel engines send a wide range of pollutants into the air, including carbon monoxide, nitrogen dioxide and tiny particles which can get deep into our lungs (referred to as particulate matter).[3] Trains, shipping and aircraft also contribute to air pollution as well as industry, agriculture and emissions from our own homes.[4]

*What can I do about it? Except for wearing one of those ominous-looking coronavirus masks . . .*

Perhaps the simplest and most effective way to avoid exposure to outdoor air pollution is to stay indoors.

*That's your solution?!*

Depending on where you live, you may be able to access daily air pollution alerts that will enable you to avoid going outside when levels are unusually high. This is recommended particularly for people with chronic cardiovascular or lung disease, but it won't be a practical option for everyone.[5]

*You don't say. I mean, most people have to get to work . . .*

Living away from busy roads and limiting the amount of time you spend in traffic are also practical steps that some are able to take to minimise their exposure to air pollution, but, again, these won't be realistic options for many people.

*Shouldn't reducing air pollution be a priority?*

Substantially reducing the health impact of air pollution for the majority of people is largely down to governments and industry. The introduction of clean technologies, the provision of affordable clean household energy and policies to encourage a shift towards low-emission vehicles are all examples of things which can work to tackle this problem.[1]

*I'll carry on farting then.*

> ### Reality check
> In some countries, such as China, where air pollution features more highly in the public consciousness, it's common for people to wear face masks when walking or cycling in big cities, particularly during periods of especially poor quality. Although some studies have shown that they can be beneficial, their effectiveness at reducing exposure to air pollution can be limited in real-life situations. Even if a mask provides a high level of filtration, a good fit is essential to really get the benefits. A proper seal is often hard to achieve and maintain in everyday use – facial hair can be particularly problematic and not everyone will tolerate the discomfort.[6]

*So basically, we're saying . . .*
Outdoor air pollution is a serious health risk but, although it's possible to take steps to reduce your exposure, practically there's a limited amount that most of us can do in our everyday lives.[4]

# Natural disasters

*I had a natural disaster at a date's house last week – I did a poo that refused to flush.*

Natural disasters can take many forms, including volcanic eruptions, earthquakes, hurricanes, floods and landslides, but they're all defined by the catastrophic impact they have on everyday life. These disasters bring great helplessness and suffering in the places where they occur, necessitating the provision of food, clothing, shelter and medical care in response.[1]

*Well, it was a pretty big poo.*

Every year, natural disasters affect millions of people and cause thousands of deaths. Between 2007 and 2016, they killed an average of just over 68,000 people annually worldwide, but figures can vary a lot from one year to the next. In 2017, there were fewer than 10,000 deaths from natural disasters, but in other years a single event can take many times that number of lives.[2]

*How common are these events? Not as common as floaters, I bet.*

Over 300 natural disasters typically occur around the world each year, with floods and storms tending to account for the vast majority. Asia typically experiences the largest proportion of the world's natural disasters and around half of the total resulting deaths. Between 2007 and 2016, earthquakes were the deadliest form of disaster, killing over 35,000 people on average per year. Storms and extreme temperature events killed the second and third highest numbers of people – just over 17,000 and over 7400 on average per year respectively.[2]

*Does climate change mean disasters are getting worse?*

It's difficult to make generalisations when it comes to disasters because their very nature means that single major events which happen very infrequently can really skew the figures when we look at averages over several years. In 2007, for example, just 17,000 people were reported to have been killed by natural disasters, but the following year a cyclone hit Myanmar which alone killed over 138,000 people.[3]

*You're right, my disaster pales in comparison. Though I did nearly die of embarrassment.*

*Reality check*
Natural disasters tend to get lots of media coverage because they're visually dramatic, out of the ordinary and take place within a short timeframe. On a global scale, there are much bigger killers which take huge numbers of lives on a daily basis. Mosquitoes cause millions of deaths every year by spreading diseases such as malaria. At an individual level, of course, where you are in the world at any one time will determine whether you're at greater risk of having your life cut short by an earthquake, a flood, a tornado or a flying insect.[4]

*So basically, we're saying . . .*
You could reduce your chances of dying in a natural disaster by moving to a part of the world where they're less common, but either way you're much more likely to be killed by something that wouldn't make for a Hollywood action movie.

# Part Ten: Beauty

# Facial attractiveness

*How pretty you are is related to longevity? That must have been hard for you to take.*

Human facial attractiveness has been the subject of a lot of research. Studies have highlighted various traits associated with attractiveness, including how masculine (for men) and feminine (for women) our faces appear and even how yellow our skin looks as a result of eating fruit and vegetables containing carotenoids (skin colour reflecting a higher carotenoid consumption is considered more attractive).[1] Unsurprisingly, age is also linked to facial attractiveness.[2]

*Tell that to the ghost of Joan Rivers.*

Another trait which has been studied in relation to physical attractiveness is facial averageness. Being told that you're average-looking may not seem like a compliment – however, it's been proven that a configuration of facial features which is close to the average of that of other people of the same sex and age range is fundamental to attractiveness. How symmetrical your face is has also been shown to play a role in perceived beauty, although researchers have argued that a symmetrical face alone won't make you attractive if you lack averageness.[3, 4]

*Is an attractive face an advantage in life?*

It's frequently been suggested that there's a so-called 'beauty premium', with attractive people tending to do better. A study of male high school graduates in the US found that being facially attractive was linked with higher earnings in later life, even after taking account of IQ, family background and personality traits which might be expected to influence career success.[5] Research has also shown that attractive people are generally judged more positively and are considered to be healthier than unattractive people.[6]

*Can we really tell much about health just from looking at faces? It sounds a bit hokey to me.*

Researchers once showed that it was possible to predict how likely people are to be overweight and suffer related health problems and premature death in adulthood based on how heavy they look in their adolescent yearbook photos.[7] In another study, participants were asked to look at headshots from a 1923 university yearbook and estimate how long each person had lived. It turned out that these estimates correlated with the actual ages at which the people had died. The research also showed, however, that this was probably explained by the study participants being able to make good estimates from the photos of how wealthy people were, rather than their perceived attractiveness or health status. We know that there's a well-established association between how financially well off people are and how long they live.[8]

*What about pictures of older people?*

In one study, researchers asked twelve young adults to look at photos of nearly 300 people taken when they were around the age of eighty-three and say how old they thought each of them was. It turned out that how old people looked was a good predictor of their chance of dying in the next seven years (irrespective of what age they really were in the photo).[9]

*OK – but do attractive people actually live longer?*

Although the results of some studies have suggested a link between attractiveness and health, others have failed to demonstrate any connection. Overall, the evidence that facial attractiveness indicates health is weak and there doesn't appear to be a link with mortality.[5, 6, 10]

*Attractiveness isn't just about the face. What about the body?*

There is some evidence that waist-to-hip ratio is related to both attractiveness and health in women but no good evidence of a link between attractiveness and health in men.[11]

*Well, in that case I'm off to do some sit-ups.*

*Reality check*
Some researchers have cast doubt on the widely documented idea of a 'beauty premium' in relation to career success. A study which looked at a nationally representative sample of people in the US found that once personality traits, intelligence and health were taken into account, the apparent link between good looks and higher income disappeared. Conversely, they actually found that people considered very unattractive tended to earn more than those who were better looking than them – suggesting that there may even be an 'ugliness premium'.[12]

*So basically, we're saying . . .*
Being a hottie won't help you live longer (although people might think you look healthier).

# Sunbathing and tanning

*I love sunshine. It makes me feel super-happy.*

Hopefully you don't go out in it too much, as being exposed to too much ultraviolet (UV) radiation either from the sun or sunbeds can cause sunburn, skin cancer and premature ageing. In the UK, almost 90 per cent of cases of melanoma (the most serious type of skin cancer) could be prevented by avoiding sunbeds and following sun safety advice.[1]

*Good job I'm half-Asian then! 'Beige don't age', as the saying goes. We're less likely to get skin cancer too.*

It's certainly true that rates of melanoma vary considerably across the globe. Australia and New Zealand suffer the greatest burden because of their predominantly fair-skinned populations, high levels of sunshine and cultural emphases on tanning.[2]

*Even if you're white, there aren't many hot sunny days in the UK to worry about.*

The heat that you can feel on a sunny day isn't actually what does the damage. Infrared rays are responsible for the feeling of warmth you get from being in the sun, while UV radiation can still burn your skin on a cool day.[1]

*How badly sunburnt do I have to be?*

The idea of being sunburnt often conjures up images of large areas of skin being really red and sore and eventually peeling off, but even if you've only gone a little pink in the sun it still counts as sunburn. People with darker skin may just experience sunburn as a feeling of itching or tenderness. If you start to notice that you're getting sunburnt, you should cover up or get out of the sun as quickly as possible.[1]

*I've never felt itchy or tender in the sun. But how much do my white relatives have to get sunburnt for it to be a problem?*

You don't have to be getting sunburnt frequently to increase your risk – just once every two years is enough to triple your risk of developing melanoma – so, it's really important to follow sun safety advice consistently.[1] You can find lots of information online from official sources on how to stay safe in the sun, including how to choose and properly apply sunscreen – most people don't put on enough.[3]

*And sunbeds are definitely bad too?*

There has been some argument among scientists over the years about the health impact of sunbed use, but the latest evidence shows clearly that using them will increase your risk of skin cancer.[4] In Europe, over 3400 cases of melanoma are attributed to sunbed use every year.[5]

*What else can be done to decrease risk?*

As well as following sun safety advice you should learn how to look out for early signs of skin cancer. Like many potentially life-limiting diseases, it's much easier to treat successfully if caught early.[1]

*Right. I slap on loads of SPF 30 every day anyhow, to make doubly sure that 'brown don't frown'.*

*Reality check*

Getting the right amount of sun isn't a straightforward matter. The latest guidelines are that there's no healthy way to get a suntan, but staying out of the sun completely isn't good for us either – instead we should be aiming for 'moderate sun exposure'. This is because our bodies rely on exposure to sunlight to make vitamin D, which is important for maintaining strong bones. In parts of the world where clouds and rain tend to be a dominant feature of the weather, vitamin D deficiency can be surprisingly common.

As we saw in Nutritional supplements, pages 140–2, in the UK, it's estimated that around 1 in 5 adults has a low level. You should try to get short bursts of sunlight each day but not enough to burn, while avoiding the hottest part of the day. If you live in a country with low levels of sunlight, or remain covered up in the sun for cultural reasons, it's advised that you take a vitamin D supplement.[6] Between October and March it is not possible to get enough vitamin D from sunlight alone in the UK.[7]

*So basically, we're saying . . .*
Follow sun safety advice, don't use sunbeds and keep an eye on your moles.

# Hair dye

*So, the big question is: will dyeing lead to dying?*

Health problems resulting from hair dye are usually in the form of allergic reactions, although questions have been raised over whether they might have cancer causing properties.[1]

*Jesus! All I want is to nuke those pesky grey hairs. Is dye likely to give me cancer, then?*

There's evidence that some ingredients of hair dye are carcinogenic in rodents when ingested, but research has found mixed results in humans.[1] One study showed an apparent link between using hair dye and the risk of bladder cancer, while a number of other studies failed to find the same result.[2] An analysis of the results of twenty separate studies looking at a possible association between hair dyeing and leukaemia, which was published in 2017, failed to prove an overall link. However, the findings did raise some questions for further research into a possible heightened risk for certain users.[3]

*So, dyeing won't lead to dying?*

A study of over 7600 women in Copenhagen who were followed for up to thirty-seven years found that there was no difference in overall death rates between those who used hair dye and those who didn't.[4] Overall, the weight of research evidence has tended to suggest that hair dye, when used as intended, does not present a serious health risk to consumers or people exposed to it through their work.[2] In

2019, however, the results of a large study were published showing that permanent hair dye use was associated with a higher risk of breast cancer risk, particularly in black women.[5] We always have to be cautious though when interpreting the findings of a single study, especially when others have failed to provide a clear picture. More research is needed before we can properly understand whether hair dye is causally linked to cancer in humans.

*It smells like poison. Could it poison me?*

Reports of people being poisoned by hair dye are rare and have only occurred as a result of people swallowing it.[2]

*#notetoself*

> *Reality check*
> Although the vast majority aren't allergic to hair dye and only a small proportion of those who have a reaction to it seek medical attention, there have been cases of people requiring hospitalisation as a result of severe allergic reactions. Medical advice doesn't always override personal preferences and cultural pressures, however. Some continue to use hair dye after finding out that they're allergic, even after being told that they face the risk of a severe reaction.[6]

*So basically, we're saying . . .*
Unless you're allergic to hair dye or you're drinking it, the jury is still out on whether it will do you any harm. People who prefer to play it super safe might wish to stick with their natural colour in the meantime.

# Cosmetics, talc and antiperspirant

*Apparently, some make-up includes crushed beetles and whale blubber, which doesn't sound very healthy . . .*

Cosmetics typically include many different ingredients, with different roles in determining the function, smell, appearance and texture of the end product. Generally, cosmetic manufacturers are much less restricted by regulators and their products require much less rigorous testing compared with manufacturers of medicines. A number of different types of chemicals which can turn up in cosmetics have caused concern and been the subject of scientific study, including investigations into their potential to cause cancer. Overall, however, there is still not enough definitive evidence to clarify whether the normal use of cosmetics poses a significant health hazard.[1]

*You'd think stuff people put on their faces would be carefully governed.*

Controls on the chemicals allowed in cosmetics vary considerably across the globe. While most high-income countries have restrictions on the inclusion of heavy metals (such as mercury, lead and arsenic) in cosmetic products, for example, similar legislation is typically absent in low-income countries.[2] The limited regulations on cosmetic ingredients in the US compared with other major industrialised nations have also frequently been raised as a cause for concern by campaigners and the media.[3–5]

*I've heard that parabens are linked to cancer . . .?*

Parabens are a group of chemicals commonly used as preservatives in cosmetics, such as make-up, moisturisers and shaving products. Questions have been raised about whether their use might increase the risk of breast cancer. This is an ongoing area of study; however, so far the scientific evidence has failed to demonstrate that parabens in cosmetics pose a hazard to human health.[6]

*What about aluminium in antiperspirant?*

Aluminium-based compounds are the active ingredient in underarm antiperspirants. They form a temporary plug in the sweat gland and that's what keeps your armpits dry. Some people have suggested that there could be a link between using aluminium-based antiperspirants and breast cancer. More research is needed to fully explore this, but the evidence so far has failed to prove a causal link.[7]

*How about lead? The idea of it being in cosmetics sounds positively Elizabethan.*

Lead is banned from cosmetics in the EU, but this level of protection doesn't apply in all parts of the world. Researchers who conducted a study in China have suggested that ingesting lead contained in some lipsticks and lip glosses could pose a potential health risk.[8]

*I'm taking it this is accidental eating, and not because the products taste yummy?*

Yes. It's been estimated that a lipstick wearer could inadvertently ingest around 1.8 kilograms of the stuff over a lifetime.[8]

*I've heard of inner beauty, but that's crazy. Any other metals we should know about?*

A study of cosmetic products in Jordan found that 8 per cent of those tested exceeded the recommended limit for at least two types of toxic heavy metals.[9]

Mercury is sometimes used in skin lightening soaps and creams which can cause a range of health problems, including kidney damage. Mercury-containing skin lightening products have been banned in many countries, although they're often still legally available to buy over the internet.[10]

Scientists have also identified potential risks of exposure to heavy metals in some costume cosmetics among people who wear body paint and dress up as part of their jobs. More research is needed, though, to fully understand the practical health implications.[11]

*Ah, so I should avoid being a human statue. Got it. What about allergies to stuff in make-up?*

Metals, such as nickel, chromium and cobalt, in cosmetics can cause allergic reactions in some people.[12]

*Are allergic reactions a big problem?*

In the US, the FDA keeps a record of reported adverse reactions to cosmetic ingredients, but manufacturers aren't obliged to pass on these kinds of complaints from consumers, so there's a lack of reliable data on the true scale of the problem.[13]

*It's a cover-up! By the way, my cleanser says it's hypoallergenic. What does that mean, exactly?*

When a cosmetic product is labelled as hypoallergenic, it simply means that the manufacturer is claiming that it will result in relatively fewer allergic reactions than other products. This doesn't provide any guarantee that you won't still have an allergic reaction from using it. In the US, there are no laws or standard definitions which govern the use of the term and manufacturers are not required to prove that a hypoallergenic product causes fewer reactions.[14]

*I see. One of the big issues with cosmetics is talc, isn't it?*

Concern about the potential health effects of using talc first arose because of its chemical similarity to asbestos, which has been shown to cause ovarian cancer. Studies into talc use among women and ovarian cancer risk have produced conflicting results.[15]

Talc is classed by the World Health Organization as 'possibly carcinogenic to humans' and the general consensus is that while there's some evidence to suggest that talc use may increase the risk of ovarian cancer, more research is needed to establish the true picture. There's currently very little evidence to suggest a link between talc use and any other form of cancer. Women concerned about the possible increased risk of ovarian cancer are advised to avoid using talc and talc-based body powder (talc-free alternatives based on cornstarch are readily available).[16, 17]

*Put simply: don't whack a load of talc on your fanny. Noted.*

*Reality check*
Although the US bans the use of far fewer cosmetic ingredients compared with the EU, there is still a legal requirement that cosmetic products are safe to be used as intended.[18] It's impossible to proactively test every product being imported into the country, however, so dangerous cosmetics may already have reached the market before a problem is picked up. In 2019, for example, several make-up products had to be recalled after FDA testing found that they contained asbestos.[19]

*So basically, we're saying . . .*
Cosmetics safety is a complex topic and the level of potential risk varies between individual products and between countries, depending on their regulations and how effectively they're enforced. Use your own judgement on this one.

# Cosmetic surgery

*Cosmetic surgery's one risk I won't be taking. I don't want to die – or, worse, end up looking like a puffer fish.*

While the chances of dying during a cosmetic procedure are low, it's certainly not unheard of. An analysis of US data from 2012 to 2017 found forty-two recorded deaths resulting from plastic surgery. Over half of these occurred in patients who had undergone abdomino-plasty (commonly known as a 'tummy tuck'). Blood clots were the most common cause of death.[1]

*There was that Brazilian doctor called 'Doctor BumBum' who was accused of murder in 2018 after performing a fatal butt lift.*

Yes – procedures to enhance the appearance of the buttocks, such as liposuction to remove fat, cosmetic filler injections, fat transfer and implants, have grown in popularity in recent years. A number of people have died as a result of undergoing cosmetic procedures on their buttocks, with cases often attracting a high level of media attention.[2]

*People from the UK seem to go abroad a lot for surgery. I know that from watching* Love Island, *to my shame.*

The risks can be higher when people travel abroad to have cosmetic procedures done more cheaply than in their home countries. Cosmetic surgery tourism, as it's known, has grown in popularity but has also resulted in some well-publicised deaths.[3]

*Why is it riskier abroad?*

Quality and safety standards may be less rigorous in countries where cosmetic surgery is less costly, and it can be very difficult to check the qualifications of those carrying out the procedure. Processes to deal effectively with complications, such as infection and post-operative bleeding, may also be lacking.[4]

*Are people just going for butt lifts?*

Breast augmentations are the most common procedures sought by cosmetic surgery tourists despite cases of catastrophic complications, including irreversible brain injury and death.[5, 6] The most common complication experienced in cases of cosmetic surgery tourism gone wrong is developing an infection.[5]

*Say I took leave of my senses and decided to have cosmetic surgery. What should I do to minimise the risks?*

Before committing to any cosmetic procedure, you should check that it will be carried out by people who have the right training, skills and insurance to do the job safely. Never make a final decision to go ahead or pay for the procedure before you've had a consultation with the person who will carry it out.

Don't be shy about asking questions, including how much experience they have of undertaking the specific procedure you're considering, what the potential complications are and what aftercare will be provided, including their approach if something goes wrong or you're unhappy with the outcome.[7]

*Never gonna happen. I still don't want to look like a puffer fish.*

*Reality check*
All types of surgery carry some risk, but even non-surgical cosmetic procedures, such as face and lip fillers, can have serious complications, including infection, scarring and blocked blood vessels in the face (which can lead to permanent blindness).[8]

*So basically, we're saying . . .*
Although the risk is small, having cosmetic work done could put you in an early grave.

# Part Eleven: Transport

# Air travel

*I hate planes. I haven't flown since getting married in Las Vegas. I've done my research, and apparently sitting in the middle of the back row is safest.*

Well, accidents in scheduled commercial flights are very rare, so you shouldn't spend too much time worrying about it. According to figures from the International Civil Aviation Organization there were just 2.6 accidents per million departures in 2018. Of those accidents, 11 were fatal, killing a total of 514 people. Figures can fluctuate substantially, because of the number of people that could potentially be killed in a single aircraft. In the previous year, there were 50 fatalities.[1]

*I guess you're right. Besides, how else was I going to get to America? Not by hot air balloon . . .*

True. EU air safety data shows that generally only a small proportion of aviation deaths are accounted for by scheduled commercial flights. The vast majority of fatalities result from accidents involving lighter aircraft, such as small aeroplanes, gliders, microlights and hot air balloons.[2]

*How about helicopters? Are they dodgy too?*

Helicopter accidents are also rare events, although, of course, most of us are much less likely to get in a helicopter than a plane in any one year. In 2017, there were 121 helicopter accidents in the US, 20 of which were fatal. In Europe, in the same year, 43 helicopter accidents occurred, of which 11 resulted in deaths. Overall, figures suggest that helicopter safety is improving. Data from 49 countries shows that the number of fatal helicopter accidents fell by 44 per cent between 2013 and 2017.[3] Despite this, the risk of dying is much greater in a helicopter than on a scheduled commercial aeroplane flight. In the US, there is roughly one helicopter fatality for every 100,000 flight hours, compared with 0.005 fatalities among scheduled US air carriers.[4, 5]

*OK. Maybe I won't panic so much next time I take a flight. I'm sure it'll be plane sailing.*

*Reality check*
Although it might seem like the safest option is never to fly at all, this isn't necessarily the case. Fear of flying could actually increase your risk of dying in a travel-related accident. In a study published in 2004, it was estimated that more Americans died in road accidents as a result of avoiding flying in the three months following the September 11th attacks in the US than were killed on the four fatal flights that day.[6]

*So basically, we're saying . . .*
Generally, flying is far less likely to kill you than travelling by road. Avoiding unnecessary trips in anything small or lightweight will maximise your chances of staying alive.

## Gordon Burns on the show that launched a career

When I presented *The Krypton Factor* we brought in a new round called Response, which was hand-eye coordination. We took the contestants to an aircraft simulator and they had to land a jumbo jet.

They'd get a theory lecture from a flight captain – how it worked, and what they had to do – and then they'd try to land the plane.

There was a dial in front of them on the set of instruments, called a 'flight director' – basically a cross which moves. If you're coming in to land and the plane is a bit too far to the left, the vertical bar moves to the right. It's saying to you, 'follow me, don't correct me', and that brings the plane back in. As long as the bar is down the centre, you know you're on the flight path.

Equally, if the horizontal bar goes up, it means 'you're flying too low, follow me up', so you pull back on the control stick until the horizontal bar comes down to the middle. If the contestant is no good, both bars can be moving at the same time.

Some people were very good at this round, and some people couldn't do it for love nor money – hand-eye coordination was just not their thing. The contestants got two practice runs before they were marked on the third attempt. They would get a computer print-out of their descent, whether it was a straight line or a wobbly line.

We once had a student from Manchester University who did it. He was called Ibrar Ul-Haq. At this time, we didn't accept anyone who could fly airplanes on *The Krypton Factor*. So, he flew it – and it was just unbelievable. You could have drawn the line of his descent with a ruler, it was just so unbelievably accurate. The captain's eyes nearly bulged out of his head! He said, 'Ooh, first time lucky.' But Ibrar's second run was exactly the same – perfect. The captain came to me and said, 'He's flown before.' I said, 'I'm sure he hasn't.'

We went and talked to him, and he absolutely assured us he'd never set foot on the flight deck of any airplane – he'd never flown at all, and that was true. He went for his third and final run, and once again you could have drawn it with a ruler. The captain said to him afterwards, 'Even some of my best pilots would never do it that well every time. You should think about a career in flying.'

When Ibrar left university, he went into pharmaceuticals – but a couple of years later he saw an ad in the paper for British Airways, who were looking for trainee pilots. So, he decided he would try, and had various aptitude tests. He sailed through those and got on the course and began to fly British Airways planes out of Manchester.

A few years later I was coming back from Rome with my family, and as we walked up the steps of the plane, Ibrar arrived at the top of the steps. I said, 'Bloody hell, you're not flying it!?' He said, 'Yep, I'm your captain back to Manchester.'

And so, the guy who began it all on *The Krypton Factor* flew this planeload of passengers from Italy to the UK. On the way off the plane, I stuck my head in the flight deck and said, 'Landing: 8 out of 10!'

And Ibrar is now a long-haul British Airways pilot, flying round the world on their biggest jets.

# Trains

*I love trains. You can gaze out of the window and take stock of your life as the countryside rolls by.*

The statistics show that although levels of rail safety vary considerably across the globe, railways are generally safer than all other forms of transport, except commercial aviation. The risk of death for an average rail passenger in the EU is very low – around 0.16 fatalities per billion passenger kilometres according to calculations by the European Railway Agency. Their analysis showed that you're roughly three times more likely to die travelling by bus or coach, and twenty-eight times more likely to die travelling by car than you are by rail.[1]

*So I'm way better off on a train than on any other ground-based form of transport?*

In general, yes. A variety of accidents can occur on the railways though, including train collisions, derailments, collisions at level crossings, and slips, trips and falls at stations. Collisions between passenger trains travelling in opposite directions at speed are thankfully very rare, while derailments are relatively common but don't usually result in serious injuries or deaths. Accidents at level crossings most frequently result from members of the public ignoring the warning of approaching trains.[1]

*Apparently, the safest seat in the event of a crash is an aisle seat travelling backwards in the middle carriage – but not opposite another passenger, otherwise they'll crash into you. By the way, how does the UK's rail safety record compare to other countries?*

Figures published in 2013 showed that the UK has one of the safest rail networks in Europe, both for passengers and workforce. Fatality rates were much higher in some countries, such as Bulgaria, Belgium, Romania, Hungary, Poland and Spain.[1] There were 437 train accidents in Great Britain in 2017–18, but the potential for physical injury was considered relatively low in the majority of cases. Only 19 of these accidents were classified as 'potentially higher risk' – 12 of which involved a passenger train, including 3 collisions between trains and 7 collisions with vehicles at level crossings. No rail passengers died as a result of a train accident.[2]

*How about the Tube?*

In 2017–18, there were fourteen train accidents on the London Underground and three passenger fatalities.[2]

*NOWHERE AND NOTHING IS SAFE!*

*Reality check*
Our ability to accurately compare rail safety across different countries is limited because the quality of appropriate data and the methods used to collect it vary considerably.[1]

In Great Britain, the vast majority of deaths on the railways are due to people taking their own lives, rather than the result of accidents. In 2017–18, there were 337 fatalities on the rail network involving members of the public, 292 of which were known or suspected suicides.[2]

*So basically, we're saying . . .*
You're much less likely to die getting from A to B if you travel by train rather than car, as long as you don't stick your head out of the train window when a tunnel's coming up.

## Arthur Smith on trains

I love trains. I sailed through my driving test – that's why I failed! I don't drive, and I quite enjoy not driving, which surprises people – especially Americans. It's like I've said to them I don't know how to put a hat on or something.

I don't really believe flying is possible, even though I've done it a lot of times. You get in a little tin box that whizzes you across the sky at 500 mph, which should be impossible. But I do believe that trains are possible. Trains are very exciting as they go through a landscape at a speed at which you can take everything in but is still much faster than humans are designed for.

When I sit in a train I look into the landscape and imagine myself in it. If there's a hill I think, 'Ooh, I'll climb up there!' And there are houses, and farms, and I think, 'I wonder who lives there?' Ninety per cent of the humans who have ever lived haven't been able to do that.

In a train, you can walk up and down the whole train. You can get a coffee, or read a book, or gaze out of the window, or if it's the weekend you can pay a £20 supplement and go First Class. And if you make enough mess on your table, no one will come and sit with you!

The only danger on a train is if you're going on a long journey and suddenly the world's most boring man, who you've been trying to avoid for years, turns out to be on the train and comes to talk to you. Then it's a kind of hell, and you have to go and sit in the toilet for a year and hope that he'll go away.

Train stations tend to be in the middle of everything – they're not like airports, stuck outside in the middle of nowhere. And trains are so smooth. You're not on a bike, banging into people, or in a car, constricted in a tiny box, or on a plane, being bumped up and down.

I used to get trains in and out of London when I was a kid, so trains were thrilling. You could meet people, if you were in the right mood. And I love trains at night, as there are always drunks in them, and they're endlessly entertaining, especially on a weekend. That was me once, probably.

I'm always on the side of the drivers when there's a train strike, although I do feel that the two most miserable words in the English language are 'rail replacement'. My heart sinks when I see them. But I think trains should be nationalised again. Thatcher flogged them all off, and some people are getting rich and trying to cut back on staff, and I applaud the unions for saying 'Fuck you!'

I never harboured a childhood ambition to be a train driver, because I always knew that I was absolutely hopeless with levers and things. I have done it – I did it for an article – but I was hopeless. I did like shovelling the coal into a steam train furnace, but I never wanted to be a train driver. I think I'd rather have been the train manager.

But I feel a bit embarrassed that I never wanted to be a train driver, as when I was a kid everyone wanted to be one.

# Motor vehicles

*Cars are really dangerous, aren't they?*

They certainly damage the health of a lot of people. In the US, almost 6.5 million vehicle crashes were reported to the police in 2017, resulting in more than 2.7 million people being injured. Over 34,000 of these crashes were fatal, killing around 37,000 people. This equates to 11.4 deaths per 100,000 people in the population.[1]

*How much is down to alcohol and speeding?*

Around 30 per cent of vehicle crash deaths in the US involve drunk driving and more than a quarter are the result of speeding.[1]

*Are more people dying as traffic increases?*

Despite the increase in vehicle ownership, British figures show that since the 1970s the number of fatalities on the roads has fallen dramatically. That figure has been broadly stable since 2010, however. In 2018, 1,782 people were killed in road traffic accidents in Britain.[2]

*I don't drive anyway, so I'll just stick to the bus.*

That's not risk-free either. In the US, over forty bus passengers die every year, and some horrifying crashes have happened around the world.[3] Twenty-five people died in 2019 in Bolivia when the bus they were travelling in plunged into a ravine.[4]

*How safe are motorbikes? I once rode on the back of Simon Le Bon from Duran Duran's motorbike and it was one of the best experiences of my life.*

Tell Simon that, over the same number of miles travelled, motor-cyclists in the US are more than twenty-five times as likely to be killed in a crash than people in cars. Around 40 per cent of those deaths occur in motorcyclists who aren't wearing a helmet.[1] It's esti-mated that in 2017, around 750 lives would have been saved if all motorcyclists in the US wore helmets.[5]

*Simon won't take any notice. He's a Wild Boy.*

*Reality check*
While the actions of other road users present a constant source of potential danger and the risks of reckless and drunk driving may seem obvious to most of us, the seemingly unre-markable things with which we distract ourselves while at the wheel are a much less apparent threat to our health. A large study in the US found some form of inattention or distrac-tion (including tiredness) was a contributing factor in 78 per cent of crashes and 65 per cent of near crashes.

As well as visual, distractions can be cognitive (thinking about something unrelated to driving the vehicle, such as what you're going to have for dinner), biomechanical (such as reaching for a coffee cup or fiddling with the stereo), or audi-tory (such as listening to a phone call). Research has shown that distractions reduce how much attention we pay to what's around us on the road ahead and that we underestimate their impact on our driving.[6]

Mobile phones (whether hand-held or hands-free), head-phones and satnavs have all been shown to cause driver distraction.[7, 8] There's also evidence that we tend to be more accepting of distractions if we consider them to be relevant to the act of driving (such as programming a satnav).[6]

*So basically, we're saying . . .*
Keep your eyes, ears and brain on the road while driving, and
don't get a motorbike (even if you're Simon Le Bon).

## Robert Llewellyn on electric cars

I first noticed that something was happening in California in 2001
when I had a very brief ride in a very fast electric car. I'd always
thought of electric vehicles as milk floats, fork lift trucks, electric
wheelchairs: essentially slow. This thing was way faster than a Ferrari:
it was brutally quick.

It was eight years later that I got my first electric car. Here are
some very important things I've learned since driving them:

Electric cars are just cars and have all the disadvantages of the cars
we have now. They cause traffic jams, they are the second most
expensive thing any of us will buy, and we only use them for between
5 and 10 per cent of the time we own them.

Now here are the advantages: they are much cheaper to run. The
total cost of ownership, including the current higher cost of buying
one, is much lower over five years than running a conventional
petrol or diesel car. It's not just fuel; electric cars need much less
servicing. My Nissan Leaf has had one service in eight years, and
even after doing 70,000 miles it didn't really need that. Nothing was
replaced or fixed.

It has an MOT every year, I've replaced tyres (two punctures) and
the rear wiper blade and that's it. It's never broken down, has the
same brake pads, same everything. I also charge it for six months of
the year from solar panels, so fuel costs are around five pence per
mile over the year. It's comically cheap and, of course, runs incredi-
bly cleanly, because when you've charged an electric car from solar
power you release exactly zero $CO_2$ per mile.

They don't use refined oil products, which means I don't give any
money to oil companies who in turn buy the crude oil from – and
I'm trying to be diplomatic here – some of the less benign regimes in

the world. That oil is refined in the UK using huge amounts of electricity, a fact not often referred to by critics of electric cars. The pollution from a petrol or diesel car is commonly only measured by what comes out of the exhaust pipe. This is only a small part of the total. That fuel has to be drilled, pumped, stored, shipped around the globe and refined, and all of those activities use huge amounts of energy with the resulting $CO_2$ and other far more toxic emissions. When the car advert says 120 grams of $CO_2$ per mile, that is not even close to any real impact.

An electric car is fuel agnostic. It can use electricity from any generating source – coal, gas, nuclear, oil, wind, solar, hydro – so as the generating capacity of the UK is slowly cleaned up, which it has been to an amazing degree, an electric car gets cleaner and cleaner.

A combustion engine car can only use one source of fuel, petrol or diesel. It's clearly not going to run out, but it's also becoming increasingly obvious that the more we can leave in the ground, the better. Globally, sales of new combustion engine cars are falling, while sales of new electric cars are rising. We are generally only aware of cars in the UK, but countries like China, Norway and especially the USA (California) are seeing incredible growth in electric car sales.

And it's not just cars – electric buses will dominate in the next few years. London and various cities in the UK are already using them and plan to buy more. The Chinese city of Shenzhen is a bit ahead of us. They are running 16,000 electric buses already. There are no diesel buses in Shenzhen any more and the transport authority is saving many millions of dollars a year in fuel costs.

Electric motorbikes, scooters, taxis and delivery vehicles are all seeing near vertical adoption around the world, not because it's 'green' or fashionable, simply because they are cheaper to run and maintain. It's economics that will drive the adoption of electric vehicles.

# Cycling

*I'd be too scared to cycle on the roads in London, but I cycled at Center Parcs. Actually, don't laugh, but I'd forgotten how to ride a bike – so I had to ride a tricycle.*

Well, as long as you're pedalling, any form of cycling is a great way to get some physical activity. Regular cycling will improve your fitness and reduce your risk of serious diseases, such as heart disease and stroke.[1]

The downside of cycling over driving is that, as you rightly suggested, it puts you at much greater risk of being killed in a road accident. Over the same distance travelled, cyclists in Britain are almost forty times more likely to be killed or seriously injured than car drivers.[2]

*How many cyclists die on average?*

Around 800 cyclists are killed on the roads every year in the US and around 50,000 are injured.[3] In Britain, there are around 100 cycling fatalities each year, almost all of which are among adults.[2]

*What increases the risk?*

Men are much more likely to be killed or injured in a cycling accident than women.[2, 4] Accident figures show that roundabouts and junctions are particularly dangerous for cyclists. You're also more likely to be fatally injured if you're cycling on a road with a high speed limit.[2]

*When do these accidents happen?*

Most cycling accidents occur during the day but they're more likely to be fatal at night. Also, you're more likely to be injured cycling in autumn and winter than the rest of the year.[2]

*How can we make it safer?*

Plenty of cycling safety advice is available online, including tips on choosing a helmet. Following safe cycling advice is a no-brainer if you want to minimise your chances of being killed on a bike; however, nothing can offer you full protection if you collide with a moving vehicle.[5, 6]

*You'd probably end up as a no-brainer if you weren't wearing a helmet. I think I'll stick to tricycling at Center Parcs.*

*Reality check*
Although you're much more vulnerable riding a bike on the roads than driving a car, some cyclists' own risk-taking behaviours can put lives in danger. In the US, it was estimated that over a fifth of cyclists killed on the roads in 2017 were in excess of the legal alcohol limit for drivers.[4] There have also been cases of pedestrians being knocked down and killed by reckless cyclists.[7]

*So basically, we're saying . . .*
Riding a bike brings plenty of health benefits but it's a relatively dangerous way to travel. Follow cycling safety advice and only ride in good light, on slower roads and sober if you want to minimise your risk of being killed.

## Jeremy Vine on cycling

*What do you enjoy most about cycling?*

It's the one moment the phone doesn't ring. OK, in London there are hazards – it's like playing a video game where you only get one life – but I accept that for the sheer joy of an hour detached from phone and screen.

*What advice would you give someone who is just starting to cycle?*

Twenty-five per cent of all accidents happen in the moment the cyclist engages with the roadspace. You wheel yourself off the pavement and get into trouble. Be aware of that, but also be aware that you should be loving it not fearing it. Sitting on a bicycle is far less dangerous than sitting on a sofa eating Pringles.

*How about advice for someone who wants to cycle to work?*

OK, now you are getting serious. The bits of kit I have, which have vastly increased my safety and presence on the road, are:

Good lights
Cameras
Mirror fitted to right handlebar
Horn

*If you could change one thing to make life safer for cyclists, what would it be?*

Segregated space for cyclists. Roadspace in cities must be crimped not widened. Private cars should not be in city centres.

# Boats

*How safe are boats, then?*

Travelling on any kind of boat comes with risks. The potential to die in an accident involving everything from a dinghy to a cruise ship has been highlighted by numerous high-profile cases in modern times.[1-4]

*Are there a lot of deaths in boat accidents?*

The European Maritime Safety Agency publishes annual figures on incidents involving ships flying a flag of one of the EU Member States or occurring within EU Member States' territorial sea and internal waters. In 2018, they reported 53 fatalities and 95 very serious casualties; 941 people were injured in total and 25 ships were lost. These figures don't include non-accidental events, such as piracy.[5]

*Actual pirates? Like oooo-arrr, me hearties, Jack Sparrow-type pirates?*

Yes, though I'm afraid they don't all look like Johnny Depp. Every year, there are around 200 recorded incidents of vessels being attacked by pirates and robbers. In 2018, almost a quarter of these occurred in the waters of Nigeria, with Indonesia a close second. It's rare for crew members to be killed by pirates and even rarer for passenger ships to be attacked. Only two incidents of passenger vessels being attacked by pirates or armed robbers were recorded between 2014 and 2018.[6]

*Phew. What about a nice spot of leisurely weekend boating? How dangerous is that?*

In 2018, the US Coast Guard recorded over 4000 recreational boating accidents resulting in 633 deaths. This equated to a fatality rate of 5.3 deaths per 100,000 registered recreational vessels.[7]

*What goes wrong?*

Recreational boating accidents can be caused by a wide range of mishaps, including running out of fuel, speeding at night, ignoring warnings of bad weather and simply not keeping a proper lookout.[8] Around three quarters of deaths occurred on vessels operated by someone with no boating safety training. Operator inattention was the most common contributing factor in accidents overall, while alcohol use was the leading contributing factor in accidents resulting in deaths. In cases where the cause of death was known, over three quarters were the result of drowning. Only a small proportion of people who drowned were known to be wearing a life jacket.[7]

*Is this partly down to men posing for selfies in speedboats?*

Accidents involving open motorboats accounted for half of the deaths. Kayaks and canoes had the second highest percentages of deaths.[7]

*Kayuck. Who wants to drown in a giant banana?*

Quite.

*Reality check*
How safe we feel on a boat doesn't necessarily reflect how safe we are. Our perception of safety on passenger ships, for example, doesn't just come down to logical things, such as how many lifeboats there are and whether there are signs of metal fatigue. Unrelated elements of a ship's design can influence how safe we feel. The results of one study showed that people feel more safe when the walls don't have a split-level design, when there's a view to the outside and when the corridors have a curved ceiling.[9]

*So basically, we're saying . . .*
There are plenty of ways to die on plenty of types of boats. Follow safety procedures, avoid areas with pirates and don't buy a speedboat.

# Walking

*Now we're talking! No wait, I misread the title. I'm not much of a walker. Unlike running, though, at least I don't whack myself in the face with my massive boobs . . .*

In an era in which gym membership is increasingly commonplace, it's easy to overlook the benefits of simple walking as a form of exercise. Walking is one of the easiest ways to increase your level of activity and improve your health.[1]

*It's a bit boring though, isn't it? Trudge, trudge, trudge.*

Organised group walks can be great for people who enjoy the social aspect and extra motivation that these events can provide, but you don't need to be walking for hours in order to benefit. Incorporating a brisk ten-minute walk into your everyday routine will boost your health and contribute to the recommended 150 minutes of weekly exercise.[1]

Walking is a particularly good way to start getting fit if you haven't exercised for a while – it's free, low-impact, easy to fit into everyday life and you can build up the speed and duration gradually to suit your own needs.[2]

*Do you need to do the much-fabled 10,000 steps?*

No, you definitely don't need to get 10,000 steps a day to receive health benefits and reduce your risk of life-limiting illnesses.[3]

The often-quoted target of 10,000 steps a day didn't come about as the result of years of scientific research but actually stemmed from a Japanese marketing campaign for pedometers in the 1960s. That's not to say that you should cut down if you're already achieving 10,000 steps, but don't fall into the trap of thinking that walking will only improve your chances of living a long life if you consistently hit that magic number.[4]

*I probably get more than that walking back and forth to the fridge.*

Many of us overestimate how much exercise we get. In England, results of a government survey show that two thirds of men and over half of women report that they're getting the recommended amount of physical activity. When this was measured objectively, however, using movement monitors, it turned out that only 6 per cent of men and 4 per cent of women actually met the recommendations.[2]

*Sounds as though it's time for me to walk to the fridge again . . .*

*Reality check*
Globally, more than 270,000 pedestrians are killed in road accidents every year. They account for a fifth of all traffic accident deaths and in some countries that figure can be as high as two thirds.[5] In the US, around 6000 pedestrians are killed in vehicle crashes every year.[6]

Hiking up mountains could also cut your life short. Every year, roughly 4 out of every 100,000 mountain hikers will die in the act. Around half of these fatalities are due to sudden cardiac death. Those who have previously suffered a heart attack or had coronary heart disease, diabetes or high cholesterol are most at risk.[7]

*So basically, we're saying . . .*
Walking is a great way to build exercise into your daily routine and most of us could improve our health by doing more of it (just don't get run over in the process).

# Part Twelve: Dangerous Sports

# Skiing and snowboarding

*I'm getting visions of mangled limbs and brain damage. Is that accurate?*

Injuries caused by skiing and snowboarding accidents lead to an estimated 7000 hospital admissions every year in the US. A study of national trauma data from 2007 to 2014 showed that around half of patients had suffered a brain injury. Injuries to the spine, chest and abdomen were also common. Sixty per cent of patients required admission to an intensive care unit. Injured snowboarders as a whole were younger than injured skiers, but males comprised the bulk of patients in both groups.[1]

*So, if I ever have a boyfriend again and he wants to go skiing, should I stop him?*

An analysis of clinical data from the US state of Utah for the period 2001–02 to 2005–06 showed that skiing and snowboarding injuries were much more common in men, with males accounting for 70 per cent of injured skiers and 88 per cent of injured snowboarders. Head injuries were common to both groups of patients and resulted in eight of the nine fatalities which occurred over the period.[2]

*What about children? My daughter's a bit of a daredevil.*

Child skiers have a greater risk than adults of both fatal and non-fatal injuries. Data from Colorado in the US over a twenty-one-year period showed that, among this group, more fatal injuries occurred in females than males. Colliding with a tree was the most common type of fatal accident in both children and adults.[3]

*Right, I'm banning her from skiing. Can I suggest snowboarding as an alternative?*

It's been estimated that snowboarders are 50–70 per cent more likely to get injured than skiers, but 30 per cent less likely to suffer a fatal injury.[4]

*It's a slippery slope. If my daughter defies me, what should I do to protect her?*

Head injury is the leading cause of death related to skiing and snowboarding, so protecting yourself with a suitable helmet is very important. Their effectiveness in reducing rates of brain injury is well-proven and there is no good evidence that people take greater risks when wearing them.[5, 6]

*I'm off to buy her a helmet. Anything else?*

Reducing your chances of serious injury shouldn't be your only health consideration. Research shows that only a very small proportion of skiers and snowboarders comply fully with sun safety advice when they're on the slopes.[7]

*Skin cancer, serious injury and death – this chapter's gone downhill rapidly.*

> *Reality check*
> The chance of being killed skiing or snowboarding is very small when you consider the number of people taking part in these activities every year. US data for the 2011–12 season showed that only 0.001 per cent of visitors to ski areas suffered an injury, with a fatality rate of 1.06 deaths per million skier days.[4]

Although we know that there are clear sex differences in the injury data, without accurate figures on the numbers of people skiing and snowboarding overall, it's not possible to calculate reliable mortality rates for male and female participants.[3]

*So basically, we're saying . . .*
Skiing and snowboarding are unlikely to kill you, but there are definitely safer pastimes. Wear a helmet to minimise the risk of brain injury, stay away from trees and don't forget the sunscreen.

# Climbing and mountaineering

*I've never climbed a mountain. I once climbed a hill, but that was only because I had a hot boyfriend I wanted to impress. And before you ask, it wasn't a molehill.*

Well, there are various forms of climbing and mountaineering, including traditional rock climbing, indoor climbing and trekking over rock, snow or ice to reach a peak or summit. The hazards and level of risk associated with these different practices vary, although the boundaries between them aren't rigid and participants often partake in more than one.[1]

*How dangerous is it overall?*

Various studies show different injury rates for different types of climbing and mountaineering, often with differences in data collection which make comparison difficult. Overall injury rates are low; however, they tend to be higher in alpine (traditional) climbing, while fatalities occur in all of the different disciplines.[1]

*OK: how likely am I to die if I go up a mountain? I don't intend to, but you never know – I might get another hot boyfriend who likes mountain climbing.*

Death rates for mountain sports vary considerably depending on the nature of the activity, the terrain, who's doing it and at what altitude.[2] It's been calculated that mountaineering comes with a higher risk of death than hang-gliding, parachuting, boxing and American football.[3]

## Climbing and mountaineering

*I can't believe mountaineering's more dangerous than being whacked in the face by Floyd Mayweather. What are the causes of death?*

Trauma, altitude sickness, hypothermia, avalanche burial and sudden cardiac death account for the bulk of deaths in the mountains.[3]

*Cheery stuff. What's altitude sickness?*

Above 4000 metres, between 28 per cent and 34 per cent of people will experience altitude sickness. This is characterised by internal fluids moving to parts of the body where they aren't meant to be.[1]

*Does it only affect certain groups?*

It can affect anyone, irrespective of age, sex and physical fitness. Not having suffered from altitude sickness previously is also no guarantee that it won't happen on a subsequent trip.[4]

*What causes sudden cardiac death?*

This is the most frequent cause of non-traumatic death in men over the age of thirty-four during mountain-based leisure activities, such as skiing and hiking. Unexpected deaths resulting from sudden cardiac arrest can be triggered by unusual levels of physical activity coupled with inadequate intake of food and fluid, particularly during the first days at high altitude.[2]

*What about those insane/courageous people (delete as applicable) who decide to climb Everest?*

Figures for the period 1921 to 2006 showed that once above base camp the death rate among climbers on Everest was 1.3 per cent. Some fatalities were the result of falls, while others had non-traumatic causes such as altitude sickness or hypothermia. A cause of death wasn't established in every case – twenty-seven people simply disappeared and their bodies were never found.[5]

*I think I'd rather go ten rounds with Floyd Mayweather.*

*Reality check*
It's impossible to develop altitude sickness in the UK. Symptoms usually develop after reaching an altitude of more than 3000 metres above sea level – more than twice the height of the UK's highest mountain, Ben Nevis.[4] Plenty of mountain deaths do occur in this country, however, from falls and other causes.[6, 7]

*So basically, we're saying . . .*
There are lots of ways to die up mountains. If you have to go up them, make sure you're properly prepared and take the appropriate safety precautions. Climbing anything is risky, but leave Mount Everest to people who aren't trying to live to a hundred and don't attempt to scale Ben Nevis in the middle of winter in a pair of flip-flops.

# Parachuting and bungee jumping

*I'm literally more likely to stick a courgette up my bum than to ever do a bungee jump.*

Fortunately, those are not the only choices. It might not seem like an appealing concept for anyone whose top priority is extended self-preservation, but you may be interested to know that every year around a million people parachute from an aircraft.[1]

*You can kill yourself though, can't you?*

Death is extremely rare, though parachuting is the most common cause of air sports-related injuries, with the majority occurring on landing.[2] Data from different studies have shown varying injury rates, but figures quoted by the British Parachute Association suggest that 1 injury occurs for every 1100 tandem jumps and around 5 injuries per 1000 solo jumps among novices.[3] The older, heavier and less fit you are, the more likely you are to experience an injury while parachuting. Women also have higher injury rates than men.[3]

*I'm old, heavy and very unfit, so I don't relish the thought of two broken legs.*

Studies from Sweden and the US suggest that two thirds of skydiving injuries are minor, half are to the lower extremities and a broken bone only occurs once in every 200,000 jumps. Just 12 per cent of injuries are classed as 'severe'.[1]

*How many people die?*

Among fully trained skydivers, one death will occur in every 100,000 jumps. Taking part in public parachuting displays will raise your risk of death to 6 in every 100,000 jumps.[3]

*I think I'd rather parade naked in the middle of Trafalgar Square than be like those crazies who parachute off a cliff.*

Ah, you're talking about BASE jumping. This is much more of a minority sport than skydiving, with around 3000 active participants. It involves throwing oneself off fixed objects with either a parachute or wingsuit (BASE stands for Building, Antenna, Span, Earth).[1]

You're between five and eight times more likely to be killed or injured BASE jumping than regular skydiving.[4] In every 10,000 BASE jumps, 4 people will be killed. The use of wingsuits is particularly associated with dying while BASE jumping. Most deaths occur as a result of hitting the ground or a cliff.[1]

*What about bungee jumping?*

Bungee jumping (and its close relation, reverse bungee jumping) will probably also be quite high on many people's list of things to avoid for maximum longevity. Although incident-free in most cases, deaths have occurred and a wide range of injuries have been reported – including life-threatening ones, such as bleeding around the brain.[5–8]

It's most commonly associated with eye injuries caused by a sudden rise in pressure in the tiny blood vessels within the eyeball (although people usually make a good recovery after treatment).[7, 9]

*Great. Well, if you need me, I'll be naked in Trafalgar Square with a courgette up my bum.*

*Reality check*
The sense of danger that comes with these kinds of activities is regarded as a large part of their appeal for many participants, rather than an undesirable side-effect. Train surfing – the practice of riding on the outside of a moving train – was once described as 'bungee jumping without a rope' by one participant. It's been responsible for numerous deaths of teenage boys and young men around the globe, yet research shows that, far from being deterred by stories of their peers being beheaded by cables, electrocuted and hit by trains, many feel that a heightened awareness of the risk of death only adds to its allure.[10, 11]

*So basically, we're saying . . .*
A thrill-seeking mentality is fundamentally incompatible with a long-term death-risk reduction strategy, but a single parachute jump is very unlikely to kill you.

# Hunting

*Is it mean of me to say that if you're hunting, you don't deserve much sympathy if you have an accident?*

Maybe a bit mean.

*OK – how likely is someone to get shot while hunting?*

Researchers looked at hospital emergency department statistics in the US between 1993 and 2008 and identified 1,841,269 visits for firearm-related injuries during that period. Of these, 35,970 (just under 2 per cent) were hunting-related. Only 0.6 per cent of these injuries were fatal. The researchers estimated that 9 firearm injuries occur per 1 million hunting days. Your chances of being fatally shot in a hunting accident are therefore pretty small.[1]

*Tell that to the animals! What causes these accidents?*

Causes of firearm-related hunting accidents include the shooter not seeing the victim, not using the weapon appropriately, swinging the weapon while shooting and mistaking the victim for game.[2]

*Really? 'No, your honour, I swear that I didn't just find him annoying.'*

Really. In 2019, an Italian man was shot dead while hunting by his own son who mistook him for a boar.[3]

*The swine! Who is most at risk?*

Studies in Europe have shown that hunters involved in accidents tend to be middle-aged men.[2] Hunters injured by firearms in the US are nearly all white.[1]

*What other dangers are involved?*

In the US, one of the most common causes of injury while hunting is falls from tree stands – platforms mounted on trees to provide a better vantage point for deer hunting. These falls often result in multiple spinal fractures.[4]

*Ouch. And are people often killed by the animal they're hunting?*

That's also a risk. Examples include cases of a rhino poacher killed by an elephant and eaten by lions and a big game hunter gored to death by a buffalo in South Africa, and a hunter killed by a polar bear in Canada.[5–7]

*What a terrible, terrible shame.*

*Reality check*
Hunting is a minority pastime, but the possibility of being killed by a wild animal is an ever-present threat in some parts of the world. Globally, it's estimated that at least 20,000 people a year are killed by snakebites.[8] There have been cases of people being killed by hippos and crocodiles, and in Australia up to four people a year are believed to be killed by bee stings.[9–11] Even something domesticated and seemingly innocuous could polish you off – over a fifteen-year period in Britain, from April 2000, seventy-four people were killed by cows.[12] People are also killed and seriously injured every year horse riding.[13]

*So basically, we're saying . . .*
Trying to kill animals could prove fatal, but you should probably be more worried about them trying to kill you.

# Motor racing

*Surely motor racing is an obvious one to avoid?*

All motor sports carry risk, but some races are more dangerous than others. Deaths are especially common in the annual Isle of Man Tourist Trophy (or TT) motorcycle races. The two-week event takes place on public roads across the island, meaning that riders don't have the benefit of purpose-built track safety features, and the risk of crashing into buildings, walls and spectators is ever-present. Whereas several seasons of Formula One can go by without a fatal crash, riders die taking part in the TT races almost every year.[1]

*Better to watch from the sidelines, I guess.*

If you're watching in person, you're probably going to want to avoid any race where there isn't a safety barrier between you and the vehicles. Spectators have also been killed in accidents at the TT races.[2] Deaths have also occurred when cars have spun off the road and ploughed into the crowd during rally events.[3]

*So as long as I avoid recognised racing venues, I'll be fine?*

Not always. Illegal street racing is responsible for a number of deaths in the US each year, although they account for only a fraction of a percent of all fatal vehicle crashes.[4] Figures from Los Angeles, where street racing has long been a particular problem, show that over half of the people killed in these crashes haven't been the ones driving the offending vehicles. Passengers, spectators, uninvolved motorists and pedestrians account for the majority of deaths.[5]

*I give up! Nowhere is safe.*

Don't worry – research conducted in Ontario found that only around 1 per cent of adults engage in street racing, although it's much more common among young drivers.[6] A US study in the 1990s found that around 60 per cent of male high school students and a third of female high school students had raced another car in the previous year.[4] It's also more prevalent among people who drive under the influence of alcohol or cannabis.[6] In comparison with other drivers involved in fatal accidents, street racers are more likely to be male, teenagers and already have a history of crashes and driving violations.[4]

*Why can't they spend their whole lives playing video games like normal teenagers?*

*Reality check*
Although racing a car round a track is inherently dangerous, decades of safety advances in some motor sports have led to substantial reductions in fatality rates.[7, 8] In a paper published in 2016, researchers calculated that you'd actually be more likely to survive a NASCAR racing crash than a traffic accident in the US.[9]

*So basically, we're saying . . .*
Put aside any fantasies of motor racing glory, and don't stand in the vicinity while others are living out theirs.

# Scuba diving

*So, should we scuba-do, or scuba-don't?*

It's estimated there are fewer than two deaths per million recreational scuba dives, and around 15 deaths per 100,000 scuba divers every year.[1, 2] In 2016, 169 deaths involving recreational scuba diving were recorded worldwide.[1]

*Who is most likely to die from scuba diving?*

The majority of scuba deaths occur in males and people over fifty years old, but we don't know how this compares with the characteristics of scuba divers as a whole. Fatalities occur at all skill levels, including among instructors.[1]

*Are most deaths because of the bends?*

Decompression sickness (or 'the bends') is responsible for some fatalities, but drowning is the most commonly recorded cause of death.[1]

*What about diving without all the gear?*

Breath-hold diving can also go fatally wrong. It includes everything from a spontaneous dive to the bottom of your local swimming pool or a casual snorkel, to spearfishing and competitive freediving. The statistics are less reliable than they are for scuba diving, but sixty deaths were recorded in 2016 worldwide.

*Who dies in breath-hold accidents?*

Fatalities peak in people aged sixty and over, and more deaths occur in males than females. Most fatal breath-hold diving accidents occur during snorkelling and spearfishing.[1]

*And they would have got away with it if it wasn't for that pesky oxygen.*

*Reality check*
While deep sea scuba diving or spearfishing might seem like treacherous activities, many people fail to recognise the risks of jumping into water in more familiar surroundings. Tombstoning – jumping from a height into water (such as off a cliff or pier) – is especially dangerous. Jumpers can overestimate the depth of the water or hit submerged rocks or other objects, causing catastrophic spine and head injuries. The shock of immersion in cold water can also make it difficult to swim and strong currents can quickly sweep people away.[3] There have been many well-publicised deaths and cases of life-changing injuries in the UK alone in recent years.[4]

*So basically, we're saying . . .*
Your chances of dying while diving are fairly small, but jumping off a cliff at the seaside is a definite no-no for the aspiring centenarian.

## Jon Holmes on scuba diving

I was about to scuba dive when a wave took me into a colony of sea urchins. They were big and black and spiny, and they went into my arms and legs. I tried to scramble out of the water because I panicked, making it worse. I started to go into shock because I didn't know if they were poisonous or not!

I was on my own, the beach was deserted, and this was only hours before my flight home. I staggered up the beach, bleeding out of my limbs, got to the diving shop, and they took one look at me and just went, 'Hospital?!'

I was put in a jeep and was taken across the island to the hospital, where a doctor spent ages pulling bits of sea urchin out of me with tweezers. Then he said, 'Well, I can't get them all out – they break off – but they're alive in you now! So, this is what's going to happen: I'll bandage you up, but over the next month or so they'll wriggle out of you. You won't even notice – they'll just dissolve and come out, but they're alive – just bear that in mind.'

So, I was full of live sea urchin spines! I had to go back through America where they ask you, 'Are you bringing anything live into the country?' And I said [puts on serious voice], 'No, no!'

If I'd had sex with my wife with the sea urchins in me, that wouldn't have just been a threesome – they were too numerous to count, so that would have been an aquatic hundredsome! And I'm all up for experimenting.

It would have been awkward if it had been sex with a stranger though – that's not a great bit of pillow talk, if sea urchins are coming out of you during sex. 'What's that?' 'Oh, it's just some sea urchin. It's in me – and now it's in you!'

# Contact sports

*I'm sorry but if you hit people for a living, can you really be surprised if your life is shorter as a result?*

I don't hit people for a living, but many cases have been highlighted in the media of boxers and mixed martial artists dying as a result of injuries sustained during a match.[1-4] Head injuries are responsible for most boxing fatalities, although it's also possible to be killed by a body shot.[5] The leading cause of death is a condition called subdural haematoma, where blood collects between the skull and the surface of the brain.[6]

*Bleurrgh. How common are boxing deaths?*

There's a surprising lack of good data around boxing deaths. The best we have is a record of fatalities which was begun during the 1940s by an anti-boxing activist, which stretches back to the eighteenth century. The most recent complete decade of data in 'The Manuel Velazquez Boxing Fatality Collection' is for 2000–09, in which 103 deaths were recorded worldwide – an average of ten a year.[7]

Unfortunately, we don't have good enough data to be able to calculate reliably how many injuries and deaths occur in a certain number of boxing or mixed martial arts matches.[8, 9] Without this information we can't accurately estimate how likely someone would be to die as a result of participating in these sports.

*Are there any long-term risks from punching or colliding with people?*

Most people taking part in combat sports won't sustain a catastrophic injury in a match, but there can be long-term risks to consider as well. Professional athletes in sports which are prone to concussion injuries have an increased risk of developing a progressive neurodegenerative disease called amyotrophic lateral sclerosis (or Lou Gehrig's disease), for example, which ultimately results in paralysis and death.[10]

*How about ice hockey fights? They can look seriously nasty.*

Although seemingly regarded by many as part of the entertainment, the routine fist fights between ice hockey players can prove deadly.[11] Ice hockey deaths have also occurred as a result of less obvious dangers, including a player's neck being accidentally slashed by a skate and others being struck in the chest or neck by the puck.[12–14]

*Sheesh. What's wrong with a nice game of tiddlywinks?*

People also die participating in other contact sports which don't involve combat. In 2018, France experienced the deaths of three rugby players in separate incidents within just five months. One of these was an under-21 player who was reported to have died as a result of a two-man tackle that broke his neck, caused a cardiac arrest and cut off the oxygen supply to his brain.[15] Deaths have also occurred as a result of players colliding in football, including Australian rules football and American football.[16–18]

*These incidents are few and far between though, right?*

Researchers have calculated that the risk of sustaining a catastrophic injury in rugby union in England is less than 1 in 100,000 each year, compared with 1 in 4000 for ice hockey players and 2 in 100,000 for American football players. There was considerable variation between nations though, with playing rugby union appearing to carry a greater risk in New Zealand, Australia and Fiji.[19]

*You know what? I'm going to stick to playing Uno.*

*Reality check*

Combat sports carry very obvious health risks, but freak incidents can also cause death in seemingly non-dangerous sports. In 2014, twenty-five-year-old Australian cricketer Phil Hughes was killed when the ball bounced up and struck him in the neck, rupturing an artery.[20] A twenty-two-year-old English hockey player died, in 2015, as a result of being accidentally struck on the head by a hockey stick during a training session.[21] In 2010, a twenty-three-year-old Brazilian futsal player died following a match after a piece of the court's wooden floor came off and struck him in the abdomen.[22]

*So basically, we're saying . . .*

Although accidents can happen in any sport, anything that involves taking blows to the head or chest is not for the risk-averse.

# Part Thirteen: Other Hazards

# Carbon monoxide

*What's carbon monoxide when it's at home?*

It's when it's in your home, or other enclosed spaces, that there's a problem. Carbon monoxide is a poisonous gas that kills around twenty-five people in England and Wales every year. It has no smell or taste, which makes it particularly dangerous because people are often unaware that they're breathing it in.[1]

*Scary. Where does it come from?*

It's given off when fuels such as gas, oil, coal and wood don't burn fully. It's also produced by barbecues, car exhausts and smoking. The most common causes of accidental carbon monoxide poisoning are household appliances, such as cookers, heaters and central heating boilers, that are incorrectly installed, poorly maintained or poorly ventilated. Blocked flues and chimneys, and burning fuel in an enclosed or unventilated space, such as running a car engine or petrol-powered generator inside a garage, can also cause exposure to carbon monoxide.[1]

*How can I tell if I'm being exposed to carbon monoxide?*

The symptoms of carbon monoxide poisoning can be similar to those of flu and food poisoning, although it doesn't cause a high temperature. The most common symptom is a headache. You may also experience dizziness, nausea and vomiting, tiredness and confusion, stomach pain, shortness of breath and difficulty breathing.

People often fall victim to carbon monoxide poisoning while they're asleep, so it's possible to be killed by it without ever being aware that you're becoming unwell.[1]

*How exactly does it kill you, then?*

When you breathe in carbon monoxide, it enters your bloodstream and prevents your blood from being able to carry oxygen around your body, causing your cells and tissue to fail.[1]

*It sounds horrible. How can I reduce my risk of dying from it?*

The main ways to reduce your risk of carbon monoxide poisoning in your own home are to ensure that any gas appliances you have are serviced annually by an appropriately qualified and registered gas engineer, have any other fossil fuel burning appliances professionally serviced every year and fit carbon monoxide detectors. If you have a chimney you should get it swept regularly by a professional.[2]

*You mean an orphan boy from a workhouse?*

It's also important to be aware of the risks of carbon monoxide poisoning outside of your own home, especially when on holiday. There have been plenty of cases of people being killed by carbon monoxide from barbecues and heaters in tents and caravans.

*That'd put a dampener on a cheery summer holiday.*

You should never take a barbecue into a tent, awning, caravan, motorhome or boat, and never use a fuel-burning heater inside a tent or awning. Similarly, you should never use a gas, petrol or diesel-powered generator in an enclosed space or where fumes from it could blow inside. When staying in holiday homes and hotels you should also be aware of the risk of faulty gas boilers and appliances. Taking a portable carbon monoxide alarm with you when you go away is the best way to protect yourself.[3]

*Reality check*
Dying from accidental carbon monoxide poisoning is relatively uncommon when compared with the big killers such as cancer and heart disease; however, it's a preventable cause of death which presents more of a danger than some more high-profile risks. An analysis of US data found that the average American is roughly five times more likely to die from accidental carbon monoxide poisoning than in a mass shooting.[4]

*So basically, we're saying . . .*
Carbon monoxide poisoning kills a relatively small number of people, but it's a cause of death which you can easily prevent by taking some simple precautions and using carbon monoxide detectors (including when you go on holiday).

# Drowning

*I can't swim. What have you got to tell me?*

The World Health Organization estimated that 360,000 people died from drowning in 2015, accounting for just under 10 per cent of total deaths across the globe and making it the third leading cause of death from unintentional injury.[1]

*That's crazy – 10 per cent? I don't know of anyone who's drowned.*

That's probably because you live in England. Low- and middle-income countries account for over 90 per cent of the world's accidental drowning deaths. In Africa, drowning mortality rates are up to twenty times higher than in the UK.[1]

*Wow. Are these all people who fell in or were some of them pushed?*

Very few. In the UK in 2017 there were 592 drowning deaths, of which 242 were suspected or confirmed accidents, 209 were suspected or confirmed suicides and 5 were suspected or confirmed to be the result of a crime. Natural causes were suspected or confirmed in 13 of the deaths, and there was no record of cause in the remaining 123 cases.[2]

*What are the main risk factors?*

Age is a major risk factor for death by drowning, with the highest rates seen in young children. Across the globe, one- to four-year-olds are most likely to die by drowning, followed by five- to nine-year-olds. A report published in 2014 showed that drowning was the leading cause of death by unintentional injury among one- to three-year-olds in Australia and the second leading cause in one- to fourteen-year-olds in the US.[1] A UK study found that children aged five to fourteen, people aged fifteen to thirty and men over eighty-five had an increased risk of drowning at inland water locations.[3]

*What's the male–female split?*

Males are much more likely than females to die by drowning or to be hospitalised for non-fatal drowning. A combination of spending more time around water and greater risk-taking behaviour among males is believed to account for this difference.[1] Males are more likely to take part in recreational activities such as swimming, boating and fishing, and to take greater risks, such as not wearing a personal flotation device and swimming alone or after consuming alcohol.[4]

*Right. Any other risk factors?*

Simply spending more time around water makes drowning more likely to happen.[1]

*No shit, Sherlock!*

Figures for accidental inland fatal drownings in the UK show that men living in areas which have a lot of rivers, canals and other open water are especially at risk.[5] The rates are also particularly high for certain water sports.

*I had a boyfriend who was into that. We had to put a bin liner down on the mattress.*

Those taking part in motorboating and scuba diving (also see pages 301–3 for scuba diving) have the highest risk of death by drowning. Angling, sailing, jet skiing and kayaking/canoeing also see high rates of accidental death. In contrast, the risk of fatally drowning while swimming indoors is very low.[5]

*It's possible to drown in the bath though, isn't it? They always warn new parents that babies can drown in just an inch of water.*

Every year in Britain, around twenty people drown in the bath. The risk is highest among the over-sixty-fives.[5]

*No more baths for me! Showers only from now on.*

Simple measures in the home can reduce the risk of drowning. In warmer countries, such as Australia, for example, installing fencing around home swimming pools has proven to be particularly effective in reducing deaths.[3]

*Surely, as a species, we should have evolved past drowning by now . . .?*

In the UK, drowning deaths peaked in the late 1970s. Since then, we've seen a gradual decline. Drowning fatalities in managed swimming pools are now very uncommon.[3]

*Some good news at last. I'm looking on the bright side and seeing this as an excuse to go shopping for a new bikini. I might go for a neon colour, so I'm easily spotted by lifeguards. I'm basically turning into Borat.*

*Reality check*
Drowning is generally not well-recorded, so we don't get a full picture from the available data; for example, it's common for death certificates to register the complication of drowning rather than drowning itself, partly because it can be difficult to determine the sequence of events.[3, 6] Also, only a very small proportion of drowning incidents are fatal. Most of the time when people get into difficulty in water they're able to get themselves out of trouble or are rescued quickly without the incident ever being recorded.[6]

*So basically, we're saying . . .*
Always swim in a lifeguard-supervised area, fence off your pool if you have one and take appropriate safety precautions if participating in any kind of leisure activity on, in or near water.[6]

# Choking

*Since becoming a parent I've discovered that grapes are a big choking hazard. I now spend much of my life cutting grapes in half. I call them the grapes of wrath.*

Although we often think of very young children as being at the greatest risk of choking on food, the over sixty-fives are several times more likely to die this way than one- to four-year-olds. A study published in 2014 showed that around 500 people aged sixty-five and over choke to death on food in the US every year. Men aged eighty-five and over have the highest risk of all.[1] In England and Wales, around 400 choking related deaths occur every year. Most of these happen in people aged sixty and over.[2]

*Ah yes – my ninety-five-year-old nan needs help to eat because she chokes so much. But why are old people more likely to choke on food?*

Fifty pairs of muscles are involved when we swallow. As we get older these can become weaker, making swallowing less easy. Difficulty with chewing can also mean that we end up trying to swallow bigger chunks of food. Most of us don't even realise that these changes are occurring, but they can increase the risk of us choking when eating.[3]

*What can people do to reduce the risk of choking, short of living on soup?*

There are steps you can take to reduce your risk of choking as you get older, such as taking small bites, chewing slowly and not talking and eating at the same time.[3]

*And cutting grapes in half. FINE.*

*Reality check*

People often use the term 'choking' when they're actually talking about strangulation. In medical terminology, choking refers to the obstruction of the airway by a foreign body. When pressure is applied to the neck, cutting off circulation or airflow from the outside, it's referred to as strangulation.

There have been cases of people dying accidentally as a result of voluntary strangulation in what's sometimes known as the 'choking game'. The aim is to achieve a brief state of euphoria caused by lack of oxygen to the brain, but it can easily go fatally wrong.[4] Other accidental deaths by strangulation have occurred when scarves or towels placed round the neck have become caught in machinery or the wheels of a motor vehicle.[5, 6]

*So basically, we're saying . . .*
Don't bite off more than you can chew and don't talk with your mouth full (especially when you get old).

# Hazardous jobs

*I'm lucky I'm a comedy writer instead of going up pylons for a living, aren't I?*

You are. In 2018–19 there were 147 fatal injuries in the workplace in Britain. Falls from a height were the most common type of fatal accident, followed by being struck by a moving vehicle. Almost a third of these deaths were in 'agriculture, forestry and fishing', while another 30 per cent occurred in the construction industry.

When the number of people working in each industry is taken into account, as well as the number of accidents, 'agriculture, forestry and fishing' and 'waste and recycling' emerge as the riskiest sectors, with fatal injury rates around eighteen and seventeen times higher than the average across all industries respectively.[1]

*Is fishing dangerous?*

Yes: commercial fishing is one of the most dangerous occupations in the US. Research shows that commercial fishermen consistently underestimate the risks they face. The degree of overconfidence varies depending on certain characteristics, including age, education and what the researchers described as risk-loving tendencies in other facets of life, such as smoking and not wearing a seatbelt.[2]

*That's in America. What about risky jobs in other countries?*

Rates of fatal injuries at work vary substantially between countries. The rate in Luxembourg is around ten times that in the UK, for example, although differences in definitions of workplace accidents and reporting systems mean that it's not possible to accurately compare rates across continents.[1]

In the US, there are over 5000 fatalities from injuries at work every year, of which transportation incidents account for around 40 per cent. The occupational category 'driver/sales workers and truck drivers' experience the largest number of fatal injuries; however, the rate of fatal injuries is highest among 'fishers and related fishing workers', followed by 'logging workers'.[3]

In Australia, the category with the highest rate of fatal injuries at work is 'machinery operators and drivers', with around 10 deaths every year per 100,000 workers.[4]

*I'm guessing this mostly affects men?*

US figures show that men are almost ten times more likely to be killed by an injury at work than women.[3]

*Right. Well I'm going to stick with writing, I think. Hopefully I won't get impaled on a pen.*

Even writing has its hazards. See the Reality check box below.

*Reality check*
As discussed in Standing (pages 91–4), although a desk-based office job might put you at less risk of dying from an injury at work, prolonged sitting and a sedentary lifestyle could still result in an early death by increasing your chances of developing a long-term health condition, such as diabetes. To reduce this risk, it's recommended that sedentary office workers should initially aim to build in two hours per day of standing and light walking while at work, eventually progressing to four hours per day.

If you work for an employer who is prepared to provide you with a standing desk and allow you to take regular breaks to move around this may be achievable, but for many people this won't feel like a realistic goal.[5, 6]

*So basically, we're saying . . .*
Fishing for a living could result in a quick premature death and sitting at a desk all day could result in a slow one.

# High blood pressure

*I know it's important to your health, but what is blood pressure?*

It's a measure of how much force your heart is using to pump blood around your body.[1] High blood pressure (also called hypertension) is the world's leading preventable risk factor for both cardiovascular disease and premature death. It's the second biggest risk factor for disease (after poor diet) in the world, and the third biggest in the UK (after smoking and poor diet).[2]

*Wow. Which diseases does it cause?*

Having high blood pressure increases your risk of heart failure, coronary artery disease, stroke and vascular dementia.[2] These links have been well-established by research, including the benefits of lowering blood pressure on the risk of cardiovascular disease and death.[3]

*I have no idea what my blood pressure measurement is. You have to use that pump thingy at the doctor's that hurts your arm, don't you?*

The only way to tell if your blood pressure is too high or too low is to get it tested, because most people won't notice any symptoms. If you have a validated blood pressure monitor this is something you can do yourself at home rather than going to your doctor. Alternatively, your pharmacist or even your workplace may offer blood pressure testing. Once you're over forty, you should get your blood pressure checked at least every five years.[1]

*What can I do about the numbers I get, though?*

Some simple lifestyle changes can help you to avoid hypertension or lower your blood pressure if it's already too high. This is mostly the kind of advice that you'd expect for improving your health generally – eat plenty of fruit and vegetables, keep your alcohol intake below recommended limits, maintain a healthy weight, and get the recommended level of physical exercise and a good night's sleep. Keeping your salt intake below the recommended limit of 5 grams a day is also important for avoiding high blood pressure.[1] One of the key ways to achieve this is to minimise the amount of processed food you eat. Processed foods, such as bread, and ultra-processed foods, such as canned soup, are often surprisingly high in salt.

*Ultra-processed? Does that mean the food's been microwaved, digested and refrozen before packaging?*

Ultra-processed food tends to be high in poor quality fat, have added sugar and salt, and provide little in terms of vitamins and fibre. They include ice cream, cookies, hamburgers, sausages and pizza. Too much as part of your regular diet can boost your chances of an early death. Having four or more servings of ultra-processed foods daily has been shown to increase mortality by 62 per cent.[4]

*Isn't smoking linked to high blood pressure too?*

Smoking doesn't *cause* high blood pressure but both it and hypertension narrow your arteries, so if you do have hypertension *and* you smoke, your risk of developing heart problems is increased dramatically.[1]

*How about drinking caffeine?*

Too much caffeine (e.g. more than four cups of coffee a day) may raise your blood pressure. It's best not to rely on caffeinated drinks as your main source of fluid intake.[1]

*I guess I should go and buy a squeezy-arm-thingy, then. It sounds like a solid investment.*

*Reality check*
Our blood pressure typically increases as we get older, so for people aged sixty and over the guidance around what constitutes an acceptable measurement tends to be a little different from those applied to the general adult population. Some research suggests that a blanket approach of 'lower blood pressure is better' may not be appropriate for older people and that low blood pressure may actually be a bigger risk factor for death than high blood pressure in this age group.[5]

*So basically, we're saying . . .*
High blood pressure is generally bad news for your health. Get your blood pressure checked regularly and follow a healthy lifestyle to reduce the risk of hypertension scuppering your quest for a long life.

# Infectious diseases

*Is 'infectious' the same as 'communicable'?*

Yes. Infectious, or communicable, diseases are those which are passed from person to person (or animal to person). They're caused by infectious organisms, such as bacteria, viruses or fungi.[1]

*Are we mainly talking colds here? 'Cause I wouldn't call them a disease. If I told a mate 'I've got a terrible disease – it's a cold' I reckon they'd laugh at me.*

Infectious diseases range from mild illnesses, such as the common cold, through to diseases with a very high fatality rate, such as Ebola. There are also many ways that you can catch an infectious disease. Different infections are spread in different ways. Direct contact with an infected person is the most obvious. Some diseases, for example, are transmitted through unprotected sexual contact, while others can be passed through the air by coughing and sneezing. Some infections can be picked up by indirect contact, such as touching a door handle that has germs on it from someone else's hand and then putting your fingers in your mouth. Insect or animal bites and consuming contaminated food or water are other common ways of becoming infected.[2]

*What about when you can't stop running to the toilet? Is that an infection or just bad luck?*

The most common cause of diarrhoeal disease in the world is campylobacter. Species of campylobacter bacteria are commonly carried by farm animals, including poultry. The main way that people become infected is by eating undercooked meat which has been contaminated by faeces during the slaughtering process. Although the illness is generally mild but unpleasant, it can be fatal in very young children, the elderly and people with weakened immune systems.[3] Another common cause of diarrhoea (and/or vomiting) is norovirus. It can also be very unpleasant and is highly contagious. It can be passed through direct or indirect contact, including eating food that's been handled by someone carrying the virus. Symptoms usually clear up after a couple of days but, like campylobacter, it can cause potentially fatal complications in vulnerable groups.[4]

*'I've got campylobacter' sounds much more impressive than 'I've got the squits'. So how do I avoid infectious diseases, then?*

Steps you can take to reduce your risk of developing an infectious disease include getting any appropriate vaccinations, including when travelling abroad; washing your hands often and avoiding eating or touching your mouth with unclean fingers; following food safety advice, particularly when handling or eating meat; practising safe sex; not sharing items such as toothbrushes and straws; and avoiding contact with wild animals.[2]

*Easy, tiger. I haven't been abroad for years. That means I'm safer, right?*

Which part of the world you're in will partly determine your risk of catching specific infectious diseases, but there's always potential for some diseases to spread from one country to another and for new diseases to develop.[5] Infections that have recently appeared or have spread to new geographical areas are known as 'emerging infectious diseases'. The natural evolution of disease-causing organisms and human behaviour can both contribute to this threat.[6, 7]

*And there are all those dodgy mutations, aren't there?*

The novel coronavirus (COVID-19), which first appeared in Wuhan, China in 2019, is a perfect example of how diseases can be passed from animals to humans and spread rapidly, causing a large number of deaths.

The influenza (flu) virus is particularly well known for its ability to change its genetic make-up. When a new variant emerges that the human immune system hasn't encountered before and is therefore unprepared to defend against, it can spread rapidly and cause disease on a very large scale. In 2009, the H1N1 swine flu virus, which passed to humans from pigs, spread around the world faster than any virus in history. This was largely thanks to the huge volume of commercial air travel.[7] Although it killed hundreds of thousands of people globally in its first year of circulation, this particular strain of flu turned out to be less deadly than at first feared.[8] The H5N1 bird flu virus, on the other hand, which can be passed to humans, has a much higher fatality rate. At the moment, it can't be transmitted easily from person to person, but if a new strain of flu were to emerge with both swine flu's ability to spread and the deadliness of bird flu, it would pose a very serious threat to our health.[7, 9]

*Note to self: avoid pigs and birds. Not that I hang out with them much now.*

As well as the threat of emerging infectious diseases, we're also facing the growing danger of antibiotic resistance. Antibiotics are vital for treating infections caused by bacteria, but over-use in both humans and animals has meant that we're increasingly seeing bacteria which have changed in response and become resistant to them. A growing list of infections, such as pneumonia and tuberculosis, are becoming harder to treat as the antibiotics we rely on become less effective. The World Health Organization has warned that without urgent action we're heading towards a post-antibiotic era, in which common infections and minor injuries can be deadly – just as they were before antibiotics became widely available.[10]

*Yikes! I think I feel some campylobacter coming on.*

*Reality check*

Outbreaks of deadly infectious diseases are very dramatic events which immediately cause fear and alarm. They attract a lot of media attention when they occur and make for good Hollywood movies. Currently, though, infectious diseases aren't what polishes most of us off.

Globally, non-communicable diseases, such as heart disease and cancer, account for almost three quarters of all deaths. This figure rises to almost 90 per cent in people aged seventy and older. In Western Europe, non-communicable diseases cause an even greater proportion of total deaths – over 90 per cent. In the US, injuries cause more deaths than infectious diseases.[11]

In sub-Saharan Africa, however, the picture is quite different. Here, non-communicable diseases account for just over a third of all deaths, with respiratory infections and tuberculosis being the leading cause of mortality. Even here, though, non-communicable diseases become the most common cause of death once people reach the age of seventy (accounting for around 70 per cent of deaths in this age group).[11]

*So basically, we're saying . . .*

Follow food safety advice, don't put your fingers in your mouth without washing them first, use condoms, get vaccinated and remember that lack of exercise, smoking and a bad diet are a bigger threat to most people's lives than scary germs.

# Mobile phones

*Please don't tell me I have to make like the Amish and bin my iPhone?*

Binning your phone would be a little extreme, but people have long had concerns about whether the radiation they produce could be harmful to health.[1] Alarmist media reports have played a part in fuelling public fear.[2]

Particularly, there's been speculation about a possible increased risk of cancer from using a mobile phone or living near a mobile phone mast (or base station). Since the 1990s, a large amount of research has been undertaken and the weight of the evidence to date suggests that neither of these is likely to increase the risk of health problems.[1]

*My mum was always worried about radiation. She refused to get a microwave and would make us sit three metres from our telly. Could phones irradiate our bodies?*

Your mobile phone sends radio waves in all directions in order to find the nearest base station, so some of them will be absorbed by your body as energy. The only proven effect of this, though, is a rise in the body's temperature of up to 0.2 degrees Celsius, which poses no known health risk.[1]

*What about brain tumours?*

Most studies have found no association between mobile use and the risk of brain tumours in people. A few studies have suggested a link, but this may be the result of methodological issues with the research. Scientists can't completely exclude the possibility of a causal link between mobile use and cancer, but currently the balance of available evidence doesn't suggest that there's a problem.[3]

*So, it's safe to live near a mast?*

Large studies have found no evidence that living near a mobile phone mast causes any unpleasant symptoms. You get much more exposure to radiation from your phone than you do from masts.[1] The strength of radio waves coming from mobile phone masts reduces rapidly as you get further away. In the UK, restrictions on public access around bigger, more powerful masts prevent people from being exposed to levels of radiation which exceed international guidelines.[4]

*What about 5G? People are properly getting their knickers in a twist about that.*

Some people have raised particular concerns about the safety of 5G mobile networks because the higher-frequency waves used require more masts which are positioned closer to the ground.[5, 6]

We may be exposed to a higher level of radiation as a result of the introduction of 5G, but this will still be well below recommended limits. No adverse health effects are anticipated on the basis of current evidence, although there's always the potential for new evidence to emerge in future which changes the scientific consensus.[7]

*So, we can't be completely confident there's no long-term risk from our phones?*

Although no convincing evidence of harm to health has been identified so far, it's an ongoing area of research. Using a mobile has only become common practice relatively recently, so it's impossible to rule out any effects of longer-term use. We can't yet say for sure if there are any effects of using one over the course of a lifetime.[1]

*What can I do if I'm worried? Except for making like the Amish, of course.*

If you're concerned about the remaining uncertainty regarding long-term mobile phone use, there are steps you can take to minimise your exposure (other than simply getting rid of your phone altogether). Using a hands-free kit will keep the amount of time you spend with the phone near your head to a minimum.

When choosing a phone, you can also compare how much radio wave energy will be absorbed into your body by different models by checking with the retailer the specific absorption rate (or SAR). Another tip is to avoid using your phone when you don't have a strong signal, as it needs to use more energy to communicate with the base station.[1]

*To be honest, if I binned my phone I'd be worried about my personal safety when out late at night.*

Like many things, it's a question of balancing risks and benefits. Phones are useful, and they *probably* won't cause you any harm.

*Reality check*
Your body absorbs up to five times more of the signal from FM radio and television masts than mobile phone base stations. This is due to their lower frequencies and the fact that a person's height makes the body an efficient receiving antenna. TV and radio signals have been a regular feature of life for a lot longer than mobile phones without any known dangers to health.[8]

The biggest known health risk from mobile phones is using one while driving, because it can make you up to four times more likely to have an accident.[1]

*So basically, we're saying . . .*
Your mobile phone is unlikely to kill you unless you're using it at the wheel (although it's too early to say for certain).

# Fairground rides and amusement parks

*I broke my arm on a bouncy castle when I was five. A bouncy castle! So, I don't trust fairground attractions. There are lots of regulations these days though, right?*

Regulations pertaining to fairground and theme park rides vary between nations. Inspection and enforcement practices can also differ between areas within the same country. Health and safety regulations can't completely eliminate the risk of injury or death from amusement park rides, however.[1] In recent years there have been examples of an entire seating unit breaking off during a ride due to corrosion, killing one man and injuring others, and a collision between roller-coaster trains resulting in amputations.[2]

*That's horrific. These rides are meant for kids.*

Yes. And it's easy to assume that even the most extreme-looking amusement park rides must be designed in such a way that they're fundamentally safe to ride on. Sadly, this doesn't always turn out to be true. In 2016, a child was decapitated by a 169-foot-tall water slide in the US, marketed as the tallest in the world, when the raft carrying him became airborne and his head struck a metal pole. Other reported injuries prior to the fatal accident included slipped discs, whiplash, broken toes and lacerations. In the aftermath of the tragedy, serious questions were asked about the qualifications of those who designed the ride.[3]

*These incidents are still pretty rare though, right?*

It's certainly important to keep in mind that a major theme park can receive millions of visitors annually, the vast majority of whom go home unscathed.

A study published in 2019 looked at global data on theme park and amusement ride accidents over a one-year period. In total, 182 accidents were reported from 38 countries, 51 of which involved a fatality. Fixed-site rides (amusement and theme parks), mobile rides and water parks had similar numbers of incidents. The number of accidents in relation to the number of people attending was highest in Latin America.[2] In Britain, 369 injuries to members of the public were recorded in one year (2017–18) as a result of 'activities of amusement parks and theme parks'. Workers sustained 61 recorded injuries in the same year.[4]

*How many people need to be hospitalised?*

US Government figures estimate that in 2018, over 42,000 people were treated in emergency departments as a result of injuries from fixed rides in amusement or theme parks, mobile rides, inflatables, rides at shopping malls or restaurants, and water slides. This equates to 12.9 injuries per 100,000 people in the US population. Despite the seemingly large number of people injured, over 97 per cent were treated and released without requiring hospitalisation.[5]

*Were most of them kids?*

Injuries happened in all age groups, but the bulk occurred in people aged from five to fourteen.[5]

*Are riders ever to blame? You know, by not keeping their hands inside the car?*

Improper rider action was reported in just 11 of the 182 reported accidents globally in 2017–18. Another 11 involved medical conditions or reactions.[2]

*Is it mainly roller coasters that could kill me? I feel that Ronan Keating needs to shoulder some responsibility here.*

Roller coasters are involved in around a third of amusement ride accidents.[2] Less obviously scary attractions can be lethal though. In recent years there have been a number of serious accidents involving inflatable amusements, such as bouncy castles and inflatable slides.

*Oh yes, don't I know it!*

Serious injuries and deaths have occurred as a result of inflatables collapsing, being blown over and, in one case in the UK, bursting.[6, 7, 8] A study based on US data from 2010 found that inflatables were involved in over 42 per cent of amusement injuries.[9] It's estimated that they were responsible for over 113,000 injuries treated in US emergency departments between 2003 and 2013. Two thirds of these were arm and leg injuries. Over the same period, 12 people died as a result of accidents involving inflatable amusements.[10]

*Wow. In that case, I was lucky to get off with just a broken arm.*

*Reality check*
Compared with driving a car, fairground and amusement park rides are relatively safe.[1] International data shows an injury rate of less than 1 per 1 million rides. According to the International Association of Amusement Parks and Attractions, the chance of being seriously injured on an amusement park ride in the US is just 1 in 17 million rides.[2]

*So basically, we're saying . . .*
The risk of death from amusement park rides and bouncy castles is small but real. The most dedicated self-preservation-ists will avoid getting on them at all.

# Part Fourteen: Stuff You Can't Do Anything About

# Genes

*I'm so fat, I can't get into my jeans.*

Maybe not, but I'm talking about the genes in *you*. Along with environmental and lifestyle factors, our genetic make-up plays a role in determining how long we live. The siblings and children of people who live an unusually long time are also more likely than their peers to reach a ripe old age and remain healthy for longer. If your parents lived to a hundred, you're more likely at age seventy to be free of diseases such as high blood pressure, heart disease and cancer.[1]

*Is there a longevity gene, then?*

No one has found a single longevity gene – rather, it appears that combined variants in multiple genes contribute to some people living longer than most.[1] Some of the gene variants which are related to longevity are involved with maintaining the body's cells and protecting them from damage caused by free radicals (unstable molecules produced naturally in the body which can damage your DNA).

Others are associated with levels of inflammation in the body, the immune system or the cardiovascular system, for example, reducing the risk of conditions such as heart disease and stroke. Our understanding of which genes affect longevity and how is still quite limited, though. Scientists continue to search for specific genes which may play a role in determining how long we can expect to live.[1-4]

*Aren't there places now where everyone is ancient?*

Around the world, there are a handful of communities, known as Blue Zones, in which it is commonplace for people to live into their nineties and beyond, such as Sardinia in Italy and Okinawa in Japan. Researchers study these populations, trying to work out why they tend to live longer. A combination of genetic and lifestyle factors, such as diet, is believed to be at work, but quantifying the role of specific individual factors is challenging.[1]

*How much of a role do genes play?*

Although the precise balance of genetic and non-genetic factors in determining the risk of chronic diseases remains open for debate, it's clear that, generally, our genes play a secondary role compared with things that our bodies are exposed to after we're born.[5, 6]

The main causes of chronic conditions like cancer and heart disease are lifestyle factors, such as smoking, diet and physical activity, and things around us, such as environmental carcinogens and air pollution.[6]

*OK, but can you put a rough figure on the extent of our genes' influence?*

Currently, we estimate that around a quarter of the variation in human lifespan is down to genetics. It appears, though, that the balance between genetic and non-genetic factors shifts over the course of a lifetime. Scientists have suggested that our lifestyles are a more important determinant of our health than our genes up until we're around seventy or eighty years old. After this point, genetics seem to play an increasingly important role in keeping us healthy.[1]

*Reality check*
While for most of us genes play a relatively small role in determining our likelihood of developing chronic illnesses, some people are born with genetic predispositions to diseases which substantially increases their risk. Inherited mutations of the BRCA 1 gene account for only a small proportion of breast cancer cases, for example, but those who carry the mutated gene have more than a 70 per cent risk of developing breast or ovarian cancer in their lifetime.[6]

*So basically, we're saying . . .*
Genes play a role in determining our chances of reaching a hundred. For most of us, though, whether we reach old age in good health is mainly down to what kind of life we live.

# Height

*My dad was six foot four and my mum is four foot ten. I clock in at five foot two. So, what determines height? Did I just inherit my mum's height gene?*

As well as your genes, your adult height is influenced by nutritional intake and development during two growth periods – the first occurring from conception to two years of age, and the second occurring during adolescence, before the onset of puberty.[1, 2]

*Ah well. I guess I'll never be a supermodel. But it could be worse: my Indonesian friend Klaas Jan is five foot four and lives in the Netherlands, where all the women are taller than him.*

Globally, there are big variations in adult height. Countries with the tallest populations are in Western Europe, while the shortest can be found in sub-Saharan Africa and South East Asia. Men are generally taller than women, but the largest differences in height between sexes occur in the countries with the tallest populations overall. Big variations also occur within countries, particularly between different ethnic and socio-economic groups.[3]

*So, how does height affect your chances of living to a hundred?*

In the early twentieth century, data collected by the insurance industry showed that taller people appeared to live longer on average than shorter people. Since then, health researchers have taken an interest in exploring the relationship between people's height and their risk of death and disease.[1]

Some studies have found that being taller is associated with a lower risk of certain diseases, including coronary heart disease, stroke and respiratory disease, while one showed that shorter people were at greater risk of dying while waiting for a lung transplant.[1, 3]

*My ex-husband is almost six foot six, the jammy bastard. But why would taller people be less likely to die?*

A few possible reasons have been put forward to explain the apparent relationship between height and health outcomes. One suggestion is that height is an indicator of development and nutrition in early childhood (as well as pre-birth factors, such as smoking in pregnancy), and that it's these which influence our risk of certain diseases in later life.[1]

We also know that height is related to social class, with those from a more privileged background tending to be taller. Social class influences a range of things which directly contribute to disease risk, including the likelihood of having been exposed to damaging traumatic experiences in childhood and lifestyle factors such as smoking. The fact that rates of smoking-related cancers are not related to height would appear to challenge this explanation, however.[1]

There's also a theory that the relationship is at least partly explained by people becoming shorter as a result of ill health, rather than the other way around. This could either be actual height loss due to compression of the discs in the spine, or apparent height loss due to an inability to stand fully erect when measured. The findings of one study, however, suggest that this explanation only plays a part in deaths from respiratory disease.[1]

*I feel a bit depressed now. I wish I'd inherited my dad's height.*

If it makes you feel better, some studies have suggested that taller people are more likely to die from cancer.[1, 4]

*Weirdly, my dad actually died of a stroke, which tall people are meant to be at lower risk of.*

With all these kinds of things, it's important to bear in mind that reduced risk doesn't mean zero risk. A non-smoker can die of lung cancer and a tall person can have a stroke.

*OK then, I won't rush out and buy a stretching rack.*

> ### Reality check
> This is an area of research in which there's quite a lot of inconsistency between the findings of different studies, particularly around the possible links between height and various cancers.[1, 5] Not all studies have supported the idea that taller people live longer and one research paper from Switzerland published in 2017 even concluded that taller women had a higher risk of death.[4]

> ### So basically, we're saying . . .
> Taller people may have a lower risk of dying overall than short people, but the research is inconsistent, and once you're an adult there's not much you can do to change your height anyway.

## Jon Holmes on being five foot four

I used to have a t-shirt that someone bought me that said, 'I may look short, but there's 12 inches of me you can't see!'

I think I was always slightly shorter than the rest of my class at school, but because it's one of those things you can't change, it's never bothered me. Of course, you could buy built-up shoes like Tom Cruise, but they're never going to be built-up enough to make me look six foot. That's stilettos! I'd look foolish, though I realise in this day and age anyone can wear anything they want . . .

I don't notice my height until I'm in close proximity to people. I'll be at a social event, talking to a group of people, all of whom are six foot, and I'll suddenly go, 'Oh shit, I actually do feel a bit short now!'

It's sometimes annoying in bars, where you don't get noticed because taller people are a bit more dominant in terms of leaning over the bar, but think about the advantages on planes. Every seat is like business class!

All my girlfriends have been a similar height or maybe a little bit taller, but not Rod Stewart-and-Leggy-What's-Her-Face tall.

I got made fun of at school, inevitably, because at school everyone's got a thing. So, the ginger kid got the ginger stuff, same for the speccy kid and the fat kid, and I was the short kid. There was a bit of teasing going on, but not any more than anyone else got for whatever their foible was. There's that cliché of compensating with humour, but I don't know how true that is – I was gobby, but I don't think I was gobby because of that. It's just how I am. I never felt bullied for being short.

It's a good job really, because in my career I was the butt of short jokes for quite a long time. But here's the beautiful thing about that: for eighteen years I was introduced on *The Now Show* with a height-related joke from Hugh Dennis. He used to get emails from listeners saying, 'How dare you be heightist! You're a bully, Hugh Dennis, picking on Jon', etc., etc.

And the joy of this was that I used to write these introductions – so the more I knew he'd get abuse, the worse I made the joke!

Ronnie Corbett said in an interview that he was worried about being short, but I think it was Bruce Forsyth who said to him, 'No, no, make it your comedy thing. Because everyone's got to have a thing.'

Hugh Dennis told me he did a documentary for BBC Two where he had to go up a mountain with a film crew. They were going to find a hermit who hadn't had any human contact, and somehow they'd set up this interview where Hugh Dennis would talk to this guy in a shack.

So, he got up there with the crew, and they started the interview, and Hugh said, 'My name's Hugh Dennis, I'm from England, and—'

And the hermit said, 'I know who you are.' He had a radio that picked up BBC World Service in the shack.

Hugh Dennis thought: 'That's amazing – I've travelled all this way to meet this guy who doesn't really have any contact with humans, in self-imposed exile, and he's connected to the world with this radio.'

Then the hermit said in broken English, 'I've got one question for you.'

There was a pause.

And the hermit asked: 'How tall Jon Holmes?!'

And I thought: 'Yeah, I'll take that!'

## Richard Osman on being six foot seven

*When I first met you, you stood up and I went, 'Oh wow, you're so tall!' And you said that everyone says that, and everyone makes comments and jokes. Does the fact that you are probably likely to live longer for being tall make up for all those jokes?*

No, because I don't think I *will* live longer! I think if you're six foot three, that's statistically when you'll live longer – the Danes and the Norwegians and stuff. I think that as soon as you get to six foot seven, which is the height that people find remarkable, once again your life expectancy goes down – or at least, the life expectancy of your knee joints and ankle joints and hips, because you're carrying six foot seven around. So, I don't think I'll live longer.

Comments about height give you an amazing radar for the worst people in the world. Everyone reacts to it – everyone, you can't help it – but in the way they react you can tell an awful lot about them. Some people are slightly taken aback and don't mention it at all, and you think, 'Ah, that's nice.' Some people get quite excited or enthusiastic about it, which is lovely.

344

And then, walking down the street, people just shout stuff at you. Being tall is a very good twat radar, in the same way I imagine being short is – you very quickly work out the cut of someone's jib.

I don't think there are any six-foot-seven hundred-year-olds in the world. If you can find one after this interview, I would love to read about him or her – especially if it's a her. What if that was your fetish, hundred-year-old six-foot-seven women? You'd be very lonely!

*What's the best thing about being tall?*

The best thing can also be the worst thing – you never go unnoticed. In life, this can be very important. If you need to be noticed, you can walk into a room and grab people's attention, but a lot of the time you don't want to. I said to my son, who's six foot six – a tiny little fella – you've got two options when you walk into the room. You've got (a) 'Who's that tall guy?' or (b) 'Who's that tall guy who looks awkward about being tall?'

Choose option (a). You can't not be tall.

Jon Holmes says you forget about being short, and you forget about being tall too – when you're at home, you forget. It's only when you walk down the street that you remember, as everyone's tiny. Or you're in a pub and there's noise and everyone's talking a foot below your head, and you think, 'I'm not getting any of this!' That's when you think, 'Of course I'm tall, of course I'm unusual!'

Everyone else in the world looks five foot seven. How tall are you? Five foot two? You look five foot seven to me. Anyone who's six foot four or five foot two, it doesn't matter. It's a matter of perspective.

*And you can see all the people who are going grey and going bald?*

Well I suppose so, but I was also blessed with the gift of terrible eyesight! So, at gigs I can see over everyone's head, but I can't see more than ten feet ahead of me, so I lose some of the advantages of being tall. Especially as I always have to stand at the back. Whenever I tweet saying, 'I'm going to this gig or this play', twenty people will go, 'Wouldn't want to be sitting behind you!'

I always sit at the back if I can, or in an aisle, so I'm not in anyone's way. I don't want tutting all the way through a play! I always get pretty bad seats wherever I go, as I don't want people having to have me sitting in front of them.

So, if a sense of shame shortens your lifespan, that's another thing about being tall.

# Race, ethnicity and country of birth

*I know there's a lot of debate about definitions, but aren't these fundamentally different things?*

Both race and ethnicity are social constructs with no genetic basis. Race is typically associated with physical characteristics, whereas ethnicity is considered to be more about culture, language and identity. Country of birth is simply an objective fact. Despite these differences, researchers and statisticians often look at them together.

*OK. Well, I'm a half-Asian Londoner, so this should be interesting.*

Inequalities between people of different racial and ethnic backgrounds across a range of health outcomes have been well established by research and government statistics.[1] A report by Public Health England published in 2017 described wide variations across a range of health indicators by both ethnicity and country of birth.[2]

*You mean, like how the Japanese live longer than the British? I reckon it's all that sushi and green tea.*

It can be closer to home than that. Compared with the UK as a whole, those born in Scotland, Ireland and Northern Ireland had higher death rates at all ages and were more likely to die before the age of seventy-five. Suicide rates also varied significantly by country of birth, with higher rates in males born in the EU Accession

347

countries, including Poland, and people born in Scotland and Ireland.[2]

*That's bleak.*

Of course, for many of us, how long we live in good health is just as important, if not more so, than how long we live overall. Scientists in England calculated how long different ethnic groups could expect to live free from disability. They found large variations which exceeded those in overall life expectancy. Chinese men fared best and could expect to live 64.7 years free from disability.

*I want to be reincarnated as a Chinese man.*

Bangladeshi men and Pakistani women could expect the shortest period of disability-free life (just 54.3 years and 55.1 years respectively). The researchers noted that while Indian women had a similar life expectancy to White British women, they had 4.3 years fewer of disability-free life.[3]

*Do white people do better than ethnic minorities overall?*

There are certainly plenty of examples of white people faring better than non-whites; for example, UK data show that white children are generally more likely to get a good start in life, with lower rates of low birthweight and infant deaths than other ethnic groups.[2] It's far from the case that white people experience better health outcomes across the board, however. When researchers calculated life expectancy figures for different ethnic groups in Scotland, using death records linked to population census data, they found that most of the larger ethnic minority groups had longer life expectancies than the white Scottish majority.[4]

*What causes inequalities, then?*

A number of causal factors are believed to underpin these kinds of inequalities, including differences in lifestyle and the tendency for people in minority groups to have poorer access to healthcare, greater socio-economic disadvantage, lower levels of education, higher levels of hazardous work and lower rates of health insurance coverage.[1]

UK Government data available in 2019 showed notable differences between ethnic groups for a wide range of health factors, including considerable variations in lifestyle, such as levels of physical activity, intake of fruit and vegetables, and smoking rates.[5]

*What about diseases? Are different races more likely to suffer from certain conditions?*

Inequalities can occur across multiple aspects of a disease pathway, culminating in different death rates between groups for the same illness. Cancers are a good example of this – researchers looking at US data from 2011 found differences in the rate of new cancer cases, the stage at which people are diagnosed, the treatment received, and the length of time people live after the diagnosis has been made. The overall burden of cancer was highest in non-Hispanic blacks, but lower in non-Hispanic Asians than non-Hispanic whites.[6]

*Do poverty and economic factors explain a lot of this?*

Yes. One of the explanations for these health inequalities is that some ethnic groups are far more likely than others to live in areas with high levels of deprivation. Lots of evidence has established a strong link between deprivation and poorer health outcomes, including lower life expectancy (see also Where you live, pages 199–201). In 2011, over half of the Bangladeshi and Pakistani ethnic populations in England lived in the top 20 per cent of the most deprived areas in the country – a much higher proportion than other ethnic groups. Unpicking the role of poverty and deprivation can be tricky, however. In England, for example, child obesity is much more common in the Bangladeshi population;

349

however, Bangladeshi children are also much more likely than average to live in deprived areas where child obesity rates are generally higher. More research is needed to understand the extent to which health inequalities based on race and ethnicity are a reflection of other underlying causal factors.[2]

*If you're a rich, upper-middle-class professional, are you likely to live a longer life?*

While we know that income and social status are linked to health and longevity, a study in the US challenged the view that socio-economic position is a fundamental cause of poor health in African Americans. The researchers showed that achieving a higher socio-economic position brought health benefits for whites which weren't experienced by African Americans. They concluded that being black was in itself a much more fundamental determinant of health than the relatively low socio-economic position with which it's typically correlated.[7]

Another piece of research in the US also found that while those in employment generally live longer than those who are unemployed, this relationship doesn't apply equally to all races. Their analysis showed that the health benefit of being in employment was less for black people than white people.[8]

*Could it be due to the racism black people experience?*

Research in the UK found cumulative exposure to racial discrimination has incremental negative long-term effects on the mental health of people in ethnic minorities.[9] Experiencing racism has been shown by a number of studies to be associated with poorer physical and mental health, with some variation in the strength of this relationship between different groups. In the US, research has shown a stronger correlation between racism and poorer mental health in Asian Americans and Latino Americans, and a stronger association with poorer physical health in Latino Americans compared with African Americans.[10]

*How are these inequalities being tackled?*

Although addressing inequalities in health outcomes between different sections of the population has long been a focus of public health work in some countries, they often remain stubbornly present in the statistics.

Researchers analysing US data from the period from 1933 to 1999 found little reason for optimism. Their work showed that nationally there had been no sustained decrease in differences between blacks and whites in either death rates or life expectancy at birth since 1945.[11]

Another analysis of US mortality data, this time from 1999 to 2014, found that while rates of premature deaths have been reduced in some ethnic groups (thanks partly to improvements in HIV treatment and public health efforts to reduce smoking), potentially avoidable causes of death (including drug poisonings, suicide and chronic liver disease) in twenty-five- to forty-nine-year-olds meant that premature death rates were still notably high in some groups, particularly American Indians and Alaska Natives.[12] Over a similar period, death rates in children and young people had generally declined overall, but were found to be particularly high among black, American Indian and Alaskan Native youth.[13]

*This is all so grim. The only good news for me is I was born in England.*

*Reality check*
In the UK, ethnicity is not recorded when deaths are registered, meaning that life expectancy estimates and mortality rates for ethnic groups can't be calculated in the same way that they are for men and women. The lack of official data on this topic means that we can't make an accurate and complete assessment of how ethnicity relates to longevity and how that relationship might be changing over time.[2]

We do know, however, that the picture of health variations between people of different races, ethnicities and countries of birth is a complex one, because some groups fare well in certain aspects and poorly in others.[2] We can't, therefore, say that one group experiences better health outcomes across the board. UK Government data available in 2019 showed, for example, that black adults were the most likely to be overweight or obese, but their rate of smoking was lower than the England average.[5] The situation is further complicated when variations in levels of premature mortality occur between sexes within the same group.[2]

*So basically, we're saying . . .*
There are significant inequalities in a broad range of health statistics based on race, ethnicity and country of origin, including variations in rates of early death. A complex mix of things probably lies behind these differences, but adopting a healthy lifestyle will help maximise your chances of a long life no matter what your colour or background.

# Biological sex

*Seeing the word 'sex' has reminded me that I haven't had any yet this decade.*

It might cheer you up to know that, historically, women have generally outlived men.[1] In 2015–17, the life expectancy at birth for females in England was 83.1 years, compared with 79.6 years for males. During the same period, men accounted for over two-thirds of premature deaths from cardiovascular diseases in the country. They were also more likely to die before the age of 75 from cancer, liver disease and respiratory disease.[2]

*An earlier death for men isn't inevitable though, is it?*

UK deaths data from 2016 showed nearly a quarter of all deaths were from causes which are considered avoidable, with 60 per cent of these occurring in males. Causes of avoidable death fit into a number of categories, including cardiovascular diseases (such as coronary heart disease and stroke), infections, injuries, respiratory diseases and drug use disorders, as well as a range of other conditions. In 2016, the leading cause of avoidable deaths in the UK was cancer (and other non-cancerous tissue growths).[3]

*Why are more men dying from avoidable causes, then?*

A number of things are believed to contribute to the disparity in longevity between men and women. Lifestyle factors certainly explain some of the variation. Men are more likely to smoke, drink alcohol at hazardous levels, become alcohol dependent and use illegal drugs.[4, 5] Research has also shown that men are more likely to engage in a combination of three or four risky behaviours than women. Risk-taking behaviour is particularly associated with traditional concepts of masculinity – whether that be a disregard for concepts of healthy living, choosing a hazardous occupation or dangerous driving.[6]

*Or not going to the doctor when your leg's hanging off?*

Evidence suggests that men are less knowledgeable about health issues and less confident about using health services. Coupled with a tendency for health to be culturally regarded as primarily a female domain, this makes men less likely than women to see a doctor or visit a pharmacy and less likely to acknowledge illness or to seek help when they have health problems. Research has highlighted that traditional notions of masculinity can be a barrier to timely medical intervention, with a tendency for men to downplay symptoms and regard seeking professional help as acceptable only once a certain threshold of illness or injury has been reached.[6]

*Wow, men are a bit hopeless, aren't they? I still want a boyfriend though.*

Unpicking the complex interplay of factors which determine men's health (and what we can do to address those things) has become a field of research in its own right, so there's a lot that we still have to learn, including why certain things seem to affect one sex more than the other. The negative impact on life expectancy of living in a deprived neighbourhood appears to be greater for men than women, for example.[7] Suicide is also much more common among men – in 2017, three quarters of recorded suicides in England were in males.[8]

*OK, now I feel a bit bad for calling men hopeless.*

Although the relationship between sex and life expectancy has been longstanding, it has varied considerably over time. The gap in expected lifespan between men and women in the UK was actually at its narrowest point in the early twentieth century. We also see variation in the size of the difference between developed countries. We shouldn't, therefore, regard this inequality between men and women as something fixed and inevitable.[7]

*I guess two world wars in the last century didn't help . . .?*

Not at the time. In 1940, life expectancy in the UK fell sharply for both sexes, but the drop was bigger for men. It was back to pre-war figures by 1944.

*How have men in the UK fared since then?*

The gap between male and female life expectancy has been narrowing since the 1970s. The shift away from physically intensive and more hazardous occupations, including mining and manufacturing, towards service sector jobs, coupled with a decrease in the smoking rate among men, are likely to be major contributory factors.[1] It's even been projected (albeit with some caution) that the gap between male and female life expectancy could disappear altogether by 2032 if this trend continues.[7]

*I'll turn fifty-two that year. Hopefully I'll have a boyfriend by then and we'll both live to a hundred.*

*Reality check*
Not all men conform – or aspire – to a stereotype of traditional maleness. When looking at patterns in data for large populations we inevitably have to make generalisations. There's huge variation, though, in health and lifestyle between people of both sexes, as well as a range of masculine identities which may seem very different from each other.

The differences in life expectancy between men and women apply across the social spectrum; however, men in professional occupations are less likely than those in unskilled jobs to have three or four unhealthy behaviours and will generally live longer.[6] Research on life expectancy in the UK between 2007 and 2011 found for the first time that men in the highest occupational group could expect to live marginally longer than an average woman, although women in the highest group still had the longest life expectancy of all.[1]

*So basically, we're saying . . .*
Women generally live longer than men, although the gap in life expectancy is gradually closing. A range of factors account for this, but if you're a man, adopting a healthy lifestyle, not putting off going to the doctor (including for mental health issues) and avoiding things which are likely to cause injuries will go a long way to helping you buck the trend.

## Angela Saini on the sexes

*Women live longer than men, on average. Why do you think this is?*

Oddly, nobody is quite sure. Scientists have only recently begun investigating it, but there does seem to be something possibly intrinsic to women's bodies that makes them on average a little more robust. I'm not a good example of this because I'm constantly catching colds, but women tend to have stronger immune systems than men, and also recover more quickly from illness. In medical school, you sometimes hear the phrase, 'women get sicker, but men die quicker'. In other words, diseases that kill men don't kill women at the same rate, so women live with pain and illness, but men just die.

## Biological sex

*If you could live another life and choose your sex, would you decide to be male or female, and why?*

I would never choose to be anyone other than who I am. For me, one of the greatest experiences of my life has been giving birth. Yes, it does destroy your body a little and you're never quite the same again afterwards, but it's so bloody worth it. To create and nurture a new little life inside your own body – I still can't quite believe I did it and I wouldn't give that up even for a ticket to the moon.

*Do you think women living longer than men compensates in part for all the inequality we experience?*

No! A few more years of an unequal life isn't really any kind of compensation at all, especially when women are known globally to do a disproportionate amount of housework and childcare, even when they are in full-time work. Whatever longevity dividend we get probably gets spent over the course of lives folding laundry.

# Sexuality

*Do gay people have different death rates to straight people?*

Research into this question hasn't always provided consistent results.[1, 2] A study published in 2016, however, which looked at over 15,500 US adults, found that sexual minorities had a higher risk of dying over a ten-year period compared with their heterosexual counterparts. This appeared to be the result of an increased risk of HIV infection and other health disadvantages experienced by sexual minorities, rather than sexual orientation in itself being a direct determinant of longevity.[3]

*What health disadvantages?*

It's well established that a range of health issues are more common among sexual minorities.[4] There's evidence that sexual minorities are more likely to smoke and abuse drugs and alcohol than heterosexual people. There's good evidence that LGB* people are more likely to suffer from mental health problems, including a higher risk of depression and anxiety disorders, and suicide attempts. LGBT people may also perceive certain health services as discriminatory and be less likely, or less able, to make full use of them as a result.[5] As we discussed in Marriage (pages 3–7), gay men and women also don't appear to experience the same health benefits from marriage as straight people.

---

* In this chapter we refer sometimes to LGB people and sometimes to LGBT people depending on which specific groups were included in the different studies.

358

*What about in later life?*

One way to measure current physical and mental well-being is to ask people to rate their own health. In the UK, LGBT men and women aged fifty and over have poorer self-rated health than heterosexuals. Studies have shown that self-rated health is a strong predictor of future illness and mortality. We also know that non-heterosexual men aged fifty and over are more likely to be living with a limiting long-term illness and more likely to have attempted suicide, while non-heterosexual women in the same age group are more likely to smoke.[4]

*Give me some good news . . . please?*

Research shows that LGB people over the age of fifty-five are more likely to exercise than their straight counterparts.[5]

Of course, all of these findings, whether good or bad, are generalisations based on comparing one cohort of people with another. At an individual level, there will be plenty of LGBT people who are much healthier than lots of straight people.

*Reality check*
Depending on where you are in the world, simply being in a sexual minority can put your life in danger. Many countries criminalise homosexuality in some way and several have laws which make same-sex relationships punishable by death.[6]

Across the globe, there are also countless examples of people having been killed in homophobic attacks.[7-9]

*So basically, we're saying . . .*
Sexual minorities generally experience a range of poorer health outcomes and risk factors which can affect longevity.

# Left-handedness

*My ex-husband is left-handed. How common is it though?*

The prevalence of left-handedness has gone up and down over the centuries, but it's believed that around 1 in 10 people are left-handed.[1, 2]

*I've heard they live shorter lives, possibly because they accidentally stab themselves with right-handed scissors . . .?*

Left-handedness appears to be less common among older people, which has led some scientists to hypothesise that left-handed people tend to have a shorter lifespan. Studies investigating this idea have found conflicting results, however.[3]

Another theory that's been put forward is that left-handed people switch to right-handedness over the years, due to cultural conditioning. There's evidence to support this hypothesis, as well as research that directly challenges the idea that right-handed people live longer.[4, 5]

*So, is there any difference at all in longevity between left- and right-handers?*

Although we can't say convincingly that right-handed people live longer, there could still be other differences with health implications. There's evidence, for example, that left-handed women tend to develop breast cancer earlier than right-handed women.[3]

*That's odd, but it probably won't affect my ex-husband.*

It's unlikely to, but it can happen. Just under 400 men in the UK are diagnosed with breast cancer each year, compared with just under 55,000 women.[6]

*Reality check*
Rather than favouring one or the other, being able to switch between hands might seem like the ideal. Research suggests, however, that there are downsides to this. Those who use their non-dominant hand for some manual activities have been found to be more gullible.[7] Being ambidextrous has also been linked with lower IQ and higher risk of schizophrenia.[8, 9]

*So basically, we're saying . . .*
Although society caters primarily for the needs of right-handers, they probably won't live any longer than their lefty counterparts.

# Adverse childhood experiences

*I definitely had a rough childhood. My dad was physically violent and emotionally abusive, plus I was severely bullied at school. Is that what you mean by adverse experiences?*

Yes. Adverse childhood experiences, or ACEs, are potentially traumatic events that occur in childhood. You hit the nail on the head: abuse and neglect, experiencing or witnessing violence in the home, growing up in a household with adults with drug or alcohol problems, and being abandoned by a parent through separation or divorce, are all recognised examples of ACEs.[1, 2]

*It's hard as most of my friends seem to have had very stable and loving childhoods.*

It's very common to have had ACEs. Studies suggest that almost half of adults in England have had one and 8 per cent have had four (in Wales, it's 14 per cent).[2] People may not necessarily think of themselves as having experienced a traumatic childhood, even though they've had multiple ACEs. You can find your own ACE score easily using freely available tools online.

*I just calculated mine. It's six. But what's the link to health?*

Numerous studies have shown a correlation between ACEs and subsequent health issues in adulthood, including risky behaviours (such as smoking and drug misuse), chronic health conditions (such as type 2 diabetes and cancer) and early death. The risks increase the more ACEs someone has had, but the relationship is particularly notable when looking at people who've had four or more ACEs.[1–4] People with four or more ACEs are also much more likely than the general population to go to prison or be violent towards others.[4]

*At least those things don't apply to me. Why do ACEs affect health?*

Researchers believe that the excessive activation of stress response systems triggered by ACEs has an impact on children's developing brains, immune systems, metabolic regulatory systems and cardio-vascular systems.

*What can I do about it if I feel ACEs are affecting my health?*

There's no doubt that prevention is better than cure when it comes to ACEs but recognising any ACEs that you have had and seeking out talking therapies to work through them can help reduce any impact they may have on your future life.

*Reality check*
ACEs don't make it inevitable that someone will go on to experience poorer health in adulthood. They just make their risk of this higher than that of the general population. Certain things can help to protect against the long-term negative impact of ACEs.[1] Safe, stable and nurturing relationships, a positive, strong support network and professional intervention where appropriate can help build the resilience necessary to minimise the negative impact of ACEs.[2, 5] Research has shown that if a child has a good relationship with one trusted adult it can mitigate the impact of adverse experiences on physical and mental health.[2]

*So basically, we're saying . . .*
Having multiple traumatic experiences in childhood increases your risk of poor health in adulthood and premature death. If you do have unresolved childhood trauma, it's never too late to get help to address it.

# Other people's actions

*My ex-husband was terrible at actions, especially the dance routine for 'YMCA'.*

I'm talking about dangerous actions.

*You haven't seen him dance.*

Specifically, things that might kill you. No matter how healthy your lifestyle or how risk-averse you are, there's always the possibility that someone else's actions will end your life. A hundred pedestrians in Britain were killed or seriously injured by drunk drivers in 2016, for example.[1] All of us are at risk of a violent death to varying degrees. Over 300,000 people are killed in intentional homicides globally every year, with tens of thousands more losing their lives as a result of unintentional homicides and law enforcement actions. On average, there are just over 7 violent deaths per 100,000 people every year.[2]

*I concede that most of these probably aren't the result of misadventure during 'The Birdie Song'. A lot probably have to do with wars and terrorism.*

The risk of being killed by terrorism varies depending on where you are in the world and can change substantially over a relatively short period of time. Between 2002 and 2018, 93 per cent of all deaths from terrorism occurred in South Asia, the Middle East, North Africa and sub-Saharan Africa. Globally, just under 16,000 people were killed by terrorists in 2018.[3]

*Thanks for the list of areas of the world to avoid. I never travel anywhere unsafe and carry a personal safety alarm with me in case I get attacked.*

The decisions of others can also affect our life expectancy in numerous other more indirect ways, many of which we've already touched on in previous chapters. The policies made by politicians in national and local government can influence all kinds of things which are associated with health longevity. Some of these will be more obvious, such as car seatbelt legislation reducing the chances of people dying in car accidents and congestion charging reducing air pollution from traffic. Other things, such as policies which affect access to education and welfare benefits or the availability of employment, can have an indirect effect on health and well-being, the impact of which might only be seen over a long period of time.[4, 5]

*My ex-husband's dancing wore me down over a long period of time. The Village People have a lot to answer for.*

> *Reality check*
> Although none of us can completely control all the factors which influence our risk of dying prematurely, it's important to take ownership of your own health within reason. Research shows that people who believe that their health is outside of their control tend to have worse outcomes, while those who are more inclined to feel that they can determine their own health are more likely to be proactive in looking after themselves and to make healthy choices.[6]

*So basically, we're saying . . .*
Directly or indirectly, there are lots of ways that other people could shorten your lifespan, but feeling powerless about your health could do just the same.

# The ageing process

*What exactly* is *ageing?*

Ageing is the progressive accumulation over time of changes to the molecular structure – and, hence, function – of our bodies. The damage from these changes results in an ever-increasing susceptibility to disease and ultimately death.[1]

*Wow, this is an uplifting last chapter! How well do we understand ageing?*

The mysteries of the ageing process have challenged scientists for decades. Big advances in knowledge about how we age continue to be made but a lot of debate remains regarding the importance of individual biological processes.[2] Researchers are constantly seeking out new insights into different processes going on in the body that contribute to ageing.

Some researchers focus on studying one particular factor, such as the role of free radicals or telomere shortening.[3] It's becoming clearer, though, that ageing is the result of a combination of several causes, rather than one individual mechanism.[1]

*How long can people live at the moment?*

Although average life expectancy has increased dramatically over the past century, the oldest age that people can reach has remained relatively unchanged.[4] According to Guinness World Records, the oldest person who ever lived was Jeanne Calment from France who was born in 1875 and died in 1997 at the age of 122 years and 164 days.[5] The oldest man ever is listed as Jiroemon Kimura from Japan. He was born in 1897 and died in 2013 at the age of 116 years and 54 days.[6] Some other claims of super-longevity can't be verified, though, so we can't rule out the possibility that longer lifespans than these have been achieved.

*I'm not sure I'd want to live that long. My spiky black chin hair would become a trip hazard. How long do you think we'll be able to live in the future though?*

Right now, there's a lot of optimism in the world of ageing research – a sense that we're entering a new era in which new discoveries are waiting to be made that will help us prevent, delay and maybe even reverse the effects of ageing. Whether the maximum lifespan of humans will be extended as a result remains an open question, though.[2] Some argue that we're already close to the maximum achievable human lifespan, while others believe that with further scientific advances we could eliminate the biological inevitability of death altogether.[1]

*What about these places where everyone lives to 150?*

As we mentioned in Genes (pages 337–9), there are some regions of the world with exceptionally high life expectancy, such as Sardinia in Italy and the island of Okinawa in Japan. These so-called 'Blue Zones' are an ongoing subject of scientific study. The hope is that by understanding what's different about the people who live in these places, lessons can be applied to the rest of us which will extend our lifespans as well.[7, 8]

*What are these lessons, apart from moving to Okinawa?*

The key lifestyle factors which have been highlighted by this research so far probably won't come as a surprise for anyone who's reached this point in the book. Building physical activity into everyday life, having ways to minimise and cope with stress, not over-eating, having a mainly plant-based diet, moderate drinking, being involved in the community, and having strong and positive family and social ties are common to Blue Zone centenarians, as well as having a sense of purpose in life. What's also become clear, however, is that the environments people inhabit in these zones tend to be conducive to practising a healthy lifestyle – it's not just about personal choices.[9]

*I've been feeding my ninety-five-year-old nan at the nursing home. She needs to be helped to go to the toilet. I'm starting to realise that being a hundred doesn't always look like much fun.*

We won't all make it to a hundred, but we can all take steps to ensure that we spend our later years in as good a state of health as possible. As life expectancy has increased, the concept of 'healthy ageing' has gained increasing attention. The World Health Organization defines healthy ageing as 'the process of developing and maintaining the functional ability that enables well-being in older age'. This means still being able to meet your basic needs; learn, grow and make decisions; be mobile; build and maintain relationships; and contribute to society. While all of the factors that will enable this to happen aren't within your control, many are.[10]

*So, what's the one thing I can do to make sure I'm still able to do all this?*

The best protector against age-related problems that we know of is physical exercise. It's currently the only thing that has demonstrated a remarkable effectiveness in reducing the risk of age-related diseases, improving quality of life and increasing lifespan in humans. Even a modest amount of exercise done regularly brings benefits. Keeping physically active (along with good nutrition) is your best bet in the battle against ageing as things stand.[2]

*I need all the help I can get. Give me some specifics.*

The best advice for people aged sixty-five and over currently is to:

- Aim to be physically active every day (even if it's just light activity).
- Do activities that improve strength, balance and flexibility at least 2 days a week.
- Do at least 150 minutes of moderate intensity activity a week or 75 minutes of vigorous intensity activity if you're already active (or a combination of both).
- Reduce the amount of time you spend sitting or lying down and break up long periods of not moving with some activity.[11]

*Thanks for that. Goodbye, then. It's been informative.*

And emotional. Good luck living to a hundred.

*Cheers. Look out for the radio announcement that says 'Ariane Sherine, creator of the Atheist Bus Campaign and author of* How to Live to 100, *has died aged forty-two after being hit by a bus.'*

*Reality check*
Not getting enough physical activity can become a vicious cycle as we enter our later years. A lack of regular exercise can combine with and exacerbate other bodily effects of ageing, such as loss of muscle and bone density, reducing our capacity to be physically active. The less we feel able to exercise, the less we do, and a spiral of decline sets in.[12]

*So basically, we're saying . . .*
Some scientists believe the day will come when the average human life expectancy far exceeds a hundred. Others are a whole lot more sceptical. Until new technology or a medical breakthrough allows you to drink from the proverbial fountain of youth, keep active and keep re-reading this book.

## Dr Aubrey de Grey on ageing

*What futuristic developments do you think could lead to us living much longer?*

That question assumes that the developments that will allow us to live much longer are futuristic – but they aren't. They are coming and coming fast. It's no accident that SENS Research Foundation has spun out half a dozen of its projects into start-up companies. The necessary developments are not futuristic: they are very foreseeable.

*You've been quoted as saying that the first person to live to 1000 may have already been born. Do you see super-long life as being something that will be the preserve of a privileged few, or do you think that a hundred years from now this kind of lifespan will be the norm?*

Definitely it will be the norm. It will result from people not getting sick however long ago they were born. And as anyone can see, the health issues of old age are a vast economic drain on society. Therefore, these therapies will – and will be seen to – pay for themselves really fast, many times over . . . so it will be inescapable, even in as tax-averse a country as the USA, that these therapies need to be paid for somehow, irrespective of the end-user's ability to pay, in order for the country not to go bankrupt really rather soon.

*If there comes a time when living well beyond a hundred does become the norm, how do you foresee us avoiding a crisis of overpopulation, if people continue to reproduce at the same rate without older people dying to free up demand for housing, food and other resources?*

The main answer to this comes from other technologies. As we progress in developing renewable energy, artificial meat, desalination, etc., we will increase the carrying capacity of the planet, i.e. the number of people who can be alive while the total amount of pollution that they generate remains manageable. By any realistic

371

assumptions about the timeframe for these technologies, there is no way that the defeat of ageing will end up being a problem.

*Do you think health promotion messages will become redundant in the future as science will fix everything we do to our bodies, or do you think we'll still need to take care of ourselves?*

It'll still be a balance between the two. But what really matters is how we behave before these therapies arrive, because that's what maximises our chance of benefiting from future medicines.

# Would you like to live to a hundred? Celebrities have their say

### Clive Anderson (aged 67)

I wouldn't say I am dying to live to a hundred.

### Sanjeev Kohli (aged 48)

I WOULD like to live to a hundred. Because I know for a fact that several people at my wake will say 'he had a good innings'. And in this sprawling cricket analogy, a century is definitely considered a 'good innings'. Ninety-three, for example, would be characterised as a disappointment, and would not guarantee selection for a strong county side.

### Josie Long (aged 38)

I think it would depend on where my body was, and also on climate change. I like the idea of living to a hundred if I can still walk and swim and think and talk. When I meet people in their eighties and nineties who are able to enjoy a slightly more ascetic but still thriving life, I'm like, 'Yeah, I would love to do that!'

But at other times I'm like, 'Sod it, why stick around for the hard bit? Just get in and get out!'

If you live to a hundred and your daughter's in her seventies, she might be like, 'All right, let me have some time on my own, Mum!'

### Jeremy Vine (aged 55)

I want to live to a hundred, so long as I am able to think straight and walk round corners. In my nineties I intend to take up dangerous sports and hope my last day will be spent going down the Cresta Run on a metal tray. Live long and die short – that's the ideal.

### Derren Brown (aged 49)

I don't know, there's so much that goes with that, isn't there? I suppose, yes – all other things being equal and pleasant, then why not? And I suppose the chances of that happening only get better and better, don't they?

I remember when I was at school, anyone who was six foot was like a giant – and now everyone's six foot! So, I guess we'll be living to 110 or 150 at some point.

### Jon Holmes (aged 51)

Would I like to live to a hundred? Often, I sort of don't want to live till the end of the day, because I get tired at around four o'clock and I think, 'Imagine going to sleep forever, that'd be brilliant!' And then I realise that I've got too much to do to do that, so I'd better carry on.

Being just over fifty, I'm aware that statistically speaking I'm more than halfway through. I could live to a hundred, but that seems quite rare, and even if I live into my nineties I'm still more than halfway through. You look back and you think, 'That went fast, didn't it? And now it's going to go even faster, because that's how it works. And that means I'll be dead soon!'

So, I sort of go, 'Ah, actually I would like to live to a hundred, because at least then I'm at the halfway point.' I also have this fascination with how technology moves on and everything moves on. You know how you talk to kids now, and they go, 'What do you mean, there wasn't an internet? How did you survive?' I think it's fascinating that certain generations didn't have things, and you try to explain that to children. Like, television at my age was just a thing, whereas my grandparents remember when it was invented.

I think living to a hundred is interesting from that point of view, because imagine what will be there. Teleporting – that had better be available. Why aren't all resources going into teleporting research?! Therefore, I kind of would like to live to a hundred, but just because I'm nosy.

And, of course, you want to see what your kids are going to do. It's fascinating watching kids, 'cause mine are six and eight now, and you know when you look at them and you can sense what they're interested in and what they're crap at, just as I was. It's quite interesting how similar they are to me – reading and writing and being creative. They don't really watch TV, they put on a play instead. I was like that.

Hopefully I'll still be alive when they do get into the world of work, but imagine how the creative industries will change. Jobs for life don't exist, so what they start off doing could be quite different to what they end up doing.

I'd quite like one of them to become a funeral director, so that way I could be looked after when the time comes. I don't want them becoming care home attendants as I don't want them wiping my arse. I know I've done it for them, but it's something children shouldn't have to do.


## Bec Hill (aged 33)

The optimist in me says yes, of course, on the proviso that my friends and family are still largely around. The pessimist in me is a bit worried about what the world will look like in a hundred years. I think if everyone knew they were going to live to a hundred, we would start to see people being a bit more respectful of the planet. I think one of the reasons that we are a bit short-sighted is because there's an element of, 'Yeah, but I won't be around!' If people knew they were going to be around longer, they'd think, 'Ugh, I'm gonna have to live through that!'

### Stewart Lee (aged 52)

I would have said yes once, without hesitation. I would like to live long to see what kind of adults my kids become. But I think we have seen the best of the world, and politics and the environment are in sudden steep decline. Who wants to live in a Brexit desert? If it weren't for the kids I'd die tomorrow and not care.

### Konnie Huq (aged 45)

As long as I was happy.

### Dr Aubrey de Grey (aged 57)

I think it makes no sense to have an opinion about that, because it would be an opinion that's dependent on one's future opinions. It's a bit like having an opinion about what time you'd like to go to the toilet the Tuesday after next. Hello, you're going to have better information on that topic nearer the time.

### Arthur Smith (aged 65)

Now, I would say I wouldn't like to live to a hundred, but of course once I get to ninety-two, in the unlikely event that I do, I would say yes. It depends I suppose how I am – given the state of the coming world, there's probably quite a lot to be said for being dead! But I've never tried it, so I don't know what it's like. And once you've tried it, you can't really not try it. It would be nice to try being dead for a bit, just so you know what it feels like.

### Angela Saini (aged 39)

I can't imagine, with the way I eat or exercise, that I would be likely to live to a hundred. Then, perhaps neither would I want to. I like that life has seasons to it, and that we all at some point have to make way for the next generation. Although I may feel differently when I reach ninety-nine years old.

## Robert Llewellyn (aged 64)

This is a really difficult question because, being a lifelong atheist and having no fear of actually being dead, I'm not really looking forward to the dying part. It's not something I spend time worrying about, but the prospect of living to a hundred doesn't fill me with deep joy. I have a very elderly aunt, she turns ninety-eight this year and is remarkably active, lives on her own but with very good support from family and social services. She is a brilliant example; however, she is also a statistical anomaly. Most people her age are unable to be as independent as she is.

If I could be as healthy, both mentally and physically, as she is, then it's a less daunting prospect, but somehow, due to the way I lived my life up until I was about twenty-eight, I think I've reduced my chances considerably. Chain smoking, bad diet, high levels of stress (live stage work), poor sleep discipline and poverty will all have taken their toll. The only thing I didn't do was hard drugs and drinking, so, you know, it all evens out.

But there's a couple of reasons why I'm happy to shuffle off well before I reach a hundred. My kids are a good start. They are both now in their twenties and getting established as independent adults. I don't want them to have to still be worrying about me in thirty-six years' time (I'm sixty-four) when they'll be in their late fifties. It doesn't seem fair.

This is based on my own experience with my parents, who, although they died relatively young (Dad seventy-five and Mum seventy-six), were super-active, fit and mentally sound until they got very ill and died. They experienced 'compressed morbidity' which strikes me as the best way to live your life. Be healthy, active, engaged in the world then in the shortest possible time drop dead. No one can really plan that, but with amazing medical discoveries and improved intervention it's becoming more possible.

My dad played tennis one morning, aged seventy-five. He slipped and fell, no serious injury, but after that he went downhill fast. We all knew he had cancer and three weeks later he popped his clogs. So, three weeks of illness after seventy-five years of health strikes me as a good plan.

My mum did yoga one morning and complained of a bad back. This time we didn't know until later, but this was also cancer-related, and four weeks later she died. I held her hand as she slipped away. Seventy-six years of remarkable health and then poof, you're gone.

Here's the thing though, a mild feeling of relief at not having to worry about them is mixed in a giant sticky pudding of guilt, but there is a bit of a relief. I still miss them and think about them regularly, but I don't have to actually do anything about it. When my kids were small, and my dad was in hospital, it was quite difficult to juggle everything. After he died I had my mum to worry about, and although she was very independent she had been married for fifty years so it was only to be expected that her offspring fretted a little. Since she died, and although I knew I was next generationally speaking, I don't have to worry about her, which I used to do all the time.

So, in turn, I don't want my kids to worry about me. Even if you don't get on with your parents, you worry about them. I do get on with my kids and I want them to live their own lives without my being a burden to them. If I can't manage compressed morbidity, then I really don't want to get to a hundred. Not if I'm bedridden, doolally and incontinent – it's really not an attractive prospect.

When I visited my mother at the John Radcliffe Hospital in the last days of her life (where she was looked after with incredible dedication), there was a woman in the same ward who, I learned from the staff, had been in hospital with various serious ailments for ten years! No thanks, living to a hundred and spending the last ten to fifteen years ill and unable to look after yourself holds no attraction.

Thinking about it, I might start chain smoking again.

## Robin Ince (aged 51)

I really would like to live to a hundred, as long as health could be maintained, and a sense of purpose, which is something that I realise with a lot of old people that I know: the moment that they no longer feel they have purpose, they die, and it's a horrible thing to see, given all of that love that is still there for them from their children – but our need for purpose is so important.

I believe that, because I have at least twice as many books as I can physically read by the time I'm eighty, that extra twenty years will really be a great advantage. 'Oh *Ulysses*, I'll finally read *Ulysses!*' I'll die opening *Ulysses*, on my hundredth birthday! 'Now, I'll begin Joyce – aaaagh!'

Will I still be touring? I think that touring is so much part of my life that I hope I'm always able to get up on stage and create something. I think it's a really important part of my existence.

## Lou Sanders (aged 40)

Depends what sort of nick I'm in and if people have come round to the idea of old people being wise and cool. If I'm stumbling around and pissing myself, I'll give it a miss. I did all that in my twenties to be fair.

## Richard Osman (aged 49)

God no! What do people normally answer to this question?

*Yes.*

But why?!

*They want to meet their great-grandkids and see what happens in the future.*

Why would you want to see what happens in the future? It's a disaster!

*But space travel . . .*

Right, I don't want to go to space, I'm too tall for space. If you ever look at those space shuttles they send people up in, they're tiny. I'd get claustrophobic. And I don't want to see the future. The future is not going to be fun.

Climate change – everything's heating up. Nothing's going to get easier. The march of social progress has ended. We know that now. It's not as though we're all going to be free and super-liberal – we're going to swing back and forth between extremes of behaviour until the end of time.

So, all we've got is box sets! That's all we've got left.

## Yomi Adegoke (aged 29)

I would like to live to a hundred, probably because I've always had really great examples of old age around me. For instance, my nan is eighty-six and she looks completely amazing. She takes great care of herself – she wakes up every morning at 7 a.m. to do star jumps and exercises, and she's just living her best life. She's constantly on cruises and going on holiday, and has led and still leads a very fulfilling life – she had a very long, happy marriage to my grandad until he passed – and so of all the kinds of phobias I have, growing old isn't one of them.

## Charlie Brooker (aged 49)

It's a tricky one. Ask me when I'm ninety-nine!

## Gordon Burns (aged 78)

I don't think I'm going to live to a hundred. Firstly, not many people do; secondly, do I really want to? Because you're usually in a bad state by the time you're a hundred, with everything failing; and thirdly, no male in my family on either side has lived beyond eighty-three. So, it's unlikely. But if I was still in fantastic physical and mental health and I'd discovered some pill that kept me young, I'd be happy to go for *two* hundred!

# And finally . . .

This book may have literally been a lifesaver for me – and perhaps it can be for you, too.

When we started writing it, I was not just obese – I was class II obese, with a BMI of 37.5. I was so fat I broke two toilet seats, split the crotches of several pairs of jeans, and kept being offered a seat on the train by kindly passengers who thought I was pregnant. I was permanently short of breath, had palpitations and couldn't even run for the bus.

My wonderful and extremely honest daughter, who was seven at the time, announced: 'You're the fattest mummy I know!'

The truth was I didn't care much about looking slim like the other mums at her school, but I *did* care desperately about being around for her. The Obesity chapter was such a wake-up call for me, with its warning 'obesity is a leading cause of poor health and death', that over the course of the next year I lost three stone, going from class II obese to merely overweight. I still need to lose another two stone to get back into the 'healthy' weight bracket, but I have confidence that I'll manage it. (If you want to keep tabs on my progress, just type my name into YouTube.)

I lost the weight by eating a 95% vegan and 5% fish diet and counting calories, with stints at both Weight Watchers and Slimming World. I also joined a gym and started lifting weights and doing cardio three times a week. I hated every sweaty and painful second, but the knowledge that I was saving my own life was a great motivator – plus I felt amazing and invincible after doing two hours straight in the gym!

I also incorporated as many of this book's other recommendations into my life as possible. I now focus on getting not just five but ten fruit and veg a day, was making a proper effort to see friends regularly before lockdown, saw my nan in the care home once a week with my daughter and mum, and still live in hope of getting a boyfriend.

In addition, I read a lot, limit myself to three hours of telly a week, do a spot of gardening and sit out in the garden in the sunlight, drink lots of green tea, have developed a serious housework addiction which means I'm always on my feet, and am thinking of getting a dog.

As a big fan of *Black Mirror*, I'd love to see what the world is like in 2080, kick back in a self-driving car and go for a wild ride in a teleporter (ideally not ending up in the plot of *The Fly*). And one thing's for sure: you and I have both got far more chance of making it to a hundred thanks to the advice in this book.

Of course, this will all be very embarrassing when I die prematurely after being hit by a giant red motor vehicle, but at least I'll have helped you gain an extra few decades. Check out the handy unscientific quiz I've created on the next few pages and work out which habits you can change to make it into triple figures.

Much love and longevity,

Ariane x

# Ariane's handy unscientific 'will you live to 100?' quiz

This quiz is just for fun but should give you a general idea of what you could change to live longer. I've mainly focused on things you can control, with a few exceptions. For each question, simply answer 'yes', 'no' or 'sort of'.

| | YES | NO | SORT OF |
|---|---|---|---|
| Are you married? | | | |
| Do you cohabit with a partner? | | | |
| Do you have regular sex? | | | |
| Do you use condoms when having sex, unless you and your partner have both been tested for STIs? | | | |
| Do you have any children? | | | |
| Are you close to your friends and family? | | | |
| Do you see your friends and family often? | | | |
| Do you use social media sparingly? | | | |
| Do you volunteer for a charity? | | | |
| Do you have close ties to your community? | | | |
| Do you regularly attend religious services? | | | |
| Do you sleep between seven and eight hours a night? | | | |
| Are you generally quite happy? | | | |
| Do you laugh a lot? | | | |
| Are you a calm and relaxed person? | | | |
| Are you in regular employment? | | | |
| Are you highly educated? | | | |
| Do you feel younger than you are? | | | |

| | | | |
|---|---|---|---|
| Do you read books regularly? | | | |
| Do you watch relatively little TV? | | | |
| Do you do 150 minutes a week of exercise that gets your heart pumping? | | | |
| Do you lift weights regularly or do resistance exercise, e.g. yoga? | | | |
| Does your work involve plenty of standing up? | | | |
| Do you usually get your five a day? | | | |
| Do you regularly eat leafy green veg? | | | |
| Do you avoid eating meat? | | | |
| Do you eat oily fish at least twice a week? | | | |
| Do you regularly consume olive oil? | | | |
| Do you often eat complex carbohydrates? | | | |
| Do you avoid simple carbohydrates? | | | |
| Do you use herbs and spices when cooking? | | | |
| Do you eat sugar sparingly? | | | |
| Do you use artificial sweeteners sparingly? | | | |
| Do you take vitamin D in the winter? | | | |
| Do you avoid processed foods? | | | |
| Is your weight in the healthy BMI range? | | | |
| Do you regularly drink green tea? | | | |
| Do you often drink black tea? | | | |
| Are you a regular coffee drinker? | | | |
| Do you drink one glass of fruit juice a day or less? | | | |
| Do you steer clear of soft drinks? | | | |
| Do you avoid energy drinks? | | | |
| Are you teetotal? | | | |
| Are you a non-smoker? | | | |
| Do you steer clear of recreational drugs? | | | |
| Do you regularly go to the doctor? | | | |
| Do you have regular dental check-ups? | | | |
| Do you attend all screening appointments? | | | |
| Are you up to date with your vaccinations? | | | |
| Can you access high-quality healthcare? | | | |
| Do you live in a good neighbourhood? | | | |
| Do you own a dog? | | | |

| | | | |
|---|---|---|---|
| Do you own an Apple Watch or other device that can send an SOS in the event of a fall? | | | |
| Is your home fitted with smoke alarms? | | | |
| Does your home have a carbon monoxide detector? | | | |
| Is your home warm? | | | |
| Is your home free from damp and mould? | | | |
| Is your home free from asbestos? | | | |
| Do you steer clear of scented candles? | | | |
| Do you avoid using air fresheners? | | | |
| Do you avoid using toxic cleaning products? | | | |
| Do you take safety precautions when doing DIY? | | | |
| Do you garden regularly and safely? | | | |
| Do you avoid exposure to weedkiller and pesticides? | | | |
| Do you regularly spend time in nature? | | | |
| Do you avoid exposure to air pollution? | | | |
| Have you never used a sunbed? | | | |
| Do you use sunscreen regularly? | | | |
| Do you leave your hair its natural colour? | | | |
| Do you avoid squirting talc between your thighs? | | | |
| Do you steer clear of cosmetic surgery? | | | |
| Do you favour planes and trains when travelling? | | | |
| Do you steer clear of travelling in cars? | | | |
| Do you avoid travelling by motorbike? | | | |
| Do you cycle in safe areas? | | | |
| Do you avoid cycling in inner cities and built-up areas? | | | |
| Do you avoid light aircraft? | | | |
| Do you avoid helicopters? | | | |
| Do you take regular walks? | | | |
| Do you avoid skiing? | | | |
| Do you steer clear of snowboarding? | | | |
| Do you avoid horse riding? | | | |
| Do you steer clear of mountain climbing? | | | |
| Do you avoid parachuting and bungee jumping? | | | |
| Do you avoid BASE jumping? | | | |
| Do you steer clear of contact with wild and exotic animals? | | | |

| | | | |
|---|---|---|---|
| Do you avoid motor racing? | | | |
| Do you avoid scuba diving, tombstone diving and breath-hold diving? | | | |
| Do you steer clear of contact sports? | | | |
| Do you exclusively swim in lifeguard-supervised areas? | | | |
| Do you cut food into small chunks, chew slowly and avoid talking and eating at the same time? | | | |
| Is your job safe and hazard-free? | | | |
| Is your blood pressure in the healthy range? | | | |
| Do you own and use a blood pressure monitor? | | | |
| Do you wash your hands before putting your fingers in your mouth? | | | |
| Do you avoid taking selfies in risky places, e.g. on the edges of cliffs? | | | |
| Do you steer clear of fairground rides? | | | |
| Are you tall? | | | |
| Was your childhood free from adverse experiences? | | | |
| Do you regularly stand up throughout the day? | | | |

Give yourself one point for every 'yes' answer, half a point for each 'sort of' answer, and zero points for every 'no'. Add them all up and find out your score:

80-100: Well done! You're doing nearly everything right and are on course to get your telegram from the Queen.

60-79: Good effort! You're going to live a very long life. Enjoy it.

40-59: You're doing quite well, but there are still plenty of things you can change if you want to live longer.

20-39: There's lots of scope for change here. The good news is, you now know what to focus on.

0-19: Whoa, thrill seeker! You're going to live a fun life, but will it also be a short one?

# Celebrity biographies

**Yomi Adegoke** is a multi-award-winning journalist and co-author of the bestselling book *Slay in Your Lane: The Black Girl Bible*. She is the women's columnist at the *Guardian* and was named one of the most influential people in London by the *Evening Standard* in 2018.

**Clive Anderson** is a television and radio presenter, comedy writer and former barrister. He began experimenting with stand-up comedy and scriptwriting during his fifteen-year legal career, before starring in *Whose Line Is It Anyway?* on BBC Radio 4, then Channel 4. For many years he presented chat shows on Channel 4 and BBC One as well as other programmes and documentaries on various channels, and he makes irregular appearances on shows such as *Have I Got News for You* and *QI*. He currently presents *Loose Ends* and *Unreliable Evidence* on BBC Radio 4 and *Mystic Britain* on the Smithsonian Channel.

**Charlie Brooker** is a satirist, broadcaster, presenter, producer and writer. He is the creator of the futuristic Netflix series *Black Mirror*, for which he has won six Emmy awards. As well as writing for television programmes including *Black Mirror*, *Brass Eye*, *The 11 O'Clock Show* and *Nathan Barley*, he has presented a number of television shows, including *Screenwipe*, *Gameswipe*, *Newswipe*, *Weekly Wipe*, *Antiviral Wipe* and *10 O'Clock Live*. He also wrote the zombie horror drama *Dead Set* and co-wrote three series of *A Touch of Cloth*.

**Derren Brown** is an illusionist, mentalist, artist and author. During a varied and notorious TV career, he has played Russian roulette live, convinced middle-managers to commit armed robbery, led the nation in a séance, stuck viewers at home to their sofas, successfully predicted the National Lottery, motivated a shy man to think he was landing a packed passenger plane at 30,000 feet, hypnotised a man to assassinate Stephen Fry and created a zombie apocalypse for an unsuspecting participant after seemingly ending the world. His last book, *Happy: Why More or Less Everything is Absolutely Fine*, explores changing concepts of happiness and is a *Sunday Times* bestseller.

**Gordon Burns** made his name nationally when he presented and scripted the popular ITV quiz show *The Krypton Factor*, which ran for eighteen years in a peak time slot and achieved audiences of up to 18 million people. He then presented the BBC's nightly news programme *North West Tonight* for fifteen years, winning the Royal Television Society's Best News Presenter award five times and the coveted BBC Ruby Television Award for the best regional news presenter in the UK.

**Dr Aubrey de Grey** is a biomedical gerontologist based in Mountain View, California, USA, and is the chief science officer of SENS Research Foundation, a California-based 501(c)(3) biomedical research charity that performs and funds laboratory research dedicated to combating the ageing process. He is also VP of new technology discovery at AgeX Therapeutics, a biotechnology start-up developing new therapies in the field of biomedical gerontology. In addition, he is editor-in-chief of *Rejuvenation Research*, the world's highest-impact peer-reviewed journal focused on intervention in ageing. He received his BA in computer science and PhD in biology from the University of Cambridge.

**Bec Hill** is an Australian-born, UK-based comedian, writer, actor and presenter. She is best known for her viral flipchart videos and ridiculous social media adventures. When she's not performing stand-up around the world to both adults and kids, she is either appearing on or writing for telly, chatting on various podcasts or winning awards. She's also been a time-traveller, the voice of several characters in Mass Effect: Andromeda and Anthem, and most recently became a Tooth Fairy.

**Jon Holmes** is a multi-award-winning writer, comedian, broadcaster and presenter. He co-created *Dead Ringers*, was the short one off *The Now Show*, and his new Radio 4 show *The Skewer* sees him up for Comedy Producer of The Year. His BBC weekend show recently won a Radio Academy Award, and other credits include TV's *Horrible Histories*. He is also an award-winning travel writer and was recently Highly Commended Travel Writer of the Year as bestowed by the travel industry. He also once had to share a bed with the actor Stratford Johns while holding a car battery. Long story.

**Konnie Huq** is a television presenter, broadcaster and writer. She is the longest-serving female presenter of the legendary children's BBC show *Blue Peter*, having presented it from 1997 until 2008. She co-wrote the second episode of the Channel 4 anthology series *Black Mirror*, 'Fifteen Million Merits'. Last year she appeared in popular television miniseries *Good Omens*, and also published her debut children's novel *Cookie and the Most Annoying Boy in the World*, which became a bestseller.

**Robin Ince** is a comedian, author, broadcaster and populariser of scientific ideas. The *Guardian* once declared him a 'becardiganed polymath', which seems about right. He is probably best known as the co-host of the Sony Gold Award-winning BBC Radio 4 series *The Infinite Monkey Cage* with Professor Brian Cox. He also co-hosts the podcast *Book Shambles*, with Josie Long, which has over 100,000 listeners a month and is part of The Cosmic Shambles Network, which he also co-created. His most recent book, *I'm a Joke and So Are You*, was described by Chortle as 'one of the best books ever written about what it means to be a comedian'.

**Sanjeev Kohli** is the co-writer and co-star of award-winning BBC Radio 4 comedy *Fags Mags and Bags*, has written for sketch shows *Chewin' the Fat* and *Goodness Gracious Me*, has presented extensively on the BBC, and has written and recorded vocals for the musical project *The Grand Gestures*. He has also appeared in the likes of *Cold Feet*, *Fresh Meat* and *Look Around You* (where he played Synthesiser Patel), as well as being the star of the video for Elbow's 'Lost Worker Bee'. He is best-known, however, for playing shopkeeper Navid in *Still Game* for nine series on the BBC and three sell-out runs at The Glasgow Hydro. He is also a keen Twitter enthusiast, who once actually tweeted his arse off and rather embarrassingly tweeted someone else's arse back on.

**Stewart Lee** began stand-up in 1988 at the age of twenty, and won the Hackney Empire new act of the year award in 1990. In 2001 he co-wrote the libretto for Richard Thomas's *Jerry Springer: The Opera*, which went on to win four Olivier awards. His most recent stand-up show is *Snowflake/Tornado*. In December 2011 he won Best Male TV Comic and Best Comedy Entertainment Performance at the British Comedy Awards and his BBC show *Comedy Vehicle* won a BAFTA in 2012.

**Robert Llewellyn** was born in 1956 and grew up in West Oxfordshire. Leaving school at sixteen, he became a hippy leather worker, a shoemaker and a farm worker before stepping on a stage. Thousands of hours of live performing eventually led to him playing the role of Kryten in the BBC Two sitcom *Red Dwarf*. Thirty-one years later he is still occasionally covered in rubber. For ten years he presented the Channel 4 series *Scrapheap Challenge*. He now produces a successful series on YouTube called the *Fully Charged Show* where he and the *Fully Charged* team explore the future of energy and transport, electric cars, renewable energy and clean technology.

**Josie Long** is a comedian. She started performing stand-up at the age of fourteen and won the BBC New Comedy Awards aged seventeen. In 2006, she won the if.comeddies Best Newcomer award at the Edinburgh Festival Fringe for her show *Kindness and Exuberance*. She has been nominated for the Edinburgh Comedy Award for Best

Show three times. Since 2012 she has been making films with the director Douglas King and their first feature, *Super November*, was nominated for a BIFA Discovery Award in 2018. She has made twenty series of the BBC Radio 4 show *Short Cuts*.

**Richard Osman** is a television presenter, producer, comedian, director and novelist, best known for being the creator and co-presenter of the BBC One quiz show *Pointless*. He has also presented the BBC Two quiz shows *Two Tribes* and *Richard Osman's House of Games* and has been a team captain on the comedy panel shows *Insert Name Here* and *The Fake News Show*. He is the creative director of Endemol UK and his debut novel *The Thursday Murder Club* is out now.

**Angela Saini** is an award-winning British science journalist and broadcaster. She presents science programmes on the BBC and her writing has appeared in *New Scientist*, the *Guardian*, the *Sunday Times*, *National Geographic* and *Wired*. Her most recent book, *Superior: The Return of Race Science*, was named a book of the year by the *Sunday Times*, *Financial Times*, *New Statesman* and the *Telegraph*. Her previous book, *Inferior: The True Power of Women and the Science that Shows It*, was published in 2017 and has been translated into twelve languages. Angela has a Masters in engineering from the University of Oxford, a second Masters in science and security from the Department of War Studies at King's College London and is a former fellow of the Massachusetts Institute of Technology.

**Lou Sanders** is one of the most original comedians in Britain. She is the former champion of *Taskmaster* (DAVE). Her other recent television appearances include *QI* (BBC Two), *Travel Man: 48 Hours in . . .* (Channel 4), *8 Out of 10 Cats Does Countdown* (Channel 4), *Hypothetical* (DAVE*)*, Aisling Bea's sitcom *This Way Up* (Channel 4), *The Russell Howard Hour* (Sky One), *Jon Richardson: Ultimate Worrier* (DAVE) and Karl Pilkington's sitcom *Sick of It* (Sky One).

**Arthur Smith** is a comedian, writer and broadcaster who has appeared on *QI*, *Have I Got News for You* and is best known as the opening bat on *Grumpy Old Men*. He appears regularly on *Loose Ends* on BBC Radio 4, presents *The Comedy Club* on Radio 4 Extra and is the self-proclaimed mayor of Balham and a regular at the Edinburgh Festival since medieval times. His book *100 Things I Meant to Tell You* is out now.

**Jeremy Vine** is a presenter, broadcaster and journalist. He is best known as the host of his own BBC Radio 2 programme which features news, opinions, interviews with live guests and popular music. He is famous for his direct presenting style, and exclusive reporting from war-torn areas throughout Africa. He also presents the long-running BBC quiz show *Eggheads*, as well as his own daily Channel 5 current affairs show, *Jeremy Vine*.

# References

## Part One: Relationships

### Marriage

1. Kiecolt-Glaser J. K., Newton T. L. Marriage and Health: His and Hers. *Psychol Bull.* 2001;127(4):472–503.
2. Elwood W. N., Irvin V. L., Sun Q., et al. Measuring the Influence of Legally Recognized Partnerships on the Health and Well-Being of Same-Sex Couples: Utility of the California Health Interview Survey. *LGBT Heal.* 2017;4(2):153–160.
3. Umberson D., Donnelly R., Pollitt A. M. How Spouses Influence Each Other's Health Habits in Same-Sex Compared to Different-Sex Marriages. *PRC Res Br.* 2018;3(11).
4. Holt-Lunstad J., Birmingham W., Jones B. Q. Is There Something Unique about Marriage? The Relative Impact of Marital Status, Relationship Quality, and Network Social Support on Ambulatory Blood Pressure and Mental Health. *Ann Behav Med.* 2008;35(2):239–44.
5. Chen Y., Kawachi I., Berkman L. F., et al. A Prospective Study of Marital Quality and Body Weight in Midlife. *Heal Psychol.* 2018;37(3): 247–256.

### Cohabitation

1. Perelli-Harris B., Styrc M. E., Addo F., et al. *Comparing the Benefits of Cohabitation and Marriage for Health in Mid-Life: Is the Relationship Similar Across Countries?* ESRC Centre for Population Change; 2017.
2. Perelli-Harris B., Styrc M. Mental Well-Being Differences in Cohabitation and Marriage: The Role of Childhood Selection. *J Marriage Fam.* 2018;80(1):239–255.
3. Monden C. Partners in Health? Exploring Resemblance in Health between Partners in Married and Cohabiting Couples. *Sociol Health Illn.* 2007;29(3):391–411.

4. Ho J. Y., Fenelon A. The Contribution of Smoking to Educational Gradients in U.S. Life Expectancy. *J Health Soc Behav*. 2015;56(3):307–322.
5. Grewen K. M., Anderson B. J., Girdler S. S., et al. Warm Partner Contact is Related to Lower Cardiovascular Reactivity. *Behav Med*. 2003;29(3):123–130.
6. Joutsenniemi K., Martelin T., Martikainen P., et al. Living Arrangements and Mental Health in Finland. *J Epidemiol Community Health*. 2006;60(6): 468–475.
7. Frisch M., Simonsen J. Marriage, Cohabitation and Mortality in Denmark: National Cohort Study of 6.5 Million Persons Followed for up to Three Decades (1982–2011). *Int J Epidemiol*. 2013;42(2):559–578.
8. Mata J., Richter D., Schneider T., et al. How Cohabitation, Marriage, Separation, and Divorce Influence BMI: A Prospective Panel Study. *Heal Psychol*. 2018;37(10):948–958.

## Divorce

1. Miller R. B., Hollist C. S., Olsen J., et al. Marital Quality and Health Over 20 Years: A Growth Curve Analysis. *J Marriage Fam*. 2013;75(3):667–680.
2. Sbarra D. A., Law R. W., Portley R. M. Divorce and Death: A Meta-Analysis and Research Agenda for Clinical, Social, and Health Psychology. *Perspect Psychol Sci*. 2011;6(5):454–474.
3. Manzoli L., Villari P., M. Pirone G., et al. Marital Status and Mortality in the Elderly: A Systematic Review and Meta-Analysis. *Soc Sci Med*. 2007;64(1):77–94.
4. Fu H., Goldman N. The Association between Health-Related Behaviours and the Risk of Divorce in the USA. *J Biosoc Sci*. 2000;32(1):63–88.
5. Richards M., Hardy R., Wadsworth M. The Effects of Divorce and Separation on Mental Health in a National UK Birth Cohort. *Psychol Med*. 1997;27(5): 1121–1128. http://www.ncbi.nlm.nih.gov/pubmed/9300516. Accessed June 27, 2019.
6. Lorenz F. O., Wickrama K. A., Conger R. D., et al. The Short-Term and Decade-Long Effects of Divorce on Women's Midlife Health. *J Health Soc Behav*. 2006;47(2):111–125.
7. Williams K., Sassler S., Nicholson L. M. For Better or For Worse? The Consequences of Marriage and Cohabitation for Single Mothers. *Soc Forces*. 2008;86(4):1481–1511.

## Sex

1. Brody S. The Relative Health Benefits of Different Sexual Activities. *J Sex Med*. 2010;7(4):1336–1361.
2. Aro A. L., Rusinaru C., Uy-Evanado A., et al. Sexual Activity as a Trigger for Sudden Cardiac Arrest. *J Am Coll Cardiol*. 2017;70(20):2599–2600.

# References

3. Levine G. N., Steinke E. E., Bakaeen F. G., et al. Sexual Activity and Cardiovascular Disease. *Circulation*. 2012;125(8):1058–1072.
4. NHS. Benefits of Love and Sex. https://www.nhs.uk/live-well/sexual-health/benefits-of-love-sex-relationships/. Accessed November 17, 2019.
5. Liu H., Waite L., Shen S., et al. Is Sex Good for Your Health? A National Study on Partnered Sexuality and Cardiovascular Risk Among Older Men and Women. *J Health Soc Behav*. 2016;57(3):276–296.

## Having children

1. Modig K., Talbäck M., Torssander J., et al. Payback Time? Influence of Having Children on Mortality in Old Age. *J Epidemiol Community Health*. 2017;71(5):424–430.
2. Ruppanner L., Perales F., Baxter J. Harried and Unhealthy? Parenthood, Time Pressure, and Mental Health. *J Marriage Fam*. 2019;81(2):308–326.

## Family and friends

1. Lubben J., Gironda M. Centrality of Social Ties to the Health and Well-Being of Older Adults. In: Berkman B., Harootyan L., eds. *Social Work and Health Care in an Aging Society: Education, Policy, Practice, and Research*. Springer Publishing Company; 2003.
2. Straus M. A., Gelles R. J., Steinmetz S. K. *Behind Closed Doors: Violence in the American Family*. Anchor Doubleday Press; 1980.
3. Shor E., Roelfs D., Yogev T. The Strength of Family Ties: A Meta-Analysis and Meta-Regression of Self-Reported Social Support and Mortality. *Soc Networks*. 2013;35(4):626–638.
4. Sies P. M., Bartoo H. Friendship, Social Support, and Health. In: L'Abate L, ed. *Low-Cost Approaches to Promote Physical and Mental Health*. Springer; 2007.
5. Department for Digital, Culture, Media and Sport. *A Connected Society: A Strategy for Tackling Loneliness – Laying the Foundations for Change*. October 2018. https://assets.publishing.service.gov.uk/government/uploads/system/uploads/attachment_data/file/750909/6.4882_DCMS_Loneliness_Strategy_web_Update.pdf.
6. Nguyen A. W., Chatters L. M., Taylor R. J., et al. Social Support from Family and Friends and Subjective Well-Being of Older African Americans. *J Happiness Stud*. 2016;17(3):959–979.

## Social media

1. Hurst G. Anxious Parents 'Creating Moral Panic' over Social Media. *The Times*. May 30, 2017. https://www.thetimes.co.uk/article/anxious-parents-creating-moral-panic-over-social-media-602tfmxx0#. Accessed December 1, 2019.

2. Bányai F., Zsila Á., Király O., et al. Problematic Social Media Use: Results from a Large-Scale Nationally Representative Adolescent Sample. *PLoS One.* 2017;12(1):e0169839.

3. Pontes H. M. Investigating the Differential Effects of Social Networking Site Addiction and Internet Gaming Disorder on Psychological Health. *J Behav Addict.* 2017;6(4):601–610.

4. Kuss D. J., Griffiths M. D. Social Networking Sites and Addiction: Ten Lessons Learned. *Int J Environ Res Public Health.* 2017;14(3):311.

5. Andreassen C. S., Pallesen S., Griffiths M. D. The Relationship between Addictive Use of Social Media, Narcissism, and Self-Esteem: Findings From a Large National Survey. *Addict Behav.* 2017;64:287–293.

6. Dobrean A., Păsărelu C.-R. Impact of Social Media on Social Anxiety: A Systematic Review. In: Durbano F., Marchesi B., eds. *New Developments in Anxiety Disorders.* InTech; 2016.

7. Mitchell L., Hussain Z. Predictors of Problematic Smartphone Use: An Examination of the Integrative Pathways Model and the Role of Age, Gender, Impulsiveness, Excessive Reassurance Seeking, Extraversion, and Depression. *Behav Sci (Basel).* 2018;8(8):E74.

8. Hormes J. M. Under the Influence of Facebook? Excess Use of Social Networking Sites and Drinking Motives, Consequences, and Attitudes in College Students. *J Behav Addict.* 2016;5(1):122–129.

9. Escobar-Viera C. G., Whitfield D. L., Wessel C. B., et al. For Better or for Worse? A Systematic Review of the Evidence on Social Media Use and Depression Among Lesbian, Gay, and Bisexual Minorities. *JMIR Ment Heal.* 2018;5(3):e10496.

10. Sagioglou C., Greitemeyer T. Facebook's Emotional Consequences: Why Facebook Causes a Decrease in Mood and Why People Still Use It. *Comput Human Behav.* 2014;35:359–363.

11. Primack B. A., Shensa A., Escobar-Viera C. G., et al. Use of Multiple Social Media Platforms and Symptoms of Depression and Anxiety: A Nationally-Representative Study among U.S. Young Adults. *Comput Human Behav.* 2017;69:1–9.

12. Kim S. E., Kim J. W., Jee Y. S. Relationship Between Smartphone Addiction and Physical Activity in Chinese International Students in Korea. *J Behav Addict.* 2015;4(3):200–205.

13. Rice E. S., Haynes E., Royce P., et al. Social Media and Digital Technology Use among Indigenous Young People in Australia: A Literature Review. *Int J Equity Health.* 2016;15:81.

14. Hampton K., Rainie L., Lu W., et al. *Social Media and the Cost of Caring.* Pew Research Center. January 15, 2015. http://www.pewinternet.org/2015/01/15/social-media-and-stress/.

15. Zhang J., Brackbill D., Yang S., et al. Efficacy and Causal Mechanism of an

Online Social Media Intervention to Increase Physical Activity: Results of a Randomized Controlled Trial. *Prev Med Reports*. 2015;2:651–657.

16. Maher C. A., Lewis L. K., Ferrar K., et al. Are Health Behavior Change Interventions that use Online Social Networks Effective? A Systematic Review. *J Med Internet Res*. 2014;16(2):e40.

17. Giustini D., Ali S. M., Fraser M., et al. Effective Uses of Social Media in Public Health and Medicine: A Systematic Review of Systematic Reviews. *Online J Public Health Inform*. 2018;10(2):e215.

## Volunteering

1. Rogers N. T., Demakakos P., Taylor M. S., et al. Volunteering is Associated with Increased Survival in Able-Bodied Participants of the English Longitudinal Study of Ageing. *J Epidemiol Community Health*. 2016;70(6): 583–588.

2. Casiday R., Kinsman E., Fisher C., et al. *Volunteering and Health: What Impact Does It Really Have? Report to Volunteering England*. Volunteering England; 2008. http://dro.dur.ac.uk/9269/.

3. Kim E. S., Konrath S. H. Volunteering is Prospectively Associated with Health Care Use among Older Adults. *Soc Sci Med*. 2016;149: 122–129.

4. Detollenaere J., Willems S., Baert S. Volunteering, Income and Health. *PLoS One*. 2017;12(3):e0173139.

5. Poulin M. J. Volunteering Predicts Health among those who Value Others: Two National Studies. *Heal Psychol*. 2014;33(2):120–129.

6. Han S., Kim K., Burr J. Stress-Buffering Effects of Volunteering on Daily Well-Being: Results from the National Study of Daily Experiences. *Innov Aging*. 2019;3(Suppl 1):S235.

7. Onyx J., Warburton J. Volunteering and Health among Older People: A Review. *Autralasian J Ageing*. 2003;22(2):65–69.

8. Papa R., Cutuli G., Principi A., et al. Health and Volunteering in Europe: A Longitudinal Study. *Res Aging*. 2019;41(7):670–696.

9. Pillemer K., Fuller-Rowell T. E., Reid M. C., et al. Environmental Volunteering and Health Outcomes over a 20-Year Period. *Gerontologist*. 2010;50(5):594–602.

10. O'Reilly D., Rosato M., Ferry F., et al. Caregiving, Volunteering or Both? Comparing Effects on Health and Mortality using Census-Based Records from almost 250,000 People aged 65 and Over. *Age Ageing*. 2017;46(5): 821–826.

11. Kumar S., Calvo R., Avendano M., et al. Social Support, Volunteering and Health around the World: Cross-National Evidence from 139 Countries. *Soc Sci Med*. 2012;74(5):696–706.

397

12. Lee H. Volunteering and Health among Older Koreans: A Longitudinal Analysis. *Innov Aging.* 2017;1(Suppl 1):1197–1198.

## Community

1. Cockerham W. C., Harnby B. W., Oates G. R. The Social Determinants of Chronic Disease. *Am J Prev Med.* 2017;5(1 Suppl 1):S5–S12.
2. Ishikawa Y., Kondo N., Kondo K., et al. Social Participation and Mortality: Does Social Position in Civic Groups Matter? *BMC Public Health.* 2016;16:394.
3. Lindström M., Rosvall M. Two Theoretical Strands of Social Capital, and Total, Cardiovascular, Cancer and Other Mortality: A Population-Based Prospective Cohort Study. *SSM – Popul Heal.* 2019;7:100337.
4. Zoorob M. J., Salerni J. L. Bowling Alone, Dying Together: The Role of Social Capital in Mitigating the Drug Overdose Epidemic in the United States. *Drug Alcohol Depend.* 2017;173:1–9.
5. Murillo R., Echeverria S., Vasquez E. Differences in Neighborhood Social Cohesion and Aerobic Physical Activity by Latino Subgroup. *SSM – Popul Heal.* 2016;2:536–541.
6. Kim E. S., Kawachi I. Perceived Neighborhood Social Cohesion and Preventive Healthcare Use. *Am J Prev Med.* 2017;53(2):e35–e40.
7. Reynolds V. A. Cancer and Psychological Distress: Examining the Role of Neighborhood Social Cohesion. 2017. Kent State University. http://rave.ohiolink.edu/etdc/view?acc_num=kent1510833570995311.
8. Lagisetty P. A., Wen M., Choi H., et al. Neighborhood Social Cohesion and Prevalence of Hypertension and Diabetes in a South Asian Population. *J Immigr Minor Heal.* 2016;18(6):1309–1316.
9. Giordano G. N., Mewes J., Miething A. Trust and All-Cause Mortality: A Multilevel Study of US General Social Survey data (1978–2010). *J Epidemiol Community Health.* 2019;73(1):50–55.
10. Robinette J. W., Charles S. T., Gruenewald T. L. Neighborhood Cohesion, Neighborhood Disorder, and Cardiometabolic Risk. *Soc Sci Med.* 2018;198:70–76.
11. Carrasco M. A., Bilal U. A Sign of the Times: To Have or to Be? Social Capital or Social Cohesion? *Soc Sci Med.* 2016;159:127–131.

## Religion

1. Ofstedal M. B., Chiu C.-T., Jagger C., et al. Religion, Life Expectancy, and Disability-Free Life Expectancy Among Older Women and Men in the United States. *Journals Gerontol Ser B.* 2019;74(8):e107–e118.
2. Suh H., Hill T. D., Koenig H. G. Religious Attendance and Biological Risk: A National Longitudinal Study of Older Adults. *J Relig Health.* 2019;58(4):1188–1202.

## References

3. Hill T. D., Rote S. M., Ellison C. G. Religious Participation and Biological Functioning in Mexico. *J Aging Health*. 2017;29(6):951–972.
4. Bonelli R. M., Koenig H. G. Mental Disorders, Religion and Spirituality 1990 to 2010: A Systematic Evidence-Based Review. *J Relig Health*. 2013;52(2):657–673.
5. Li S., Okereke O. I., Chang S. C., et al. Religious Service Attendance and Lower Depression Among Women: A Prospective Cohort Study. *Ann Behav Med*. 2016;50(6):876–884.
6. Schuurmans-Stekhoven J. B. Auspicious or Suspicious: Does Religiosity Really Promote Elder Well-Being? Examining the Belief-as-Benefit Effect among Older Japanese. *Arch Gerontol Geriatr*. 2019;81:129–134.
7. Linardakis M., Papadaki A., Smpokos E., et al. Are Religiosity and Prayer Use Related with Multiple Behavioural Risk Factors for Chronic Diseases in European Adults Aged 50+ Years? *Public Health*. 2015;129(5):436–443.
8. Faries M. D., McClendon M., Jones E. J. Destroying God's Temple? Physical Inactivity, Poor Diet, Obesity, and Other 'Sin' Behaviors. *J Relig Health*. 2020;59(1):522–534.
9. Park C. L., Aldwin C. M., Choun S., et al. Spiritual Peace Predicts 5-Year Mortality in Congestive Heart Failure Patients. *Heal Psychol*. 2016;35(3):203–210.
10. Kim J., Smith T. W., Kang J. H. Religious Affiliation, Religious Service Attendance, and Mortality. *J Relig Health*. 2015;54(6):2052–2072.
11. Vitorino L. M., Lucchetti G., Leão F. C., et al. The Association between Spirituality and Religiousness and Mental Health. *Sci Rep*. 2018;8(1):17233.
12. Portnoff L., McClintock C., Lau E., et al. Spirituality Cuts in Half the Relative Risk for Depression: Findings from the United States, China, and India. *Spiritual Clin Pract*. 2017;4(1):22–31.
13. Wang L., Koenig H. G., He Z., et al. Religiosity and Telomere Length: Moderating Effect of Religiosity on the Relationship Between High-Risk Polymorphisms of the *Apolipoprotein E* and *TOMM40* Gene and Telomere Length. *J Appl Gerontol*. 2019: 733464819865415.
14. VanderWeele T. J., Shields A. E. Religiosity and Telomere Length: One Step Forward, One Step Back. *Soc Sci Med*. 2016;163:176–178.
15. Shammas M. A. Telomeres, Lifestyle, Cancer, and Aging. *Curr Opin Clin Nutr Metab Care*. 2011;14(1):28–34.
16. Morton K. R., Lee J. W., Martin L. R. Pathways from Religion to Health: Mediation by Psychosocial and Lifestyle Mechanisms. *Psycholog Relig Spiritual*. 2017;9(1):106–117.

## Part Two: Well-Being

*Sleep*
1. Alvarez G. G., Ayas N. T. The Impact of Daily Sleep Duration on Health: A Review of the Literature. *Prog Cardiovasc Nurs.* 2004;19(2):56–59.
2. Itani O., Jike M., Watanabe N., et al. Short Sleep Duration and Health Outcomes: A Systematic Review, Meta-Analysis and Meta-Regression. *Sleep Med.* 2017;32:246–256.
3. Jike M., Itani O., Watanabe N., et al. Long Sleep Duration and Health Outcomes: A Systematic Review, Meta-Analysis and Meta-Regression. *Sleep Med Rev.* 2018;39:25–36.
4. Tsou M.-T. Association Between Sleep Duration and Health Outcome in Elderly Taiwanese. *Int J Gerontol.* 2011;5(4):200–205.
5. Cooper C. B., Neufeld E. V., Dolezal B. A., et al. Sleep Deprivation and Obesity in Adults: A Brief Narrative Review. *BMJ Open Sport Exerc Med.* 2018;4(1):e000392.
6. Citoni G. The Relationship between Sleep Time and Self-Rated Health: An Analysis based on Italian Survey Data. *Epidemiol Biostat Public Heal.* 2014;11(1):e9469-1– e9469-10.
7. Hall M. H., Smagula S. F., Boudreau R. M., et al. Association between Sleep Duration and Mortality is Mediated by Markers of Inflammation and Health in Older Adults: The Health, Aging and Body Composition Study. *Sleep.* 2015;38(2):189–195.
8. Beattie L., Kyle S. D., Espie C. A., et al. Social Interactions, Emotion and Sleep: A Systematic Review and Research Agenda. *Sleep Med Rev.* 2015;24:83–100.
9. Lechner M., Breeze C. E., Ohayon M. M., et al. Snoring and Breathing Pauses During Sleep: Interview Survey of a United Kingdom Population Sample Reveals a Significant Increase in the Rates of Sleep Apnoea and Obesity over the last 20 Years – Data from the UK Sleep Survey. *Sleep Med.* 2019;54:250–256.
10. NHS. Snoring. https://www.nhs.uk/conditions/Snoring/. Accessed November 21, 2019.
11. NHS. Lifespan Linked to Sleep. https://www.nhs.uk/news/lifestyle-and-exercise/lifespan-linked-to-sleep/. Accessed November 21, 2019.

*Happiness*
1. Lawrence E. M., Rogers R. G., Wadsworth T. Happiness and Longevity in the United States. *Soc Sci Med.* 2015;145:115–119.
2. Veenhoven R. Healthy Happiness: Effects of Happiness on Physical Health and the Consequences for Preventive Health Care. *J Happiness Stud.* 2008;9(3):449–469.

# References

3. Koopmans T. A., Geleijnse J. M., Zitman F. G., et al. Effects of Happiness on All-Cause Mortality During 15 Years of Follow-Up: The Arnhem Elderly Study. *J Happiness Stud.* 2008;11(1):113–124.
4. Liu B. L., Floud S., Pirie K., et al. Does Happiness Itself Directly Affect Mortality? The Prospective UK Million Women Study. *Lancet.* 2016;387(10021):874–881.
5. Grover S., Helliwell J. F. How's Life at Home? New Evidence on Marriage and the Set Point for Happiness. *J Happiness Stud.* 2019;20(2):373–390.

## Sense of humour

1. Linge-Dahl L. M., Heintz S., Ruch W., et al. Humor Assessment and Interventions in Palliative Care: A Systematic Review. *Front Psychol.* 2018;9:890.
2. Greengross G., Martin R. A. Health among Humorists: Susceptibility to Contagious Diseases among Improvisational Artists. *Humor.* 2018;31(3):491–505.
3. Svebak S. Health and Sense of Humour: Mortality. *Ugeskr Laeger.* 2008;170(51):4199–4201.
4. Boyle G. J., Joss-Reid J. M. Relationship of Humour to Health: A Psychometric Investigation. *Br J Health Psychol.* 2004;9(1):51–66.
5. Romundstad S., Svebak S., Holen A., et al. A 15-Year Follow-Up Study of Sense of Humor and Causes of Mortality: The Nord-Trøndelag Health Study. *Psychosom Med.* 2016;78(3):345–353.
6. Svebak S., Romundstad S., Holmen J. A 7-Year Prospective Study of Sense of Humor and Mortality in an Adult County Population: The Hunt-2 Study. *Int J Psychiatry Med.* 2010;40(2):125–146.
7. Stewart S., Thompson D. R. Does Comedy Kill? A Retrospective, Longitudinal Cohort, Nested Case-Control Study of Humour and Longevity in 53 British Comedians. *Int J Cardiol.* 2015;180:258–261.
8. Stewart S., Wiley J., McDermott C., et al. Is the Last 'Man' Standing in Comedy the Least Funny? A Retrospective Cohort Study of Elite Stand-Up Comedians Versus Other Entertainers. *Int J Cardiol.* 2016;220:789–793.
9. McBride A. Comedians: Fun and Dysfunctionality. *Br J Psychiatry.* 2004;185(2):177.

## Stress

1. Song H., Fang F., Arnberg F. K., et al. Stress Related Disorders and Risk of Cardiovascular Disease: Population Based, Sibling Controlled Cohort Study. *BMJ.* 2019;365:I1255.
2. HSE. *Work-Related Stress, Anxiety or Depression Statistics in Great Britain, 2019.* October 30, 2019. http://www.hse.gov.uk/statistics/causdis/stress.pdf.

3. Kivimäki M., Leino-Arjas P., Luukkonen R., et al. Work Stress and Risk of Cardiovascular Mortality: Prospective Cohort Study of Industrial Employees. *BMJ*. 2002;325:857.

4. WHO. Stress at the Workplace. https://www.who.int/occupational_health/topics/stressatwp/en/. Accessed November 26, 2019.

5. NHS. 10 Stress Busters. https://www.nhs.uk/conditions/stress-anxiety-depression/reduce-stress/. Accessed November 26, 2019.

6. NHS. Struggling with Stress? https://www.nhsinform.scot/healthy-living/mental-wellbeing/stress/struggling-with-stress. Accessed November 26, 2019.

7. Juul L., Pallesen K. J., Piet J., et al. Effectiveness of Mindfulness-Based Stress Reduction in a Self-Selecting and Self-Paying Community Setting. *Mindfulness*. 2018;9:1288–1298.

8. Mental Health Foundation. How to Manage and Reduce Stress. https://www.mentalhealth.org.uk/publications/how-manage-and-reduce-stress. Accessed November 26, 2019.

## Employment

1. Local Government Association. *Health, Work and Health Related Worklessness: A Guide for Local Authorities*. May 2016. https://www.local.gov.uk/sites/default/files/documents/health-work-and-health-re-904.pdf. Accessed September 3, 2019.

2. NHS. Unemployment and Job Insecurity Linked to Increased Risk of Suicide. February 11, 2015. https://www.nhs.uk/news/mental-health/unemployment-and-job-insecurity-linked-to-increased-risk-of-suicide/. Accessed September 3, 2019.

3. Roelfs D. J., Shor E., Davidson K. W., et al. Losing Life and Livelihood: A Systematic Review and Meta-Analysis of Unemployment and All-Cause Mortality. *Soc Sci Med*. 2011;72(6):840–854.

4. Mustard C. A., Bielecky A., Etches J., et al. Mortality Following Unemployment in Canada, 1991–2001. *BMC Public Health*. 2013;13(1):441.

5. Health Development Agency. *Worklessness and Health: What Do We Know about the Causal Relationship? Evidence Review Summary*. 2005. http://www.employabilityinscotland.com/media/83147/worklessness-and-health-what-do-we-know-about-the-relationship.pdf. Accessed September 3, 2019.

6. Montgomery S., Udumyan R., Magnuson A., et al. Mortality Following Unemployment During an Economic Downturn: Swedish Register-Based Cohort Study. *BMJ Open*. 2013;3(7):e003031.

7. Gulliford J., Shannon D., Taskila T., et al. *Sick of Being Unemployed: The Health Issues of Out of Work Men and How Support Services are Failing to Address Them*. Men's Health Forum. June 2014. https://www.

menshealthforum.org.uk/sites/default/files/pdf/mhf-unemploy-ment2014_final_pdf.pdf. Accessed September 3, 2019.

8. Clemens T., Boyle P., Popham F. Unemployment, Mortality and the Problem of Health-Related Selection: Evidence from the Scottish and England & Wales (ONS) Longitudinal Studies. *Heal Stat Q.* 2009;(43):7–13.

9. Kim T. J., Von dem Knesebeck O. Is an Insecure Job Better for Health than having No Job at All? A Systematic Review of Studies Investigating the Health-Related Risks of both Job Insecurity and Unemployment. *BMC Public Health.* 2015;15(1):985.

10. The Marmot Review. *Fair Society, Healthy Lives.* February 2010. http://www.insti-tuteofhealthequity.org/resources-reports/fair-society-healthy-lives-the-marmot-review/fair-society-healthy-lives-full-report-pdf.pdf. Accessed September 3, 2019.

## Education

1. PHE. *Health Profile for England: 2017, Chapter 6: Social Determinants of Health, 3. Child Development and Educational Attainment.* July 13, 2017. https://www.gov.uk/government/publications/health-profile-for-england/chapter-6-social-determinants-of-health#child-development-and-educa-tional-attainment.

2. Alicandro G., Frova L., Sebastiani G., et al. Differences in Education and Premature Mortality: A Record Linkage Study of Over 35 Million Italians. *Eur J Public Health.* 2018;28(2):231–237.

3. Albert C., Davia M. A. Education is a Key Determinant of Health in Europe: A Comparative Analysis of 11 Countries. *Health Promot Int.* 2011;26(2):163–170.

4. Sasson I. Trends in Life Expectancy and Lifespan Variation by Educational Attainment: United States, 1990–2010. *Demography.* 2016;53(2):269–293.

5. Scottish Public Health Observatory. Education. https://www.scotpho.org.uk/life-circumstances/education/introduction. Accessed November 29, 2019.

6. Ho J. Y., Fenelon A. The Contribution of Smoking to Educational Gradients in U.S. Life Expectancy. *J Health Soc Behav.* 2015;56(3):307–322.

7. McGill N. Education Attainment Linked to Health throughout Lifespan: Exploring Social Determinants of Health. *Nations Health.* 2016;46(6):1–19.

## Social class

1. WHO. Social Determinants of Health. https://www.who.int/social_determi-nants/thecommission/finalreport/key_concepts/en/. Accessed January 13, 2020.

2. Ramsay S., Morris R., Whincup P., et al. Are Social Inequalities in Mortality in Britain Narrowing? Time Trends from 1978 to 2005 in a Population-Based Study of Older Men. *J Epidemiol Community Health.* 2008;62(1):75–80.

3. The Marmot Review. *Fair Society, Healthy Lives.* February 2010. http://www. instituteofhealthequity.org/resources-reports/fair-society-healthy-lives-the-marmot-review/fair-society-healthy-lives-full-report-pdf.pdf.         Accessed September 3, 2019.

4. Rose G., Marmot M. G. Social Class and Coronary Heart Disease. *Br Heart J.* 1981;45(1):13–19.

5. Marmot M. Social Determinants of Health Inequalities. *Lancet.* 2005;365(9464):1099–1104.

6. Falkstedt D., Lundberg I., Hemmingsson T. Childhood Socio-Economic Position and Risk of Coronary Heart Disease in Middle Age: A Study of 49,321 Male Conscripts. *Eur J Public Health.* 2011;21(6):713–718.

7. Ramsay S. E., Whincup P. H., Morris R. W., et al. Are Childhood Socio-Economic Circumstances Related to Coronary Heart Disease Risk? Findings from a Population-Based Study of Older Men. *Int J Epidemiol.* 2007;36(3):560–566.

8. Tang K. L., Rashid R., Godley J., et al. Association between Subjective Social Status and Cardiovascular Disease and Cardiovascular Risk Factors: A Systematic Review and Meta-Analysis. *BMJ Open.* 2016;6(3):e010137.

9. Agarwal A., Jindal D., Ajay V. S., et al. Association between Socioeconomic Position and Cardiovascular Disease Risk Factors in Rural North India: The Solan Surveillance Study. *PLoS One.* 2019;14(7):e0217834.

## Subjective age

1. Rubin D. C., Berntsen D. People over Forty Feel 20% Younger than their Age: Subjective Age across the Lifespan. *Psychon Bull Rev.* 2006;13(5):776–780.

2. Kotter-Grühn D., Kornadt A. E., Stephan Y. Looking Beyond Chronological Age: Current Knowledge and Future Directions in the Study of Subjective Age. *Gerontology.* 2015;62(1):86–93.

3. Stephan Y., Sutin A. R., Terracciano A. Determinants and Implications of Subjective Age Across Adulthood and Old Age. In: Ryff C. D., Krueger R. F., eds. *The Oxford Handbook of Integrative Health Science.* 1st ed. Oxford University Press; 2018.

4. Westerhof G. J., Miche M., Brothers A. F., et al. The Influence of Subjective Aging on Health and Longevity: A Meta-Analysis of Longitudinal Data. *Psychol Aging.* 2014;29(4):793–802.

5. Shellito N., Prasad S., Velasco Roldan S., et al. The Role of Sense of Control on the Association between Health and Subjective Age. *Innov Aging.* 2018;2(Suppl 1):1006–1007.

6. Gabrian M. Subjective Aging: Measurement Issues, Developmental Consequences, and Malleability in Midlife and Early Old Age. 2015. The

Faculty of Behavioral and Cultural Studies, Heidelberg University. http://www.ub.uni-heidelberg.de/archiv/21415.

## Puzzles and memory games

1. Prince M., Guerchet M., Prina M. *The Epidemiology and Impact of Dementia: Current State and Future Trends.* WHO. 2015. https://www.who.int/mental_health/neurology/dementia/dementia_thematicbrief_epidemiology.pdf.

2. Hardy J. L., Nelson R. A., Thomason M. E., et al. Enhancing Cognitive Abilities with Comprehensive Training: A Large, Online, Randomized, Active-Controlled Trial. *PLoS One.* 2015;10(9):e0134467.

3. Torous J., Staples P., Fenstermacher E., et al. Barriers, Benefits, and Beliefs of Brain Training Smartphone Apps: An Internet Survey of Younger US Consumers. *Front Hum Neurosci.* 2016;10:180.

4. Simons D. J., Boot W. R., Charness N., et al. Do 'Brain-Training' Programs Work? *Psychol Sci Public Interes.* 2016;17(3):103–186.

5. DiMarco L. Y., Marzo A., Muñoz-Ruiz M., et al. Modifiable Lifestyle Factors in Dementia: A Systematic Review of Longitudinal Observational Cohort Studies. *J Alzheimer's Dis.* 2014;42(1):119–135.

6. NHS. Vascular dementia. https://www.nhs.uk/conditions/vascular-dementia /. Accessed November 5, 2019.

7. Vemuri P., Lesnick T. G., Przybelski S. A., et al. Association of Lifetime Intellectual Enrichment with Cognitive Decline in the Older Population. *JAMA Neurol.* 2014;71(8):1017–1024.

8. Hughes T. F., Chang C. C., Vander Bilt J. Engagement in Reading and Hobbies and Risk of Incident Dementia: The MoVIES Project. *Am J Alzheimers Dis Other Demen.* 2010;25(5):432–438.

9. Pillai J. A., Hall C. B., Dickson D. W., et al. Association of Crossword Puzzle Participation with Memory Decline in Persons who Develop Dementia. *J Int Neuropsychol Soc.* 2011;17(6):1006–1013.

10. Fissler P., Küster O. C., Laptinskaya D., et al. Jigsaw Puzzling Taps Multiple Cognitive Abilities and is a Potential Protective Factor for Cognitive Aging. *Front Aging Neurosci.* 2018;10:299.

## TV viewing and reading

1. Grøntved A., Hu F. B. Television Viewing and Risk of Type 2 Diabetes, Cardiovascular Disease, and All-Cause Mortality: A Meta-Analysis. *JAMA.* 2011;305(23):2448–2455.

2. Basterra-Gortari F. J., Bes-Rastrollo M., Gea A., et al. Television Viewing, Computer Use, Time Driving and All-Cause Mortality: The SUN Cohort. *J Am Heart Assoc.* 2014;3(3):e000864.

3.  Burazeri G., Goda A., Kark J. D. Television Viewing, Leisure-Time Exercise and Acute Coronary Syndrome in Transitional Albania. *Prev Med.* 2008;47(1):112–115.

4.  Lindstrom H. A., Fritsch T., Petot G., et al. The Relationships between Television Viewing in Midlife and the Development of Alzheimer's Disease in a Case-Control Study. *Brain Cogn.* 2005;58(2):157–165.

5.  Matthews C. E., George S. M., Moore S. C., et al. Amount of Time Spent in Sedentary Behaviors and Cause-Specific Mortality in US adults. *Am J Clin Nutr.* 2012;95(2):437–445.

6.  Sudore R. L., Yaffe K., Satterfield S., et al. Limited Literacy and Mortality in the Elderly: The Health, Aging, and Body Composition Study. *J Gen Intern Med.* 2006;21(8):806–812.

7.  Jacobs J., Hammerman-Rozenberg R., Cohen A., et al. Reading Daily Predicts Reduced Mortality among Men from a Cohort of Community-Dwelling 70-Year-Olds. *J Gerontol B Psychol Sci Soc Sci.* 2008;63(2):S73–S80.

8.  Hughes T. F., Chang C. C., Vander Bilt J., et al. Engagement in Reading and Hobbies and Risk of Incident Dementia: The MoVIES Project. *Am J Alzheimers Dis Other Demen.* 2010;25(5):432–438.

9.  Gottlieb S. Mental Health may Help Prevent Dementia. *BMJ.* 2003;236:1418.

10.  Yates L. A., Ziser S., Spector A., et al. Cognitive Leisure Activities and Future Risk of Cognitive Impairment and Dementia: Systematic Review and Meta-Analysis. *Int Psychogeriatrics.* 2016;28(11):1791–1806.

## Part Three: Exercise

*Aerobic exercise*

1.  Penedo, F. J., Dahn J. R. Exercise and Well-Being: A Review of Mental and Physical Health Benefits associated with Physical Activity. *Curr Opin Psychiatry.* 2005;18(2):189–193.

2.  Lazzer S., Rejc E., Del Torto A. Benefits of Aerobic Exercise Training with Recommendations for Healthy Aging. *Annales Kinesiologiae.* 2018;8(2):111–124.

3.  Santos-Parker J. R., LaRocca T. J., Seals D. R. Aerobic Exercise and Other Healthy Lifestyle Factors that Influence Vascular Aging. *Adv Physiol Educ.* 2014;38(4):296–307.

4.  Kemi O. J., Wisløff U. High-Intensity Aerobic Exercise Training Improves the Heart in Health and Disease. *J Cardiopulm Rehabil Prev.* 2010;30(1):2–11.

5.  Mandsager K., Harb S., Cremer P., et al. Association of Cardiorespiratory Fitness With Long-Term Mortality among Adults Undergoing Exercise Treadmill Testing. *JAMA Netw Open.* 2018;1(6):e183605.

# References

6. NHS. Exercise: Physical Activity Guidelines for Adults Aged 19 to 64. https://www.nhs.uk/live-well/exercise/. Accessed June 21, 2019.
7. Farrell S. W., Finley C. E., Haskell W. L., et al. Is There a Gradient of Mortality Risk among Men with Low Cardiorespiratory Fitness? *Med Sci Sport Exerc*. 2015;47(9):1825–1832.
8. Montoya Arizabaleta A. V., Orozco Buitrago L., Aguilar de Plata A. C., et al. Aerobic Exercise During Pregnancy Improves Health-Related Quality of Life: A Randomised Trial. *J Physiother*. 2010;56(4):253–258.
9. Shigematsu R., Chang M., Yabushita N., et al. Dance-Based Aerobic Exercise may Improve Indices of Falling Risk in Older Women. *Age Ageing*. 2002; 31(4):261–266.

## Strength exercise

1. Ruiz J. R., Sui X., Lobelo F., et al. Association between Muscular Strength and Mortality in Men: Prospective Cohort Study. *BMJ*. 2008;337(7661):92–95.
2. Metter E. J., Talbot L. A., Schrager M., et al. Skeletal Muscle Strength as a Predictor of All-Cause Mortality in Healthy Men. *J Gerontol A Biol Sci Med Sci*. 2002;57(10):B359–B365.
3. Newman A. B., Kupelian V., Visser M., et al. Strength, But Not Muscle Mass, is Associated with Mortality in the Health, Aging and Body Composition Study Cohort. *J Gerontol A Biol Sci Med Sci*. 2006;61(1):72–77.
4. Rantanen T., Harris T., Leveille S. G., et al. Muscle Strength and Body Mass Index as Long-Term Predictors of Mortality in Initially Healthy Men. *J Gerontol A Biol Sci Med Sci*. 2000;55(3):M168–M173.
5. NHS. Exercise: Physical Activity Guidelines for Adults Aged 19 to 64. https://www.nhs.uk/live-well/exercise/. Accessed November 21, 2019.
6. NHS. Exercise: How to Improve your Strength and Flexibility. https://www.nhs.uk/live-well/exercise/how-to-improve-strength-flexibility/. Accessed November 21, 2019.
7. Lazzer S., Rejc E., Del Torto A. Benefits of Aerobic Exercise Training with Recommendations for Healthy Aging. *Annales Kinesiologiae*. 2018;8(2): 111–124.

## Standing

1. Biddle S. J. H., Bennie J. A., Bauman A. E., et al. Too Much Sitting and All-Cause Mortality: Is there a Causal Link? *BMC Public Health*. 2016;16:635.
2. Puig-Ribera A., Bort-Roig J., Giné-Garriga M., et al. Impact of a Workplace 'Sit Less, Move More' Program on Efficiency-Related Outcomes of Office Employees. *BMC Public Health*. 2017;17:455.

3. Van Uffelen J. G., Wong J., Chau J. Y., et al. Occupational Sitting and Health Risks: A Systematic Review. *Am J Prev Med*. 2010;39(4):379–388.

4. Stamatakis E., Rogers K., Ding D., et al. All-Cause Mortality Effects of Replacing Sedentary Time with Physical Activity and Sleeping using an Isotemporal Substitution Model: A Prospective Study of 201,129 Mid-Aged and Older Adults. *Int J Behav Nutr Phys Act*. 2015;12:121.

5. Van der Ploeg H. P., Chey T., Ding D., et al. Standing Time and All-Cause Mortality in a Large Cohort of Australian Adults. *Prev Med*. 2014;69:187–191.

6. Sjögren P., Fisher R., Kallings L., et al. Stand Up for Health: Avoiding Sedentary Behaviour might Lengthen your Telomeres: Secondary Outcomes from a Physical Activity RCT in Older People. *Br J Sports Med*. 2014;48(19):1407–1409.

7. Australian Government Department of Health. Australia's Physical Activity and Sedentary Behaviour Guidelines and the Australian 24-Hour Movement Guidelines. https://www1.health.gov.au/internet/main/publishing.nsf/content/health-pubhlth-strateg-phys-act-guidelines#apaadult. Accessed November 21, 2019.

8. Mansfield L., Hall J., Smith L., et al. 'Could you Sit Down Please?' A Qualitative Analysis of Employees' Experiences of Standing in Normally-Seated Workplace Meetings. *PLoS One*. 2018;13(6):e0198483.

## Part Four: Food

### *Five a day*

1. Aune D., Giovannucci E., Boffetta P., et al. Fruit and Vegetable Intake and the Risk of Cardiovascular Disease, Total Cancer and All-Cause Mortality: A Systematic Review and Dose-Response Meta-Analysis of Prospective Studies. *Int J Epidemiol*. 2017;46(3):1029–1056.

2. NHS. Why 5 A Day? https://www.nhs.uk/live-well/eat-well/why-5-a-day/. Accessed June 19, 2019.

3. Liu R. H. Health-Promoting Components of Fruits and Vegetables in the Diet. *Adv Nutr*. 2013;4(3):384S–392S.

4. Ledoux T. A., Hingle M. D., Baranowski T. Relationship of Fruit and Vegetable Intake with Adiposity: A Systematic Review. *Obes Rev*. 2011;12(5):e143–e150.

5. Oyebode O., Gordon-Dseagu V., Walker A., et al. Fruit and Vegetable Consumption and All-Cause, Cancer and CVD Mortality: Analysis of Health Survey for England Data. *J Epidemiol Community Health*. 2014;68(9):856–862.

6. Slavin J. L., Lloyd B. Health Benefits of Fruits and Vegetables. *Adv Nutr*. 2012;3(4):506–516.

7. Hyson D. A. A Review and Critical Analysis of the Scientific Literature Related to 100% Fruit Juice and Human Health. *Adv Nutr.* 2015;6(1):37–51.
8. NHS. 5 A Day portion sizes. https://www.nhs.uk/live-well/eat-well/5-a-day-portion-sizes/. Accessed June 19, 2019.
9. Offringa L. C., Stanton M. V., Hauser M. E., et al. Fruits and Vegetables Versus Vegetables and Fruits: Rhyme and Reason for Word Order in Health Messages. *Am J Lifestyle Med.* 2019;13(3):224–234.
10. Lascari A. D. Carotenemia: A Review. *Clin Pediatr (Phila).* 1981;20(1):25–29.

## Leafy green vegetables

1. Gupta S., Prakash J. Studies on Indian Green Leafy Vegetables for their Antioxidant Activity. *Plant Foods Hum Nutr.* 2009;64(1):39–45.
2. Farha W., El-Aty A., Rahman M., et al. Analytical Approach, Dissipation Pattern and Risk Assessment of Pesticide Residue in Green Leafy Vegetables: A Comprehensive Review. *Biomed Chromatogr.* 2018;32(1):e4134.
3. Slavin J. L., Lloyd B. Health Benefits of Fruits and Vegetables. *Adv Nutr.* 2012;3(4):506–516.
4. Brkić D., Bošnir J., Bevardi M., et al. Nitrate in Leafy Green Vegetables and Estimated Intake. *Afr J Tradit Complement Altern Med.* 2017;14(3):31–41.
5. Latté K. P., Appel K. E., Lampen A. Health Benefits and Possible Risks of Broccoli: An Overview. *Food Chem Toxicol.* 2011;49(12):3287–3309.
6. Chen G. C., Koh W. P., Yuan J. M., et al. Green Leafy and Cruciferous Vegetable Consumption and Risk of Type 2 Diabetes: Results from the Singapore Chinese Health Study and Meta-Analysis. *Br J Nutr.* 2018;119(9):1057–1067.
7. Li M., Fan Y., Zhang X., et al. Fruit and Vegetable Intake and Risk of Type 2 Diabetes Mellitus: Meta-Analysis of Prospective Cohort Studies. *BMJ Open.* 2014;4:e005497.
8. Jia X., Zhong L., Song Y., et al. Consumption of Citrus and Cruciferous Vegetables with Incident Type 2 Diabetes Mellitus based on a Meta-Analysis of Prospective Study. *Prim Care Diabetes.* 2016;10(4):272–280.
9. Van den Driessche J. J., Plat J., Mensink R. P. Effects of Superfoods on Risk Factors of Metabolic Syndrome: A Systematic Review of Human Intervention Trials. *Food Funct.* 2018;9(4):1944–1966.

## Meat

1. NHS. Meat in your diet. https://www.nhs.uk/live-well/eat-well/meat-nutrition/. Accessed November 8, 2019.
2. Virtanen H. E. K., Voutilainen S., Koskinen T. T., et al. Dietary Proteins and Protein Sources and Risk of Death: The Kuopio Ischaemic Heart Disease Risk Factor Study. *Am J Clin Nutr.* 2019;109(5):1462–1471.

3. Rohrmann S., Overvad K., Bueno-de-Mesquita H. B., et al. Meat Consumption and Mortality: Results from the European Prospective Investigation into Cancer and Nutrition. *BMC Med.* 2013;11(63).

4. Abete I., Romaguera D., Vieira A. R., et al. Association between Total, Processed, Red and White Meat Consumption and All-Cause, CVD and IHD Mortality: A Meta-Analysis of Cohort Studies. *Br J Nutr.* 2014;112(5):762–775.

5. Larsson S. C., Orsini N. Red Meat and Processed Meat Consumption and All-Cause Mortality: A Meta-Analysis. *Am J Epidemiol.* 2014;179(3):282–289.

6. Pan A., Sun Q., Bernstein A. M., et al. Red Meat Consumption and Mortality: Results from 2 Prospective Cohort Studies. *Arch Intern Med.* 2012;172(7):555–563.

7. Sinh R., Cross A. K., Graubard B. I., et al. Meat Intake and Mortality: A Prospective Study of over Half a Million People. *Arch Intern Med.* 2009;169(6):562–571.

8. Patrick K. Bacon, Salami and Sausages: How Does Processed Meat Cause Cancer and How Much Matters? Cancer Research UK. April 26, 2019. https://scienceblog.cancerresearchuk.org/2019/04/26/bacon-salami-and-sausages-how-does-processed-meat-cause-cancer-and-how-much-matters/. Accessed February 9, 2020.

9. NHS. Food Poisoning Bug in Chicken. October 7, 2009. https://www.nhs.uk/news/food-and-diet/food-poisoning-bug-in-chicken/. Accessed November 8, 2019.

## Fish and shellfish

1. NHS. Fish and Shellfish. https://www.nhs.uk/live-well/eat-well/fish-and-shellfish-nutrition/. Accessed October 27, 2019.

2. WHO. Mercury and Health. March 31, 2017. https://www.who.int/news-room/fact-sheets/detail/mercury-and-health. Accessed October 25, 2019.

3. Silbernagel S. M., Carpenter D. O., Gilbert S. G., et al. Recognizing and Preventing Overexposure to Methylmercury from Fish and Seafood Consumption: Information for Physicians. *J Toxicol.* 2011: 983072.

4. Cantoral A., Batis C., Basu N. National Estimation of Seafood Consumption in Mexico: Implications for Exposure to Methylmercury and Polyunsaturated Fatty Acids. *Chemosphere.* 2017;174:289–296.

5. Kim H. U. Oroesophageal Fish Bone Foreign Body. *Clin Endosc.* 2016;49(4):318–326.

6. D'Costa H., Bailey F., McGavigan B., et al. Perforation of the Oesophagus and Aorta after Eating Fish: An Unusual Cause of Chest Pain. *Emerg Med J.* 2003;20(4):385–386.

7. NHS. Winter Vomiting Virus 'Found in Most Oysters.' November 29, 2011. https://www.nhs.uk/news/food-and-diet/winter-vomiting-virus-found-in-most-oysters/. Accessed October 27, 2019.
8. Smith A. J., McCarthy N., Saldana L., et al. A Large Foodborne Outbreak of Norovirus in Diners at a Restaurant in England between January and February 2009. *Epidemiol Infect.* 2012;140(9):1695–1701.
9. NIHR. Omega-3 Supplements Do Not Prevent Heart Disease, Stroke or Death. November 6, 2018. https://discover.dc.nihr.ac.uk/content/signal-000670/omega-3-supplements-do-not-prevent-heart-disease-stroke-or-death. Accessed October 27, 2019.

## Dairy products

1. Hess J. M., Jonnalagadda S. S., Slavin J. L. Dairy Foods: Current Evidence of their Effects on Bone, Cardiometabolic, Cognitive, and Digestive Health. *Compr Rev Food Sci Food Saf.* 2016;15(2):251–268.
2. Lisk R., Yeong K. Reducing Mortality from Hip Fractures: A Systematic Quality Improvement Programme. *BMJ Qual Improv Reports.* 2014;3(1):u205006.w2103.
3. Bian S., Hu J., Zhang K., et al. Dairy Product Consumption and Risk of Hip Fracture: A Systematic Review and Meta-Analysis. *BMC Public Health.* 2018;18(1):165.
4. Mazidi M., Mikhailidis D. P., Sattar N., et al. Consumption of Dairy Product and its Association with Total and Cause Specific Mortality: A Population-Based Cohort Study and Meta-Analysis. *Clin Nutr.* 2018;38(6):2833–2845.
5. Lu W., Chen H., Niu Y., et al. Dairy Products Intake and Cancer Mortality Risk: A Meta-Analysis of 11 Population-Based Cohort Studies. *Nutr J.* 2016;15(1):91.
6. Soedamah-Muthu S. S., De Goede J. Dairy Consumption and Cardiometabolic Diseases: Systematic Review and Updated Meta-Analyses of Prospective Cohort Studies. *Curr Nutr Rep.* 2018;7(4):171–182.
7. Gao D., Ning N., Wang C., et al. Dairy Products Consumption and Risk of Type 2 Diabetes: Systematic Review and Dose-Response Meta-Analysis. *PLoS One.* 2013;8(9):e73965.
8. Triggle N. Yoghurts (Even Organic Ones) 'Full of Sugar'. September 19, 2018. https://www.bbc.co.uk/news/health-45565364. Accessed June 27, 2019.
9. De Goede J., Soedamah-Muthu S. S., Pan A., et al. Dairy Consumption and Risk of Stroke: A Systematic Review and Updated Dose-Response Meta-Analysis of Prospective Cohort Studies. *J Am Heart Assoc.* 2016;5(5):e002787.

## Fats and oils

1. NHS. Fat: The Facts. https://www.nhs.uk/live-well/eat-well/different-fats-nutrition/. Accessed October 25, 2019.
2. Willett W. C. Harvard Health Letter – Ask the Doctor: Coconut Oil and Health. August 22, 2018. https://www.health.harvard.edu/staying-healthy/coconut-oil. Accessed March 7, 2020.
3. Malik V. Is there a place for coconut oil in a healthy diet? January 14, 2019. https://www.health.harvard.edu/blog/is-there-a-place-for-coconut-oil-in-a-healthy-diet-2019011415764. Accessed March 7, 2020.
4. BDA. Trans fats. https://www.bda.uk.com/foodfacts/TransFats.pdf. Accessed October 25, 2019.
5. Hooper L., Summerbell C. D., Thompson R., et al. Reduced or Modified Dietary Fat for Preventing Cardiovascular Disease. *Cochrance Database Syst Rev.* 2011;7:CD002137.
6. PREDIMED Study Investigators. Dietary Fat Intake and Risk of Cardiovascular Disease and All-Cause Mortality in a Population at High Risk of Cardiovascular Disease. *Am J Clin Nutr.* 2015;102(6):1563–1573.
7. Shai I., Schwarzfuchs D., Henkin Y., et al. Weight Loss with a Low-Carbohydrate, Mediterranean, or Low-Fat Diet. *N Engl J Med.* 2008;359:229–241.
8. BBC. Which Oils are Best to Cook With? July 28, 2015. https://www.bbc.co.uk/news/magazine-33675975. Accessed October 25, 2019.
9. Falade A. O., Oboh G., Okoh A. I. Potential Health Implications of the Consumption of Thermally-Oxidized Cooking Oils: A Review. *Polish J Food Nutr Sci.* 2017;67(2):95–105.
10. Rekhadevi P. V., Subramanyam R. Evaluation of the Deleterious Health Effects of Consumption of Repeatedly Heated Vegetable Oil. *Toxicol Rep.* 2016;3:636–643.

## Carbs

1. NHS. The Truth about Carbs. https://www.nhs.uk/live-well/healthy-weight/why-we-need-to-eat-carbs/. Accessed July 12, 2019.
2. NHS. Low-Carb or Low-Fat Diet? Both Work Well. February 21, 2018. https://www.nhs.uk/news/food-and-diet/low-carb-or-low-fat-diet-both-work-well/. Accessed July 12, 2019.
3. NHS. Low-Carb Diet 'Could Increase Long-Term Weight Loss'. November 15, 2018. https://www.nhs.uk/news/obesity/low-carb-diet-could-increase-long-term-weight-loss/. Accessed February 1, 2020.
4. NHS. Top Diets Review. https://www.nhs.uk/live-well/healthy-weight/top-diets-review/. Accessed July 12, 2019.

# References

## Vegetarianism and veganism

1. Key T. J., Appleby P. N., Rosell M. S. Health Effects of Vegetarian and Vegan Diets. *Proc Nutr Soc.* 2006;65(1):35–41.
2. Dinu M., Abbate R., Gensini G. F., et al. Vegetarian, Vegan Diets and Multiple Health Outcomes: A Systematic Review with Meta-Analysis of Observational Studies. *Crit Rev Food Sci Nutr.* 2017;57(17): 3640–3649.
3. Orlich M. J., Singh P. N., Sabaté J., et al. Vegetarian Dietary Patterns and Mortality in Adventist Health Study 2. *JAMA Intern Med.* 2013;173(13):1230–1238.
4. Seidelmann S. B., Claggett B., Cheng S., et al. Dietary Carbohydrate Intake and Mortality: A Prospective Cohort Study and Meta-Analysis. *Lancet Public Heal.* 2018;3(9):PE419–E428.
5. Virtanen H. E. K., Voutilainen S., Koskinen T. T., et al. Dietary Proteins and Protein Sources and Risk of Death: The Kuopio Ischaemic Heart Disease Risk Factor Study. *Am J Clin Nutr.* 2019;109(5):1462–1471.
6. Song M., Fung T. T., Hu F. B., et al. Association of Animal and Plant Protein Intake with All-Cause and Cause-Specific Mortality. *JAMA Intern Med.* 2016;176(10):1453–1463.
7. Appleby P. N., Crowe F. L., Bradbury K. E., et al. Mortality in Vegetarians and Comparable Nonvegetarians in the United Kingdom. *Am J Clin Nutr.* 2016;103(1):218–230.
8. Craig W. J. Health Effects of Vegan Diets. *Am J Clin Nutr.* 2009;89(5): 1627S–1633S.

## Herbs, spices and salt

1. Yashin A., Yashin Y., Xia X., et al. Antioxidant Activity of Spices and their Impact on Human Health: A Review. *Antioxidants.* 2017;6(3):70.
2. Rakhi N., Tuwani R., Mukherjee J., et al. Data-Driven Analysis of Biomedical Literature Suggests Broad-Spectrum Benefits of Culinary Herbs and Spices. *PLoS One.* 2018;13(5):e0198030.
3. Jiang T. A. Health Benefits of Culinary Herbs and Spices. *J AOAC Int.* 2019;102(2):395–411.
4. Liguori I., Russo G., Curcio F., et al. Oxidative Stress, Aging, and Diseases. *Clin Interv Aging.* 2018;13:757–772.
5. Tapsell L. C., Hemphill I., Cobiac L., et al. Health Benefits of Herbs and Spices: The Past, The Present, The Future. *Med J Aust.* 2006;185(S4): S1–S24.
6. Jin Z. Y., Waller G., Zhou J. Y., et al. Consumption of Garlic and its Interactions with Tobacco Smoking and Alcohol Drinking on Esophageal Cancer in a Chinese Population. *Eur J Cancer Prev.* 2019;28(4):278–286.

7. Hishikawa N., Takahashi Y., Amakusa Y., et al. Effects of Turmeric on Alzheimer's Disease with Behavioral and Psychological Symptoms of Dementia. *Ayu*. 2012;33(4):499–504.
8. Mishra S., Palanivelu K. The Effect of Curcumin (Turmeric) on Alzheimer's Disease: An Overview. *Ann Indian Acad Neurol*. 2008;11(1):13–19.
9. Wong M. M., Arcand J., Leung A. A., et al. The Science of Salt: A Regularly Updated Systematic Review of Salt and Health Outcomes (December 2015 – March 2016). *J Clin Hypertens*. 2017;19(3):322–332.
10. Huang D. Dietary Antioxidants and Health Promotion. *Antioxidants*. 2018;7(1):E9.
11. Kaefer C. M., Milner J. A. The Role of Herbs and Spices in Cancer Prevention. *J Nutr Biochem*. 2008;19(6):347–361.

## Sugar

1. NHS. How Much Sugar is Good for Me? https://www.nhs.uk/common-health-questions/food-and-diet/how-much-sugar-is-good-for-me/. Accessed July 12, 2019.
2. BHF. Watch: What are Free Sugars? Heart Matters. https://www.bhf.org.uk/informationsupport/heart-matters-magazine/nutrition/sugar-salt-and-fat/free-sugars. Accessed January 18, 2020.
3. Harvard Medical School. Harvard Men's Health Watch – The Sweet Danger of Sugar. November 5, 2019. https://www.health.harvard.edu/heart-health/the-sweet-danger-of-sugar. Accessed March 7, 2020.
4. NHS. The Truth about Carbs. https://www.nhs.uk/live-well/healthy-weight/why-we-need-to-eat-carbs/. Accessed July 12, 2019.
5. NHS. How Does Sugar in our Diet Affect our Health? https://www.nhs.uk/live-well/eat-well/how-does-sugar-in-our-diet-affect-our-health/. Accessed January 18, 2020.
6. NHS. Top Diets Review. https://www.nhs.uk/live-well/healthy-weight/top-diets-review/. Accessed July 12, 2019.

## Artificial sweeteners

1. NHS. The Truth about Sweeteners. https://www.nhs.uk/live-well/eat-well/are-sweeteners-safe/. Accessed January 11, 2020.
2. Saheer P. A., Parmar P., Majid S. A., et al. Effect of Sugar-Free Chewing Gum on Plaque and Gingivitis Among 14–15-Year-Old School Children: A Randomized Controlled Trial. *Indian J Dent Res*. 2019;30(1):61–66.
3. Claxton L., Taylor M., Kay E. Oral Health Promotion: The Economic Benefits to the NHS of Increased Use of Sugarfree Gum in the UK. *Br Dent J*. 2016;220(3):121–127.

## References

4. Carocho M., Morales P., Ferreira I. C. F. R. Sweeteners as Food Additives in the XXI Century: A Review of What Is Known, and What Is to Come. *Food Chem Toxicol.* 2017;107(Pt A):302–317.

5. Mishra A., Ahmed K., Froghi S., et al. Systematic Review of the Relationship between Artificial Sweetener Consumption and Cancer in Humans: Analysis of 599,741 Participants. *Int J Clin Pract.* 2015;69(12):1418–1426.

6. Miller P. E., Perez V. Low-Calorie Sweeteners and Body Weight and Composition: A Meta-Analysis of Randomized Controlled Trials and Prospective Cohort Studies. *Am J Clin Nutr.* 2014;100(3):765–777.

7. NHS. Sweeteners have 'Few Health Benefits', Study Finds. January 3, 2019. https://www.nhs.uk/news/food-and-diet/sweeteners-have-few-health-bene-fits-study-finds/. Accessed January 11, 2020.

8. Azad M. B., Abou-Setta A. M., Chauhan B. F., Rabbani R. Nonnutritive Sweeteners and Cardiometabolic Health: A Systematic Review and Meta-Analysis of Randomized Controlled Trials and Prospective Cohort Studies. *CMAJ.* 2017;189(28):E929–E939.

9. Purohit V., Mishra S. The Truth about Artificial Sweeteners: Are they Good for Diabetics? *Indian Heart J.* 2018;70(1):197–199.

10. Lohner S., Toews I., Meerpohl J. J. Health Outcomes of Non-Nutritive Sweeteners: Analysis of the Research Landscape. *Nutr J.* 2017;16(1):55.

11. Khamverdi Z., Vahedi M., Abdollahzadeh S., et al. Effect of a Common Diet and Regular Beverage on Enamel Erosion in Various Temperatures: An In-Vitro Study. *J Dent.* 2013;10(5):411–416.

## Probiotics

1. NHS. Probiotics. https://www.nhs.uk/conditions/probiotics/. Accessed July 20, 2019.

2. Li J., Zhao F., Wang Y., et al. Gut Microbiota Dysbiosis Contributes to the Development of Hypertension. *Microbiome.* 2017;5(1):14.

3. Nguyen T. T., Kosciolek T., Eyler L. T., et al. Overview and Systematic Review of Studies of Microbiome in Schizophrenia and Bipolar Disorder. *J Psychiatr Res.* 2018;99:50–61.

4. Cohen P. A. Probiotic Safety: No Guarantees. *JAMA Intern Med.* 2018;178(12):1577–1578.

5. Parker E. A., Roy T., D'Adamo C. R., et al. Probiotics and Gastrointestinal Conditions: An Overview of Evidence from the Cochrane Collaboration. *Nutrition.* 2018;45:125–134.

6. Lynch S. V., Pedersen O. The Human Intestinal Microbiome in Health and Disease. *N Engl J Med.* 2016;375(24):2369–2379.

## Nutritional supplements

1. WHO. Malnutrition. February 16, 2018. https://www.who.int/news-room/fact-sheets/detail/malnutrition. Accessed January 16, 2020.
2. WHO. Micronutrient Deficiencies: Iron Deficiency Anaemia. https://www.who.int/nutrition/topics/ida/en/. Accessed January 16, 2020.
3. Pandey A. C., Topol E. J. Dispense with Supplements for Improving Heart Outcomes. *Ann Intern Med.* 2019;171(3):216–217.
4. Gahche J., Bailey R., Burt V., et al. Dietary Supplement Use Among U.S. Adults Has Increased Since NHANES III (1988–1994). *NCHS Data Brief.* 2011;(61):1–8.
5. Wooltorton E. Too Much of a Good Thing? Toxic Effects of Vitamin and Mineral Supplements. *CMAJ.* 2003;169(1):47–48.
6. Chen F., Du M., Blumberg J. B., et al. Association Among Dietary Supplement Use, Nutrient Intake, and Mortality Among U.S. Adults: A Cohort Study. *Ann Intern Med.* 2019;170(9):604–613.
7. NHS. Dietary Supplements 'Do Not Help Improve Health Outcomes' April 9, 2019. https://www.nhs.uk/news/food-and-diet/dietary-supplements-do-not-help-improve-health-outcomes/. Accessed January 16, 2020.
8. NICE. Vitamin D: Supplement Use in Specific Population Groups. August 2017. https://www.nice.org.uk/guidance/ph56/chapter/2-Who-should-take-action. Accessed January 16, 2020.
9. The Vegan Society. Vitamin B12. https://www.vegansociety.com/resources/nutrition-and-health/nutrients/vitamin-b12. Accessed January 16, 2020.

## Obesity

1. WHO. Obesity and Overweight. https://www.who.int/en/news-room/fact-sheets/detail/obesity-and-overweight. Accessed November 7, 2019.
2. NHS. Obesity. https://www.nhs.uk/conditions/obesity/. Accessed November 7, 2019.
3. IHME. Global Burden of Disease. http://www.healthdata.org/gbd. Accessed November 7, 2019.
4. PHE. Adult Obesity: Applying All Our Health. June 17, 2019. https://www.gov.uk/government/publications/adult-obesity-applying-all-our-health/adult-obesity-applying-all-our-health. Accessed November 7, 2019.
5. PHE. *A Guide to Delivering and Commissioning Tier 2 Adult Weight Management Services.* June 2017. https://assets.publishing.service.gov.uk/government/uploads/system/uploads/attachment_data/file/737905/Tier2_adult_weight_management_services__guide.pdf.
6. Gudzune K. A., Doshi R. S., Mehta A. K., et al. Efficacy of Commercial Weight-Loss Programs: An Updated Systematic Review. *Ann Intern Med.* 2015;162(7):501–512.

7. Jolly K., Lewis A., Beach J., et al. Comparison of Range of Commercial or Primary Care Led Weight Reduction Programmes with Minimal Intervention Control for Weight Loss in Obesity: Lighten Up Randomised Controlled Trial. *BMJ*. 2011;343:d6500.
8. NHS. Start Losing Weight. https://www.nhs.uk/live-well/healthy-weight/start-losing-weight/. Accessed November 7, 2019.

## Part Five: Drink

### Green tea

1. Kunyama S., Shimazu T., Ohmon K., et al. Green Tea Consumption and Mortality Due to Cardiovascular Disease, Cancer, and All Causes in Japan: The Ohsaki study. *JAMA*. 2006;296(10):1255–1265.
2. Schneider C., Segre T. Green Tea: Potential Health Benefits. *Am Fam Physician*. 2009;79(7):591–594.
3. Choan E., Segal R., Jonker D., et al. A Prospective Clinical Trial of Green Tea for Hormone Refractory Prostate Cancer: An Evaluation Of The Complementary/Alternative Therapy Approach. *Urol Oncol*. 2005;23(2):108–113.
4. Hayat K., Iqbal H., Malik U., et al. Tea and its Consumption: Benefits and Risks. *Crit Rev Food Sci Nutr*. 2015;55(7):939–954.

### Black tea

1. Tang J., Zheng J. S., Fang L., et al. Tea Consumption and Mortality of All Cancers, CVD and All Causes: A Meta-Analysis of Eighteen Prospective Cohort Studies. *Br J Nutr*. 2015;114(5):673–683.
2. Zhang H., Qi R., Mine Y. The Impact of Oolong and Black Tea Polyphenols on Human Health. *Food Biosci*. 2019;29:55–61.
3. Yan Y., Sui X., Yao B., et al. Is there a Dose-Response Relationship between Tea Consumption and All-Cause, CVD, and Cancer Mortality? *J Am Coll Nutr*. 2017;36(4):281–286.
4. Singh B. N., Rawat A. K. S., Bhagat R. M., et al. Black Tea: Phytochemicals, Cancer Chemoprevention, and Clinical Studies. *Crit Rev Food Sci Nutr*. 2017;57(7):1394–1410.
5. McKay D. L., Blumberg J. B. The Role of Tea in Human Health: An Update. *J Am Coll Nutr*. 2002;21(1):1–13.

### Coffee

1. Freedman N. D., Park Y., Abnet C. C., et al. Association of Coffee Drinking with Total and Cause-Specific Mortality. *N Engl J Med*. 2012;366(20): 1891–1904.

2. Cano-Marquina A., Tarín J. J., Cano A. The Impact of Coffee on Health. *Maturitas.* 2013;75(1):7–21.
3. Ding M., Bhupathiraju S. N., Satija A., et al. Long-Term Coffee Consumption and Risk of Cardiovascular Disease. *Circulation.* 2014;129(6):643–659.
4. Turnbull D., Rodricks J. V., Mariano G. F., et al. Caffeine and Cardiovascular Health. *Regul Toxicol Pharmacol.* 2017;89:165–185.
5. Wikoff D., Welsh B. T., Henderson R., et al. Systematic Review of the Potential Adverse Effects of Caffeine Consumption in Healthy Adults, Pregnant Women, Adolescents, and Children. *Food Chem Toxicol.* 2017;109(Pt 1):585–648.
6. Cappelletti S., Piacentino D., Fineschi V., et al. Caffeine-Related Deaths: Manner of Deaths and Categories at Risk. *Nutrients.* 2018;10(5):E611.
7. Mitchell D. C., Knight C. A., Hockenberry J., et al. Beverage Caffeine Intakes in the U.S. *Food Chem Toxicol.* 2014;63:136–142.
8. Shilo L., Sabbah H., Hadari R., et al. The Effects of Coffee Consumption on Sleep and Melatonin Secretion. *Sleep Med.* 2002;3(3):271–273.

### *Fruit juice and smoothies*

1. Keevil J. G., Osman H. E., Reed J. D., et al. Grape Juice, but not Orange Juice or Grapefruit Juice, Inhibits Human Platelet Aggregation. *J Nutr.* 2000;130(1):53–56.
2. Basu A., Penugonda K. Pomegranate Juice: A Heart-Healthy Fruit Juice. *Nutr Rev.* 2009;67(1):49–56.
3. Hyson D. A. A Review and Critical Analysis of the Scientific Literature Related to 100% Fruit Juice and Human Health. *Adv Nutr.* 2015;6(1):37–51.
4. Committee on Nutrition. The Use and Misuse of Fruit Juice in Pediatrics. *Pediatrics.* 2001;107(5):1210–1213.
5. Abrams S. A., Daniels S. R. Fruit Juice and Child Health. *Pediatrics.* 2017;139(4):e20170041.
6. NHS. Water, Drinks and your Health. https://www.nhs.uk/live-well/eat-well/water-drinks-nutrition/. Accessed June 19, 2019.
7. Imamura F., O'Connor L., Ye Z., et al. Consumption of Sugar Sweetened Beverages, Artificially Sweetened Beverages, and Fruit Juice and Incidence of Type 2 Diabetes: Systematic Review, Meta-Analysis, and Estimation of Population Attributable Fraction. *Br Joural Sport Med.* 2016;50(8):496–504.
8. Eshak E. S., Iso H., Mizoue I., et al. Soft Drink, 100% Fruit Juice, and Vegetable Juice Intakes and Risk of Diabetes Mellitus. *Clin Nutr.* 2013;32(2):300–308.

9. Auerbach B., Littman A., Tinker L., et al. Associations of 100% Fruit Juice Versus Whole Fruit with Hypertension and Diabetes Risk in Postmenopausal Women: Results from the Women's Health Initiative. *Prev Med.* 2017;105:212–218.

## Soft drinks and energy drinks

1. Ni Mhurchu C., Eyles H., Genc M., et al. Twenty Percent Tax on Fizzy Drinks could Save Lives and Generate Millions in Revenue for Health Programmes in New Zealand. *N Z Med J.* 2014;127(1389):92–95.
2. Hodge A. M., Bassett J. K., Milne R. L., et al. Consumption of Sugar-Sweetened and Artificially Sweetened Soft Drinks and Risk of Obesity-Related Cancers. *Public Health Nutr.* 2018;21(9):1618–1626.
3. Briggs A., Mytton O., Kehlbacher A., et al. Health Impact Assessment of the UK Soft Drinks Industry Levy: A Comparative Risk Assessment Modelling Study. *Lancet Public Heal.* 2016;2(1):e15–22.
4. Goryakin Y., Monsivais P., Suhrcke M. Soft Drink Prices, Sales, Body Mass Index and Diabetes: Evidence from a Panel of Low-, Middle- and High-Income Countries. *Food Policy.* 2017;73:88–94.
5. Wikoff D., Welsh B. T., Henderson R., et al. Systematic Review of the Potential Adverse Effects of Caffeine Consumption in Healthy Adults, Pregnant Women, Adolescents, and Children. *Food Chem Toxicol.* 2017;109(Pt 1):585–648.
6. Mitchell D. C., Knight C. A., Hockenberry J., et al. Beverage Caffeine Intakes in the U.S. *Food Chem Toxicol.* 2014;63:136–142.
7. NHS. Warnings Issued over Energy Drinks. October 15, 2014. https://www.nhs.uk/news/food-and-diet/warnings-issued-over-energy-drinks/. Accessed June 19, 2019.
8. NHS. Water, Drinks and your Health. https://www.nhs.uk/live-well/eat-well/water-drinks-nutrition/. Accessed June 19, 2019.
9. Gibson S. Sugar-Sweetened Soft Drinks and Obesity: A Systematic Review of the Evidence from Observational Studies and Interventions. *Nutr Res Rev.* 2008;21(2):134–147.

## Water

1. NHS. Water, Drinks and your Health. https://www.nhs.uk/live-well/eat-well/water-drinks-nutrition/. Accessed October 25, 2019.
2. NHS. Can Fizzy Water Make You Fat? May 15, 2017. https://www.nhs.uk/news/lifestyle-and-exercise/can-fizzy-water-make-you-fat/. Accessed January 9, 2020.
3. Brown C. J., Smith G., Shaw L., et al. The Erosive Potential of Flavoured Sparkling Water Drinks. *Int J Paediatr Dent.* 2007;17(2):86–91.

4. NHS. Six to Eight Glasses of Water 'Still Best.' July 13, 2011. https://www. nhs.uk/news/food-and-diet/six-to-eight-glasses-of-water-still-best/. Accessed January 9, 2020.

5. Stetson D. Myth of 8 Glasses of Water a Day. December 11, 2015. https:// www.med.umich.edu/1libr/Gyn/ObgynClinic/8GlassesWaterMyth.pdf. Accessed January 9, 2020.

6. Mentes J. Oral Hydration in Older Adults: Greater Awareness is Needed in Preventing, Recognizing, and Treating Dehydration. *Am J Nurs.* 2006;106(6):40–49.

7. WHO. Drinking-Water. June 14, 2019. https://www.who.int/en/news-room /fact-sheets/detail/drinking-water. Accessed January 9, 2020.

## Part Six: Vices

### Alcohol

1. WHO. Every Day, About 800 People in Europe Die from Alcohol-Attributable Causes. January 11, 2019. http://www.euro.who.int/en/health-topics/disease-prevention/alcohol-use/news/news/2019/01/every-day,-about-800-people-in-europe-die-from-alcohol-attributable-causes. Accessed June 21, 2019.

2. PHE. Local Alcohol Profiles for England. https://fingertips.phe.org.uk/ profile/local-alcohol-profiles. Accessed June 21, 2019.

3. NHS. The Risks of Drinking Too Much. https://www.nhs.uk/live-well/alcohol-support/the-risks-of-drinking-too-much/. Accessed June 21, 2019.

4. NHS. Statistics on Alcohol, England, 2018. May 1, 2018. https://digital.nhs. uk/data-and-information/publications/statistical/statistics-on-alcohol/2018/ part-6. Accessed June 21, 2019.

5. Møller L. Q&A – How Can I Drink Alcohol Safely? http://www.euro.who. int/en/health-topics/disease-prevention/alcohol-use/data-and-statistics/ q-and-a-how-can-i-drink-alcohol-safely. Accessed June 21, 2019.

6. NHS. New Alcohol Advice Issued: Why have the Guidelines been Revised? June 8, 2016. https://www.nhs.uk/news/food-and-diet/new-alcohol-advice-issued/#why-have-the-guidelines-been-revised. Accessed June 21, 2019.

7. Brierley-Jones L., Ling J., Mccabe K. E., et al. Habitus of Home and Traditional Drinking: A Qualitative Analysis of Reported Middle-Class Alcohol Use. *Sociol Health Illn.* 2014;36(7):1054–1076.

### Smoking

1. WHO. Tobacco. July 26, 2019. https://www.who.int/news-room/fact-sheets /detail/tobacco. Accessed November 20, 2019.

2. NHS. What are the Health Risks of Smoking? https://www.nhs.uk/common-health-questions/lifestyle/what-are-the-health-risks-of-smoking/. Accessed November 20, 2019.

3. NHS. Quit Smoking. https://www.nhs.uk/live-well/quit-smoking/. Accessed November 20, 2019.

4. NHS. E-cigarettes/Vapes. https://www.nhs.uk/smokefree/help-and-advice/e-cigarettes. Accessed November 20, 2019.

5. CDC. Smoking & Tobacco Use: Tobacco-Related Mortality. https://www.cdc.gov/tobacco/data_statistics/fact_sheets/health_effects/tobacco_related_mortality/index.htm. Accessed November 20, 2019.

6. Cancer Research UK. Smoking and Cancer: How Does Smoking Cause Cancer? https://www.cancerresearchuk.org/about-cancer/causes-of-cancer/smoking-and-cancer/shisha-and-other-types-of-tobacco. Accessed November 20, 2019.

## Drugs

1. NHS. The Effects of Drugs. https://www.nhs.uk/live-well/healthy-body/the-effects-of-drugs/. Accessed August 5, 2019.

2. Gossop M., Stewart D., Treacy S., et al. A Prospective Study of Mortality among Drug Misusers during a 4-Year Period after Seeking Treatment. *Addiction.* 2002;97(1):39–47.

3. Mathers B. M., Degenhardt L., Bucello C., et al. Mortality Among People who Inject Drugs: A Systematic Review and Meta-Analysis. *Bull World Health Organ.* 2013;91(2):102–123.

4. National Institute on Drug Abuse. Health Consequences of Drug Misuse: Cardiovascular Effects. https://www.drugabuse.gov/publications/health-consequences-drug-misuse/cardiovascular-effects. Accessed August 5, 2019.

5. National Institute on Drug Abuse. Health Consequences of Drug Misuse. https://www.drugabuse.gov/related-topics/health-consequences-drug-misuse. Accessed August 5, 2019.

6. Hopkins R. E., Dobbin M., Pilgrim J. L. Unintentional Mortality Associated with Paracetamol and Codeine Preparations, With and Without Doxylamine, in Australia. *Forensic Sci Int.* 2018;282:122–126.

7. U.S. Department of Health and Human Services. About the Epidemic: What is the U.S. Opioid Epidemic? https://www.hhs.gov/opioids/about-the-epidemic/index.html. Accessed August 5, 2019.

8. Johnson C. F., Barnsdale L., McAuley A. *Investigating the Role of Benzodiazepines in Drug-Related Mortality: A Systematic Review Undertaken on Behalf of The Scottish National Forum on Drug-Related Deaths.* NHS Health Scotland. February 9, 2016. https://www.scotpho.org.uk/media/1159/scotpho160209-investigating-the-role-of-benzodiazepines-in-drug-related-mortality.pdf. Accessed August 5, 2019.

## Part Seven: Healthcare

### Going to the doctor

1. Taber J. M., Leyva B., Persoskie A. Why do People Avoid Medical Care? A Qualitative Study Using National Data. *J Gen Intern Med.* 2015;30(3):290–297.

2. NHS. *Emerging Evidence on the NHS Health Check: Findings and Recommendations – A report from the Expert Scientific and Clinical Advisory Panel.* February 2017.

3. Cancer Research UK. *Saving Lives, Averting Costs: An Analysis of the Financial Implications of Achieving Earlier Diagnosis of Colorectal, Lung and Ovarian Cancer.* September 2014. https://www.cancerresearchuk.org/sites/default/files/saving_lives_averting_costs.pdf.

4. May M. T. Better to Know: The Importance of Early HIV Diagnosis. *Lancet Public Heal.* 2017;2(1):PE6–E7.

5. Cheatham C. T., Barksdale D. J., Rodgers S. G. Barriers to Health Care and Health-Seeking Behaviors Faced by Black Men. *J Am Acad Nurse Pract.* 2008;20(11):555–562.

6. Conrad D., White A. *Promoting Men's Mental Health.* Radcliffe Publishing; 2010.

7. Conrad D., White A. *Men's Health: How to Do It.* Radcliffe Publishing; 2007.

8. House J., Marasli P., Lister M., et al. Male Views on Help-Seeking for Depression: A Q Methodology Study. *Psycholgy Psychother.* 2018;91(1):117–140.

9. Sagar-Ouriaghli I., Godfrey E., Bridge L., et al. Improving Mental Health Service Utilization among Men: A Systematic Review and Synthesis of Behavior Change Techniques within Interventions Targeting Help-Seeking. *Am J Mens Health.* 2019;13(3):1557988319857009.

10. Seidler Z. E., Dawes A. J., Rice S. M., et al. The Role of Masculinity in Men's Help-Seeking for Depression: A Systematic Review. *Clin Psychol Rev.* 2016;49:106–118.

11. Reynolds L. M., Bissett I. P., Porter D., et al. The 'Ick' Factor Matters: Disgust Prospectively Predicts Avoidance in Chemotherapy Patients. *Ann Behav Med.* 2016;50(6):935–945.

12. Beck J., Greenwood D. A., Blanton L., et al. 2017 National Standards for Diabetes Self-Management Education and Support. *Diabetes Care.* 2017;40(10):1409–1419.

13. WHO. World Bank and WHO: Half the World Lacks Access to Essential Health Services, 100 Million Still Pushed into Extreme Poverty Because of Health Expenses. December 13, 2017. https://www.who.int/news-room/

detail/13-12-2017-world-bank-and-who-half-the-world-lacks-access-to-essential-health-services-100-million-still-pushed-into-extreme-poverty-because-of-health-expenses.

## Going to the dentist

1. Kim J. K., Baker L. A., Davarian S., et al. Oral Health Problems and Mortality. *J Dent Sci.* 2013;8(2):115–120.
2. Jansson L., Lavstedt S., Frithiof L. Relationship Between Oral Health and Mortality Rate. *J Clin Periodontol.* 2002;29(11):1029–1034.
3. Humphrey L. L., Fu R., Buckley D. I., et al. Periodontal Disease and Coronary Heart Disease Incidence: A Systematic Review And Meta-Analysis. *J Gen Intern Med.* 2008;23(12):2079–2086.
4. NHS. The Health Risks of Gum Disease. https://www.nhs.uk/live-well/healthy-body/health-risks-of-gum-disease/. Accessed November 4, 2019.
5. Dhadse P., Gattani D., Mishra R. The Link Between Periodontal Disease and Cardiovascular Disease: How Far We Have Come in Last Two Decades? *J Indian Soc Periodontol.* 2010;14(3):148–154.
6. Lafon A., Pereira B., Dufour T., et al. Periodontal Disease and Stroke: A Meta-Analysis of Cohort Studies. *Eur J Neurol.* 2014;21(9):1155–1161.
7. American Dental Association. Gum Disease Can Raise your Blood Sugar Level. *JADA.* 2013;144(7):860.
8. Millership S. E., Cummins A. J., Irwin D. J. Infection Control Failures in a Dental Surgery: Dilemmas in Incident Management. *J Public Health.* 2007;29(3):303–307.
9. NHS. Local anaesthesia. https://www.nhs.uk/conditions/local-anaesthesia/. Accessed November 4, 2019.
10. Reuter N. G., Westgate P. M., Ingram M., et al. Death Related to Dental Treatment: A Systematic Review. *Oral Surg Oral Med Oral Pathol Oral Radiol.* 2017;123(2):194–204.e10.

## Screening

1. NHS. NHS Screening. https://www.nhs.uk/conditions/nhs-screening/. Accessed July 21, 2019.
2. NHS. Diagnosing Cancer Earlier and Faster. https://www.england.nhs.uk/cancer/early-diagnosis/. Accessed February 2, 2020.
3. Andermann A., Blancquaert I., Beauchamp S., et al. Revisiting Wilson and Jungner in the Genomic Age: A Review of Screening Criteria Over the Past 40 Years. *Bull World Health Organ.* 2008;86(4):317–319.
4. Stang A., Jöckel K. H. The Impact of Cancer Screening on All-Cause Mortality: What Is the Best We Can Expect? *Dtsch Arztebl Int.* 2018;115(29–30):481–486.

5. NHS. *NHS Bowel Cancer Screening Programme: Bowel Scope Screening*. 2019. https://assets.publishing.service.gov.uk/government/uploads/system/uploads/attachment_data/file/708698/Bowel_scope_leaflet.pdf.
6. Zwink N., Holleczek B., Stegmaier C., et al. Complication Rates in Colonoscopy Screening for Cancer. *Dtsch Arztebl Int.* 2017;114(18):321–327.

## Vaccination and immunisation

1. NHS. Why Vaccination is Safe and Important. https://www.nhs.uk/conditions/vaccinations/why-vaccination-is-safe-and-important/. Accessed February 9, 2020.
2. Oxford Vaccine Group. Vaccine Ingredients. https://vk.ovg.ox.ac.uk/vk/vaccine-ingredients. Accessed February 9, 2020.
3. WHO. Immunization Coverage. https://www.who.int/news-room/fact-sheets/detail/immunization-coverage. Accessed July 22, 2019.
4. NHS. Vaccinations. December 6, 2019. https://www.nhs.uk/conditions/vaccinations/. Accessed July 22, 2019.
5. NHS. Travel Vaccinations. https://www.nhs.uk/conditions/travel-vaccinations/. Accessed July 22, 2019.
6. NHS. The Flu Vaccine. https://www.nhs.uk/conditions/vaccinations/flu-influenza-vaccine/. Accessed July 22, 2019.
7. NHS. Bird Flu. https://www.nhs.uk/conditions/bird-flu/. Accessed July 22, 2019.
8. NHS. How the Flu Vaccine Works. https://www.nhs.uk/conditions/vaccinations/how-flu-vaccine-works/. Accessed July 22, 2019.

## Access to quality healthcare

1. Taylor V. M. Cultural Context of Medicine. In: Goldman L., Schafer A., eds. *Goldman's Cecil Medicine*. 24th ed. Saunders; 2011:15–17.
2. WHO. Uneven Access to Health Services Drives Life Expectancy Gaps: WHO. April 4, 2019. https://www.who.int/news-room/detail/04-04-2019-uneven-access-to-health-services-drives-life-expectancy-gaps-who. Accessed January 20, 2020.
3. WHO. Low Quality Healthcare is Increasing the Burden of Illness and Health Costs Globally. July 5, 2018. https://www.who.int/news-room/detail/05-07-2018-low-quality-healthcare-is-increasing-the-burden-of-illness-and-health-costs-globally. Accessed January 20, 2020.
4. WHO. Health care-associated infections. https://www.who.int/gpsc/country_work/gpsc_ccisc_fact_sheet_en.pdf. Accessed January 20, 2020.
5. Sunshine J. E., Meo N., Kassebaum N., et al. Association of Adverse Effects of Medical Treatment with Mortality in the United States: A Secondary Analysis of the Global Burden of Diseases, Injuries, and Risk Factors Study. *JAMA Netw Open.* 2019;2(1):e187041.

6. All-Party Parliamentary Group For Diabetes. *Levelling up: Tackling Variation in Diabetes Care*. All-Party Parliamentary Group for Diabetes. November 2016. https://diabetes-resources-production.s3-eu-west-1.amazonaws.com/diabetes-storage/migration/pdf/0914A_APPG_Report_2016_HC_Nov10.pdf.

7. Appleby J., Raleigh V., Frosini F., et al. *Variations in Health Care: The Good, the Bad and the Inexplicable*. The King's Fund. April 2011. https://www.kingsfund.org.uk/sites/default/files/field/field_publication_file/Variations-in-health-care-good-bad-inexplicable-report-The-Kings-Fund-April-2011.pdf.

8. Greiner A. L. Medical Care in Remote Areas. In: Ciottone G, ed. *Ciottone's Disaster Medicine*. 2nd ed. Elsevier; 2016:334–336.

9. Evans D. B, Hsu J., Boerma T. Universal Health Coverage and Universal Access. *Bulletin of the World Heath Organization*. 2013;91:546–546A.

10. Oertelt-Prigione S. Immune Response: The Impact of Biological Sex and Gender. In: Legato M., ed. *Principles of Gender-Specific Medicine: Gender in the Genomic Era*. 3rd ed. Academic Press; 2017:309–321.

## Part Eight: Home

### *Where You Live*

1. CIA. The World Factbook – Country Comparison: Life Expectancy at Birth. https://www.cia.gov/library/publications/the-world-factbook/rankorder/2102rank.html. Accessed January 22, 2020.

2. The Marmot Review. *Fair Society, Healthy Lives*. February 2010. http://www.instituteofhealthequity.org/resources-reports/fair-society-healthy-lives-the-marmot-review/fair-society-healthy-lives-full-report-pdf.pdf.          Accessed September 3, 2019.

3. Raleigh V. What is Happening to Life Expectancy in the UK? The King's Fund. October 22, 2019. https://www.kingsfund.org.uk/publications/whats-happening-life-expectancy-uk. Accessed January 22, 2020.

4. Gaskin D. J., Roberts E. T., Chan K. S., et al. No Man is an Island: The Impact of Neighborhood Disadvantage on Mortality. *Int J Environ Res Public Health*. 2019;16(7):E1265.

5. WHO. Neighborhood Environments and Urban Form. https://www.who.int/sustainable-development/housing/health-risks/neighborhood-environments/en/. Accessed January 22, 2020.

6. Hobbs M., Griffiths C., Green M. A., et al. Fast-food Outlet Availability and Obesity: Considering Variation by Age and Methodological Diversity in 22,889 Yorkshire Health Study Participants. *Spat Spatiotemporal Epidemiol*. 2019;28:43–53.

7. Small Arms Survey. Direct Conflict Deaths. http://www.smallarmssurvey.org/de/armed-violence/conflict-av/direct-conflict-deaths.html. Accessed January 22, 2020.
8. Small Arms Survey. Broader Impacts of Armed Conflict. http://www.smallarmssurvey.org/de/armed-violence/conflict-armed-violence/broader-impacts-of-armed-conflict.html. Accessed January 22, 2020.
9. The Geneva Declaration. *Global Burden of Armed Violence 2015: Every Body Counts*. 2015. http://www.genevadeclaration.org/measurability/global-burden-of-armed-violence/global-burden-of-armed-violence-2015.html.
10. Wall T. The Private Renters Trapped in Britain's New Slums. *Guardian*. April 13, 2019. https://www.theguardian.com/society/2019/apr/13/trapped-britain-new-slums-poverty-austerity-social-housing. Accessed January 22, 2020.
11. Dayen D. Why the Poor Get Trapped in Depressed Areas. *The New Republic*. March 18, 2016. https://newrepublic.com/article/131743/poor-get-trapped-depressed-areas. Accessed January 22, 2020.

## Pet ownership

1. McNicholas J., Gilbey A., Rennie A., et al. Pet Ownership and Human Health: A Brief Review of Evidence and Issues. *BMJ*. 2005;331:1252–1254.
2. Smith B. The 'Pet Effect': Health Related Aspects of Companion Animal Ownership. *Aust Fam Physician*. 2012;41(6):439–442.
3. Matchock R. L. Pet Ownership and Physical Health. *Curr Opin Psychiatry*. 2015;28(5):386–392.
4. Cutt H., Giles-Corti B., Knuiman M., et al. Dog Ownership, Health and Physical Activity: A Critical Review of the Literature. *Health Place*. 2007;13(1):261–272.
5. Thorpe R. J. Jr, Kreisle R. A., Glickman L. T., et al. Physical Activity and Pet Ownership in Year 3 of the Health ABC Study. *J Aging Phys Act*. 2006;14(2):154–168.
6. Antonacopoulos N. M. D., Pychyl T. A. An Examination of the Potential Role of Pet Ownership, Human Social Support and Pet Attachment in the Psychological Health of Individuals Living Alone. *Anthrozoös*. 2010;23(1):37–54.
7. PHE. Reptiles Pose a Risk of Salmonella Infection. September 29, 2015. https://www.gov.uk/government/news/reptiles-pose-a-risk-of-salmonella-infection. Accessed November 6, 2019.
8. NHS. Toxoplasmosis. https://www.nhs.uk/conditions/toxoplasmosis/. Accessed November 6, 2019.
9. BBC News. Czech Man Mauled to Death by Lion He Kept in Back Yard. March 5, 2019. https://www.bbc.co.uk/news/world-europe-47454610. Accessed November 6, 2019.

10. BBC News. Snake Owner Daniel Brandon Killed by his Pet Python. January 24, 2018. https://www.bbc.co.uk/news/uk-england-hampshire-42801983. Accessed November 6, 2019.

## Home accidents and falls

1. Adams S. Britain's Homes 'Twice as Lethal as its Roads'. *Telegraph*. January 4, 2013. https://www.telegraph.co.uk/news/health/news/9780923/Britains-homes-twice-as-lethal-as-its-roads.html. Accessed August 10, 2019.

2. RoSPA. Home Safety Facts and Figures. https://www.rospa.com/home-safety/advice/general/facts-and-figures/. Accessed August 10, 2019.

3. RoSPA. Home Accident Statistics in Scotland. https://www.rospa.com/Home-Safety/UK/Scotland/Research/Statistics. Accessed August 10, 2019.

4. Building Safer Communities. *Strategic assessment of unintentional harm*. April 2017. http://www.bsc.scot/publications.html. Accessed August 10, 2019.

5. NHS. Falls. https://www.nhs.uk/conditions/falls/. Accessed August 10, 2019.

6. PHE. *A Structured Literature Review to Identify Cost-Effective Interventions to Prevent Falls in Older People Living in the Community*. 2018.

7. Lisk R., Yeong K. Reducing Mortality from Hip Fractures: A Systematic Quality Improvement Programme. *BMJ Qual Improv Reports*. 2014;3(1):u205006.w2103.

8. NHS. Physical Activity Guidelines for Older Adults. https://www.nhs.uk/live-well/exercise/physical-activity-guidelines-older-adults/. Accessed August 10, 2019.

9. Jain M. J., Mavani K. J. A Comprehensive Study of Worldwide Selfie-Related Accidental Mortality: A Growing Problem of the Modern Society. *Int J Inj Contr Saf Promot*. 2017;24(4):544–549.

## Fire risks

1. Home Office. Detailed Analysis of Fires, England; April 2017 to March 2018. https://assets.publishing.service.gov.uk/government/uploads/system/uploads/attachment_data/file/738435/infographic-detailed-analysis-fires-attended-fire-rescue-england-1718-hosb1718.pdf. Accessed August 10, 2019.

2. HSE. Fire Safety. http://www.hse.gov.uk/toolbox/fire.htm. Accessed August 10, 2019.

3. Communities and Local Government. *Fire Safety in the Home*. 2015. https://assets.publishing.service.gov.uk/government/uploads/system/uploads/attachment_data/file/564803/Fire-Safety-in-the-Home.pdf. Accessed August 10, 2019.

4. Rohde D., Corcoran J., Sydes M., et al. The Association between Smoke Alarm Presence and Injury and Death Rates: A Systematic Review and Meta-Analysis. *Fire Saf J*. 2016;81:58–63.

5. Istre G. R., Mallonee S. Smoke Alarms and Prevention of House-Fire: Related Deaths and Injuries. *West J Med.* 2000;173(2):92–93.
6. Home Office. *Fire and Rescue Incident Statistics, England: Year Ending December 2018.* 2019. https://assets.publishing.service.gov.uk/government/uploads/system/uploads/attachment_data/file/800492/fire-and-rescue-incident-dec18-hosb0619.pdf. Accessed August 10, 2019.

## Damp, cold and mould

1. WHO Europe. Damp and Mould: Health Risks, Prevention and Remedial Action. 2009. http://www.euro.who.int/__data/assets/pdf_file/0003/78636/Damp_Mould_Brochure.pdf. Accessed September 3, 2019.
2. NHS. Can Damp and Mould Affect my Health? https://www.nhs.uk/common-health-questions/lifestyle/can-damp-and-mould-affect-my-health/. Accessed September 3, 2019.
3. NHS. How Do I Get Rid of Damp and Mould? https://www.nhs.uk/common-health-questions/lifestyle/how-do-i-get-rid-of-damp-and-mould/. Accessed September 3, 2019.
4. PHE. Health Risks of Cold Homes: Data Sources. January 15, 2019. https://www.gov.uk/government/publications/health-risks-of-cold-homes-data-sources. Accessed September 3, 2019.
5. Hajat S., Gasparrini A. The Excess Winter Deaths Measure: Why Its Use is Misleading for Public Health Understanding of Cold-Related Health Impacts. *Epidemiology.* 2016;27(4):486–491.
6. Evans J., Hyndman S., Stewart-Brown S., et al. An Epidemiological Study of the Relative Importance of Damp Housing in Relation to Adult Health. *J Epidemiol Community Health.* 2000;54(9):677–686.
7. Department for Business, Energy & Industrial Strategy. *Annual Fuel Poverty Statistics in England, 2019 (2017 Data).* June 13, 2019. https://assets.publishing.service.gov.uk/government/uploads/system/uploads/attachment_data/file/808534/Annual_Fuel_Poverty_Statistics_Report_2019__2017_data_.pdf. Accessed September 3, 2019.

## Asbestos

1. British Lung Foundation. What is Asbestos? https://www.blf.org.uk/support-for-you/asbestos-related-conditions/what-is-asbestos. Accessed September 2, 2019.
2. HSE. *Asbestos-Related Disease Statistics in Great Britain, 2019.* http://www.hse.gov.uk/statistics/causdis/asbestos-related-disease.pdf. Accessed March 8, 2020.
3. HSE. Asbestos Related Disease. http://www.hse.gov.uk/statistics/causdis/asbestos.htm. Accessed September 2, 2019.

4. HSE. *Mesothelioma Mortality by Occupation.* http://www.hse.gov.uk/statistics/causdis/mesothelioma/mesothelioma-mortality-by-occupation-2002-2015.pdf. Accessed September 2, 2019.
5. WHO. Asbestos. https://www.who.int/ipcs/assessment/public_health/asbestos/en/. Accessed September 2, 2019.
6. Dartford Borough Council. What To Do if you have Asbestos. https://www.dartford.gov.uk/by-category/environment-and-planning2/Environmental-Health-Homepage/pollution/what-to-do-if-you-have-asbestos.   Accessed September 2, 2019.
7. United States Environmental Protection Agency. Protect Your Family from Exposures to Asbestos. https://www.epa.gov/asbestos/protect-your-family-exposures-asbestos. Accessed September 2, 2019.

## Scented candles and air fresheners

1. Petry T., Vitale D., Joachim F. J., et al. Human Health Risk Evaluation of Selected VOC, SVOC and Particulate Emissions from Scented Candles. *Regul Toxicol Pharmacol.* 2014;69(1):55–70.
2. Steinemann A. Ten Questions Concerning Air Fresheners and Indoor Built Environments. *Build Environ.* 2017;111:279–284.
3. Bridges B. Fragrance: Emerging Health and Environmental Concerns. *Flavour Fragr J.* 2002;17(5):361–371.
4. Karr G., Albinet A., Quivet E., et al. Scented Candles and Incenses as Indoor Air Fresheners: Health Risk Assessment from Real Emission Measurements. International Conference on Indoor Air Quality and Climate (Indoor Air 2016). Ghent; 2016. https://hal-ineris.archives-ouvertes.fr/ineris-01863023/.
5. Apte K., Salvi S. Household Air Pollution and its Effects on Health. *F1000Res.* 2016;5:F1000.
6. WHO. Indoor Air Pollution. November 2014. https://www.who.int/features/qa/indoor-air-pollution/en/. Accessed November 18, 2019.

## Cleaning products

1. Svanes Ø., Bertelsen R. J., Lygre S. H. L., et al. Cleaning at Home and at Work in Relation to Lung Function Decline and Airway Obstruction. *Am J Respir Crit Care Med.* 2018;197(9):1157–1163.
2. Dumas O., Donnay C., Heederik D. J., et al. Occupational Exposure to Cleaning Products and Asthma in Hospital Workers. *Occup Environ Med.* 2012;69(12):883–889.
3. McKenzie L. B., Ahir N., Stolz U., et al. Household Cleaning Product-Related Injuries Treated in US Emergency Departments in 1990–2006. *Pediatrics.* 2010;126(3):509–516.

## DIY

1. RoSPA. Do DIY Safely this Bank Holiday. May 23, 2018. https://www.rospa. com/media-centre/press-office/press-releases/detail/?id=1578. Accessed June 27, 2019.
2. Smeaton Z. A Catalogue of DIY Disasters. BBC News Magazine. August 10, 2005. http://news.bbc.co.uk/1/hi/magazine/4134074.stm. Accessed June 27, 2019.
3. Vallmuur K., Eley R., Watson A. Falls from Ladders in Australia: Comparing Occupational and Non-Occupational Injuries Across Age Groups. *Aust N Z J Public Health*. 2016;40(6):559–563.
4. Janík M., Straka Ľ., Novomeský F., et al. Circular Saw-Related Fatalities: A Rare Case Report, Review of the Literature, and Forensic Implications. *Leg Med*. 2016;18:52–57.
5. Judge C., Eley R., Miyakawa-Liu M., et al. Characteristics of Accidental Injuries from Power Tools Treated at Two Emergency Departments in Queensland. *Emerg Med Australas*. 2019;31(3):436–443.
6. Royal College of Surgeons. Don't Cut your Summer Short with a Gardening or DIY Accident this Bank Holiday Weekend, Surgeons Warn. May 24, 2018. https://www.rcseng.ac.uk/news-and-events/media-centre/press-releases/gardening-and-diy-accidents/. Accessed June 27, 2019.
7. Macera C. A. Housework Will Not Prevent Death in Middle Age but Sports and DIY Might. *Clin J Sport Med*. 2012;22(6):521–522.

## Gardening

1. Buck D. *Gardens and Health: Implications for Policy and Practice*. The King's Fund; 2016. https://www.kingsfund.org.uk/sites/default/files/field/field_ publication_file/Gardens_and_health.pdf.
2. NHS. Can DIY and Gardening Help You Live Longer? October 29, 2013. https://www.nhs.uk/news/lifestyle-and-exercise/can-diy-and-gardening-help-you-live-longer/. Accessed November 4, 2019.
3. Brooks-Pollock T. Gardener 'Died After Brushing Past Poisonous Plant' in Millionaire's Garden. *Telegraph*. November 6, 2004. https://www.telegraph. co.uk/news/uknews/law-and-order/11213530/Gardener-died-after-brushing -past-poisonous-plant-in-millionaires-garden.html. Accessed October 31, 2019.
4. NHS. Do I Need a Tetanus Jab (Vaccine) After an Accident or Injury? https: //www.nhs.uk/common-health-questions/accidents-first-aid-and-treatments/ do-i-need-a-tetanus-jab-vaccine-after-an-accident-or-injury/.     Accessed November 4, 2019.
5. NHS. Vaccinations. https://www.nhs.uk/conditions/vaccinations/. Accessed July 22, 2019.

6.  RoSPA. Do DIY Safely this Bank Holiday. May 23, 2018. https://www.rospa.com/media-centre/press-office/press-releases/detail/?id=1578. Accessed June 27, 2019.
7.  Judge C., Eley R., Miyakawa-Liu M., et al. Characteristics of Accidental Injuries from Power Tools Treated at Two Emergency Departments in Queensland. *Emerg Med Australas*. 2019;31(3):436–443.
8.  Australian Institute of Health and Welfare. *DIY Injuries Fact Sheet*. 2017. https://www.braininjuryaustralia.org.au/wp-content/uploads/AIHWdiyinjury2014.pdf.
9.  Bhogal G., Tomlins P. J., Murray P. Penetrating Ocular Injuries in the Home. *J Public Health*. 2007;29(1):72–74.
10. Royal College of Surgeons. Don't Cut your Summer Short with a Gardening or DIY Accident this Bank Holiday Weekend, Surgeons Warn. May 24, 2018. https://www.rcseng.ac.uk/news-and-events/media-centre/press-releases/gardening-and-diy-accidents/. Accessed November 4, 2019.

# Part Nine: Environment

## *Weedkiller and pesticides*

1.  Kim K. H., Kabir E., Jahan S. A. Exposure to Pesticides and the Associated Human Health Effects. *Sci Total Environ*. 2017;575:525–535.
2.  US Department of Health and Human Services. Glyphosate & Glyphosate Formulations. https://ntp.niehs.nih.gov/whatwestudy/topics/glyphosate/index.html. Accessed January 9, 2020.
3.  European Food Safety Authority. Conclusion on the Peer Review of the Pesticide Risk Assessment of the Active Substance Glyphosate. *EFSA J*. 2015;13(11):4302.
4.  NHS. How to wash fruit and vegetables. https://www.nhs.uk/live-well/eat-well/how-to-wash-fruit-and-vegetables/. Accessed January 9, 2020.
5.  Food Standards Agency. Pesticides in Food: Legislation. https://www.food.gov.uk/business-guidance/pesticides-in-food#legislation. Accessed January 9, 2020.
6.  Blair A., Ritz B., Wesseling C., et al. Pesticides and Human Health. *Occup Environ Med*. 2015;72(2):81–82

## *Nature*

1.  World Health Organization. Environmental Health in Emergencies: Natural Events. https://www.who.int/environmental_health_emergencies/natural_events/en/. Accessed November 6, 2019.
2.  Richardson M., Cormack A., McRobert L., et al. 30 Days Wild: Development and Evaluation of a Large-Scale Nature Engagement Campaign to Improve Well-Being. *PLoS One*. 2016;11(2):e0149777.

3. Gladwell V. F., Brown D. K., Wood C., et al. The Great Outdoors: How a Green Exercise Environment can Benefit All. *Extrem Physiol Med*. 2013;2:3.

4. Frumkin H., Bratman G. N., Breslow S. J., et al. Nature Contact and Human Health: A Research Agenda. *Env Heal Perspect*. 2017;125(7):075001.

5. Elsworthy E. Over-Reliance on Screens can be 'Damaging', Psychologist Warns. *Independent*. March 2, 2018. https://www.independent.co.uk/news/uk/home-news/screen-time-damaging-psychologist-study-six-hours-average-a8237441.html. Accessed January 4, 2020.

6. Thompson Coon J., Boddy K., Stein K., et al. Does Participating in Physical Activity in Outdoor Natural Environments have a Greater Effect on Physical and Mental Wellbeing than Physical Activity Indoors? A Systematic Review. *Env Sci Technol*. 2011;45(5):1761–1772.

7. Shanahan D. F., Bush R., Gaston K. J., et al. Health Benefits from Nature Experiences Depend on Dose. *Sci Rep*. 2016;6:28551.

8. Van Heezik Y., Brymer E. Nature as a Commodity: What's Good for Human Health Might Not Be Good for Ecosystem Health. *Front Psychol*. 2018;9:1673.

9. Shanahan D. F., Fuller R. A., Bush R. A., et al. The Health Benefits of Urban Nature: How Much Do We Need? *Bioscience*. 2015;65(5):476–485.

10. Pretty J., Peacock J., Sellens M., et al. The Mental and Physical Health Outcomes of Green Exercise. *Int J Env Heal Res*. 2005;15(5):319–337.

11. Brown D. K., Barton J. L., Gladwell V. F. Viewing Nature Scenes Positively Affects Recovery of Autonomic Function Following Acute-Mental Stress. *Environ Sci Technol*. 2013;47(11):5562–5569.

## *Air pollution*

1. WHO. Mortality and Burden of Disease from Ambient Air Pollution. https://www.who.int/gho/phe/outdoor_air_pollution/burden_text/en/. Accessed December 27, 2019.

2. PHE. *Associations of Long-Term Average Concentrations of Nitrogen Dioxide with Mortality (2018): COMEAP Summary*. August 22, 2018. https://www.gov.uk/government/publications/nitrogen-dioxide-effects-on-mortality/associations-of-long-term-average-concentrations-of-nitrogen-dioxide-with-mortality-2018-comeap-summary.

3. DEFRA. Causes of Air Pollution. https://uk-air.defra.gov.uk/air-pollution/causes. Accessed December 27, 2019.

4. PHE. *Review of Interventions to Improve Outdoor Air Quality and Public Health*. 2019. https://assets.publishing.service.gov.uk/government/uploads/system/uploads/attachment_data/file/795185/Review_of_interventions_to_improve_air_quality.pdf.

5. Laumbach R., Meng Q., Kipen H. What can Individuals Do to Reduce Personal Health Risks from Air Pollution? *J Thorac Dis*. 2015;7(1):96–107.

6. Cherrie J. W., Apsley A., Cowie H., et al. Effectiveness of Face Masks used to Protect Beijing Residents Against Particulate Air Pollution. *Occup Environ Med.* 2018;75(6):446–452.

## Natural disasters

1. WHO. Environmental Health in Emergencies: Natural Events. https://www. who.int/environmental_health_emergencies/natural_events/en/. Accessed November 6, 2019.
2. Below R., Wallemacq P. *Annual Disaster Statistical Review 2017.* Centre for Research on the Epidemiology of Disasters; 2018. https://www.cred.be/ annual-disaster-statistical-review-2017.
3. Vos F., Rodriguez J., Below R., et al. *Annual Disaster Statistical Review 2009 The Numbers and Trends.* Centre for Research on the Epidemiology of Disasters; 2010. https://www.who.int/hac/techguidance/ems/annual_disaster_statistical_review_2009.pdf?ua=1.
4. WHO. Mosquito-Borne Diseases. https://www.who.int/neglected_diseases/vector_ecology/mosquito-borne-diseases/en/. Accessed November 6, 2019.

# Part Ten: Beauty

## Facial attractiveness

1. Foo Y. Z., Simmons L. W., Rhodes G. Predictors of Facial Attractiveness and Health in Humans. *Sci Rep.* 2017;7:39731.
2. Little A. C. Facial Attractiveness. *WIREs Cogn Sci.* 2014;5(6):621–634.
3. Simmons L. W., Rhodes G., Peters M., et al. Are Human Preferences for Facial Symmetry Focused on Signals of Developmental Instability? *Behav Ecol.* 2004;15(5):864–871.
4. Trujillo L. T., Jankowitsch J. M., Langlois J. H. Beauty is in the Ease of the Beholding: A Neurophysiological Test of the Averageness Theory of Facial Attractiveness. *Cogn Affect Behav Neurosci.* 2014;14(3):1061–1076.
5. Scholz J. K., Sicinski K. Facial Attractiveness and Lifetime Earnings: Evidence from a Cohort Study. *Rev Econ Stat.* 2015;97(1):14–28.
6. De Jager S., Coetzee N., Coetzee V. Facial Adiposity, Attractiveness, and Health: A Review. *Front Psychol.* 2018;9:2562.
7. Reither E. N., Hauser R. M., Swallen K. C. Predicting Adult Health and Mortality from Adolescent Facial Characteristics in Yearbook Photographs. *Demography.* 2009;46(1):27–41.
8. Re D. E., Tskhay K. O., Tong M.-O., et al. Facing Fate: Estimates of Longevity from Facial Appearance and their Underlying Cues. *Arch Sci Psychol.* 2015;3(1):30–36.

9. Dykiert D., Bates T. C., Gow A. J., et al. Predicting Mortality from Human Faces. *Psychosom Med.* 2012;74(6):560–566.
10. Rhodes G., Zebrowitz L. A., Clark A., et al. Do Facial Averageness and Symmetry Signal Health? *Evol Hum Behav.* 2001;22(1):31–46.
11. Weeden J., Sabini J. Physical Attractiveness and Health in Western Societies: A Review. *Psychol Bull.* 2005;131(5):635–653.
12. Kanazawa S., Still M. C. Is There Really a Beauty Premium or an Ugliness Penalty on Earnings? *J Bus Psychol.* 2018;33:249–262.

## Sunbathing and tanning

1. Cancer Research UK. How Does the Sun and UV Cause Cancer? https://www.cancerresearchuk.org/about-cancer/causes-of-cancer/sun-uv-and-cancer/how-does-the-sun-and-uv-cause-cancer. Accessed December 23, 2019.
2. Karimkhani C., Green A. C., Nijsten T., et al. The Global Burden of Melanoma: Results from the Global Burden of Disease Study 2015. *Br J Dermatol.* 2017;177(1):134–140.
3. NHS. Sunscreen and Sun Safety. https://www.nhs.uk/live-well/healthy-body/sunscreen-and-sun-safety/. Accessed December 23, 2019.
4. Suppa M., Gandini S. Sunbeds and Melanoma Risk: Time to Close the Debate. *Curr Opin Oncol.* 2019;31(2):65–71.
5. Suppa M., Gandini S., Bulliard J. L., et al. Who, Why, Where: An Overview of Determinants of Sunbed Use in Europe. *J Eur Acad Dermatology Vereology.* 2019;33(S2):6–12.
6. NHS. New NICE Guidelines on Sun Exposure Warn 'Tanning is Unsafe'. February 10, 2016. https://www.nhs.uk/news/cancer/new-nice-guidelines-on-sun-exposure-warn-tanning-is-unsafe/. Accessed December 23, 2019.
7. NICE. Sunlight Exposure: Risks and Benefits. February 2016. https://www.nice.org.uk/guidance/ng34. Accessed December 23, 2019.

## Hair dye

1. Kim K. H., Kabir E., Jahan S. A. The Use of Personal Hair Dye and its Implications for Human Health. *Environ Int.* 2016;89–90:222–227.
2. Nohynek G. J., Fautz R., Benech-Kieffer F., et al. Toxicity and Human Health Risk of Hair Dyes. *Food Chem Toxicol.* 2004;42(4):517–543.
3. Towle K. M., Grespin M. E., Monnot A. D. Personal Use of Hair Dyes and Risk of Leukemia: A Systematic Literature Review and Meta-Analysis. *Cancer Med.* 2017;6(10):2471–2486.
4. Vedel-Krogh S., Nielsen S., Schnohr P., et al. Morbidity and Mortality in 7,684 Women According to Personal Hair Dye Use: The Copenhagen City Heart Study followed for 37 Years. *PLoS One.* 2016;11(3):e0151636.

5. Eberle C. E., Sandler D. P., Taylor K. W., et al. Hair Dye and Chemical Straightener Use and Breast Cancer Risk in a Large US Population of Black and White Women. *Int J Cancer.* 2019:10.1002/ijc.32738.
6. McFadden J. P., White I. R., Frosch P. J., et al. Allergy to Hair Dye. *BMJ.* 2007;334(7587):220.

## Cosmetics, talc and antiperspirant

1. Pines A. Cosmetics and Women's Health. *Maturitas.* 2017;100:113.
2. Michalek I. M., Benn E. K. T., Dos Santos F. L. C., et al. A Systematic Review of Global Legal Regulations on the Permissible Level of Heavy Metals in Cosmetics with Particular Emphasis on Skin Lightening Products. *Environ Res.* 2019;170:187–193.
3. Faber S. On Cosmetics Safety, U.S. Trails More Than 40 Nations. EWG. March 20, 2019. https://www.ewg.org/news-and-analysis/2019/03/cosmetics-safety-us-trails-more-40-nations. Accessed October 16, 2019.
4. Campaign for Safe Cosmetics. Chemicals of Concern. http://www.safecosmetics.org/get-the-facts/chem-of-concern/. Accessed October 16, 2019.
5. Cunningham V. 10 Toxic Beauty Ingredients to Avoid. HuffPost. January 23, 2014.https://www.huffpost.com/entry/dangerous-beauty-products_b_4168587?guccounter=2. Accessed October 17, 2019.
6. US Food & Drug Administration. Cosmetics Safety Q&A: Parabens. https://www.fda.gov/cosmetics/resources-consumers-cosmetics/cosmetics-safety-qa-parabens. Accessed October 17, 2019.
7. National Cancer Institute. Antiperspirants/Deodorants and Breast Cancer. August 9, 2016. https://www.cancer.gov/about-cancer/causes-prevention/risk/myths/antiperspirants-fact-sheet. Accessed March 7, 2020.
8. Zhao D., Li J., Li C., et al. Lead Relative Bioavailability in Lip Products and their Potential Health Risk to Women. *Environ Sci Technol.* 2016;50(11):6036–6043.
9. Ababneh F. A., Al-Momani I. F. Assessments of Toxic Heavy Metals Contamination in Cosmetic Products. *Environ Forensics.* 2018;19(2):134–142.
10. WHO. *Mercury in Skin Lightening Products.* 2019. https://www.who.int/ipcs/assessment/public_health/mercury_flyer.pdf. Accessed October 17, 2019.
11. Perez A. L., Nembhard M., Monnot A., et al. Child and Adult Exposure and Health Risk Evaluation Following the Use of Metal- and Metalloid-Containing Costume Cosmetics Sold in the United States. *Regul Toxicol Pharmacol.* 2017;84:54–63.
12. Brzóska M. M., Galażyn-Sidorczuk M., Borowska S. Metals in Cosmetics. In: Chen J. K., Thyssen J. P., eds. *Metal Allergy.* Springer International Publishing; 2018:177–196.

13. Kwa M., Welty L. J., Xu S. Adverse Events Reported to the US Food and Drug Administration for Cosmetics and Personal Care Products. *JAMA Intern Med*. 2017;177(8):1202–1204.
14. US Food & Drug Administration. 'Hypoallergenic' Cosmetics. https://www.fda.gov/cosmetics/cosmetics-labeling-claims/hypoallergenic-cosmetics. Accessed October 17, 2019.
15. Jacob S. L., Cornell E., Kwa M., et al. Cosmetics and Cancer: Adverse Event Reports Submitted to the Food and Drug Administration. *JNCI Cancer Spectr*. 2018;2(2):pky012.
16. NHS. Talc and Ovarian Cancer: What the Most Recent Evidence Shows. March 8, 2016. https://www.nhs.uk/news/cancer/talc-and-ovarian-cancer-what-the-most-recent-evidence-shows/. Accessed October 17, 2019.
17. American Cancer Society. Talcum Powder and Cancer. http://www.cancer.org/cancer/cancer-causes/talcum-powder-and-cancer.html. Accessed October 17, 2019.
18. US Food & Drug Administration. Cosmetics Safety Q&A: Contaminants. https://www.fda.gov/cosmetics/resources-consumers-cosmetics/cosmetics-safety-qa-contaminants. Accessed October 17, 2019.
19. US Food & Drug Administration. FDA Advises Consumers to Stop Using Certain Cosmetic Products. https://www.fda.gov/cosmetics/cosmetics-recalls-alerts/fda-advises-consumers-stop-using-certain-cosmetic-products. Accessed October 17, 2019.

## Cosmetic surgery

1. Bucknor A., Egeler S. A., Chen A. D., et al. National Mortality Rates after Outpatient Cosmetic Surgery and Low Rates of Perioperative Deep Vein Thrombosis Screening and Prophylaxis. *Plast Reconstr Surg*. 2018;142(1):90–98.
2. Rapkiewicz A. V., Kenerson K., Hutchins K. D., et al. Fatal Complications of Aesthetic Techniques: The Gluteal Region. *J Forensic Sci*. 2018;63(5):1406–1412.
3. Izundu C. C. Second Brit dies after 'Brazilian Butt Lift' Surgery. BBC News. October 4, 2018. https://www.bbc.co.uk/news/health-45731191. Accessed October 16, 2019.
4. Lee J. C., Morrison K. A., Chang M. M., et al. Abstract: Is Cosmetic Surgery Tourism Worth It? A Cost Analysis of Nontuberculous Mycobacterium Surgical Site Infections Contracted Abroad. *Plast Reconstr Surg Glob Open*. 2016;4(9 Suppl):28–29.
5. Klein H. J., Simic D., Fuchs N., et al. Complications after Cosmetic Surgery Tourism. *Aesthetic Surg J*. 2017;37(4):474–482.
6. Brightman L., Ng S., Ahern S., et al. Cosmetic Tourism for Breast Augmentation: A Systematic Review. *ANZ J Surg*. 2018;88(9):842–847.

7. NHS. Cosmetic Procedures – Choosing Who will do your Cosmetic Procedure. https://www.nhs.uk/conditions/cosmetic-procedures/choosing-who-will-do-your-procedure/. Accessed October 16, 2019.
8. NHS. Cosmetic Procedures – Face and Lip Fillers (Dermal Fillers). https://www.nhs.uk/conditions/cosmetic-procedures/dermal-fillers/.        Accessed October 16, 2019.

## Part Eleven: Transport

### Air travel

1. ICAO. *State of Global Aviation Safety.* 2019. https://www.icao.int/safety/Documents/ICAO_SR_2019_29082019.pdf.
2. EUROSTAT. Air Safety Statistics in the EU. July 2019. https://ec.europa.eu/eurostat/statistics-explained/index.php/Air_safety_statistics_in_the_EU. Accessed December 27, 2019.
3. IHSF. Continuing Decrease for Helicopter Accidents in Key Regions Around the World. 2018. http://www.ihst.org/Default.aspx?tabid=1507&mid=2918&newsid2918=64036&language=en-US. Accessed December 27, 2019.
4. Federal Aviation Administration. Fact Sheet – General Aviation Safety. July 30, 2018. https://www.faa.gov/news/fact_sheets/news_story.cfm?newsId=21274. Accessed March 7, 2020.
5. NTSB. NTSB News Release: U.S. Aviation Fatalities Increased in 2018. November 14, 2019. https://www.ntsb.gov/news/press-releases/Pages/NR20191114.aspx. Accessed March 7, 2020.
6. Gigerenzer G. Dread Risk, September 11, and Fatal Traffic Accidents. *Psychol Sci.* 2004;15(4):286–287.

### Trains

1. International Railway Safety Council. Railway Safety: Safety Statistics. https://international-railway-safety-council.com/safety-statistics/. Accessed January 9, 2020.
2. Office of Rail and Road. Rail Safety. https://dataportal.orr.gov.uk/statistics/health-and-safety/rail-safety/. Accessed January 9, 2020.

### Motor vehicles

1. National Highway Traffic Safety Administration. *Quick Facts 2017.* July 2019. https://crashstats.nhtsa.dot.gov/Api/Public/ViewPublication/812747.
2. Department for Transport. *Reported Road Casualties in Great Britain: Main Results 2018.* July 25, 2019. https://assets.publishing.service.gov.uk/

government/uploads/system/uploads/attachment_data/file/820562/
Reported_road_casualties_-_Main_Results_2018.pdf.

3. United States Department of Transportation. Transportation Fatalities by Mode. https://www.bts.gov/content/transportation-fatalities-mode. Accessed February 5, 2020.

4. BBC News. Bolivia Crash: Bus Plunges into Ravine Killing 25. April 23, 2019. https://www.bbc.co.uk/news/world-latin-america-48021650. Accessed February 5, 2020.

5. National Highway Traffic Safety Administration. *Traffic Safety Facts 2017 Data*. August 2019. https://crashstats.nhtsa.dot.gov/Api/Public/ViewPublication/812785.

6. RoSPA. *Driver Distraction Factsheet*. July 2017. https://www.rospa.com/rospaweb/docs/advice-services/road-safety/drivers/driver-distraction.pdf.

7. RoSPA. *Mobile Phones and Driving Factsheet*. July 2018. https://www.rospa.com/media/documents/road-safety/mobile-phones-and-driving-factsheet.pdf.

8. RoSPA. *Satellite Navigation (Sat Nav) Devices Factsheet*. April 2018. https://www.rospa.com/rospaweb/docs/advice-services/road-safety/vehicles/satnav.pdf.

## Cycling

1. NHS. Cycling for Beginners. https://www.nhs.uk/live-well/exercise/cycling-for-beginners/. Accessed October 17, 2019.

2. RoSPA. *Cycling Accidents*. November 2017. https://www.rospa.com/rospaweb/docs/advice-services/road-safety/cyclists/cycling-accidents-factsheet.pdf. Accessed October 17, 2019.

3. National Highway Traffic Safety Administration. *Quick Facts 2017*. July 2019. https://crashstats.nhtsa.dot.gov/Api/Public/ViewPublication/812747. Accessed October 17, 2019.

4. National Highway Traffic Safety Administration. *Traffic Safety Facts 2017 Data: Bicyclists and Other Cyclists*. July 2019. https://crashstats.nhtsa.dot.gov/Api/Public/ViewPublication/812765. Accessed October 17, 2019.

5. NHS. *Cycle Safe*. https://www.uhb.nhs.uk/Downloads/pdf/CycleSafeLeaflet.pdf. Accessed October 17, 2019.

6. RoSPA. *Cycle Helmets*. March 2018. https://www.rospa.com/rospaweb/docs/advice-services/road-safety/cyclists/cycle-helmets-factsheet.pdf. Accessed October 17, 2019.

7. BBC News. 'Death by Dangerous Cycling' Law Considered. August 12, 2018. https://www.bbc.co.uk/news/uk-45154708. Accessed October 17, 2019.

# References

## Boats

1. BBC News. Costa Concordia Wreck Raised from Under-Sea Platform. July 14, 2014. https://www.bbc.co.uk/news/world-europe-28288823. Accessed January 15, 2020.

2. BBC News. Charlotte Brown: Man Guilty of First Date Speedboat Death. July 26, 2018. https://www.bbc.co.uk/news/uk-england-london-44924244. Accessed January 15, 2020.

3. Dangerfield A. Marchioness Survivors and Victims' Families Recall Thames Disaster. August 20, 2014. BBC News. https://www.bbc.co.uk/news/uk-england-london-28839099. Accessed January 15, 2020.

4. Mrad M. Tragedy as British Man, 46, is Crushed to Death after Trying to Secure a Dinghy in Rough Waters. *Daily Mail.* April 28, 2019. https://www.dailymail.co.uk/news/article-6968475/Tragedy-British-man-46-crushed-death-trying-secure-dingy-rough-waters.html. Accessed January 15, 2020.

5. European Maritime Safety Agency. *Annual Overview of Marine Casualties and Incidents 2019.* 2019. https://www.iims.org.uk/wp-content/uploads/2019/11/EMSA-Annual-Overview-of-Marine-Casualties-and-Incidents-2019.pdf.

6. ICC International Maritime Bureau. *Piracy and Armed Robbery Against Ships: Report for the Period 1 January – 31 December 2018.* January 2019. https://www.icc-ccs.org/reports/2018_Annual_IMB_Piracy_Report.pdf.

7. U.S. Department of Homeland Security, United States Coast Guard. *2018 Recreational Boating Statistics.* August 19, 2019. https://www.iims.org.uk/wp-content/uploads/2019/08/USCG-Recreational-Boating-Statistics-2018.pdf.

8. Griffin S. Top 11 Causes of Boating Accidents. *Boating Safety.* March 1, 2019. https://www.boatingsafetymag.com/boatingsafety/top-11-causes-boating-accidents. Accessed January 15, 2020.

9. Ahola M., Mugge R. Safety in Passenger Ships: The Influence of Environmental Design Characteristics on People's Perception of Safety. *Appl Ergon.* 2017;59(Pt A):143–152.

## Walking

1. NHS. Walking for Health. https://www.nhs.uk/live-well/exercise/walking-for-health/. Accessed January 9, 2020.

2. De Moor D. *Walking Works.* Walking for Health. October 2013. https://www.walkingforhealth.org.uk/sites/default/files/Walking works_LONG_AW_Web.pdf.

3. Kraus W. E., Janz K. F., Powell K. E., et al. Daily Step Counts for Measuring Physical Activity Exposure and its Relation to Health. *Med Sci Sport Exerc.* 2019;51(6):1206–1212.

4. Tudor-Locke C., Craig C. L., Brown W. J., et al. How Many Steps/Day are Enough? For Adults. *Int J Behav Nutr Phys Act.* 2011; 8: 79.

5. United Nations Road Safety Collaboration. Pedestrian Safety: A Road Safety Manual for Decision-Makers and Practitioners. https://www.who.int/road-safety/projects/manuals/pedestrian/en/. Accessed January 9, 2020.
6. National Highway Traffic Safety Administration. Pedestrian Safety. https://www.nhtsa.gov/road-safety/pedestrian-safety. Accessed January 9, 2020.
7. Burtscher M., Pachinger O., Schocke M. F., et al. Risk Factor Profile for Sudden Cardiac Death during Mountain Hiking. *Int J Sports Med.* 2007;28(7):621–624.

## Part Twelve: Dangerous Sports

### Skiing and snowboarding

1. De Roulet A., Inaba K., Strumwasser A., et al. Severe Injuries Associated with Skiing and Snowboarding: A National Trauma Data Bank Study. *J Trauma Acute Care Surg.* 2017;82(4):781–786.
2. Wasden C. C., McIntosh S. E., Keith D. S., et al. An Analysis of Skiing and Snowboarding Injuries on Utah Slopes. *J Trauma.* 2009;67(5):1022–1026.
3. Xiang H., Stallones L., Smith G. A. Downhill Skiing Injury Fatalities among Children. *Inj Prev.* 2004;10(2):99–102.
4. Flanagan O. Danger on the Slopes: How Risky is Skiing? *Significance.* January 7, 2014. https://www.statslife.org.uk/sports/1157-danger-on-the-slopes-how-risky-is-skiing. Accessed December 29, 2019.
5. Kwiatkowski T. Safety Helmets for Skiers and Snowboarders – Efficacy, Safety and Fitting Principles: Review of Literature. *Przegl Lek.* 2015;72(8):428–431.
6. Haider A. H., Saleem T., Bilaniuk J. W., et al. An Evidence-Based Review: Efficacy of Safety Helmets in the Reduction of Head Injuries in Recreational Skiers and Snowboarders. *J Trauma Acute Care Surg.* 2012;73(5): 1340–1347.
7. Buller D. B., Andersen P. A., Walkosz B. J., et al. Compliance with Sunscreen Advice in a Survey of Adults Engaged in Outdoor Winter Recreation at High-Elevation Ski Areas. *J Am Acad Dermatol.* 2012;66(1):63–70.

### Climbing and mountaineering

1. Heggie T. W, Caine D. J., eds. *Epidemiology of Injury in Adventure and Extreme Sports.* Kargel; 2012. https://www.karger.com/Book/Home/256975.
2. Burtscher M., Ponchia A. The Risk of Cardiovascular Events During Leisure Time Activities at Altitude. *Prog Cardiovasc Dis.* 2010;52(6):507–511.
3. Windsor J. S., Firth P. G., Grocott M. P., et al. Mountain Mortality: A Review of Deaths that Occur during Recreational Activities in the Mountains. *Postgrad Med J.* 2009;85(1004):316–321.

4. NHS. Altitude Sickness. https://www.nhs.uk/conditions/Altitude-sickness/. Accessed November 7, 2019.
5. Firth P. G., Zheng H., Windsor J. S., et al. Mortality on Mount Everest, 1921–2006: Descriptive Study. *BMJ*. 2008;337:a2654.
6. Lake District Search & Mountain Rescue Association. *Mountain Accidents 2015*. http://www.ldsamra.org.uk/documents/LDSAMRAAnnualReport 2015.pdf.
7. Morris H. Lake District Mountains to be Graded like Ski Runs after Rise in Hiker Deaths. *Telegraph*. May 9, 2018. https://www.telegraph.co.uk/travel/ destinations/europe/united-kingdom/england/cumbria/lake-district/articles/ mountain-walks-graded-like-ski-pistes/. Accessed November 7, 2019.

## Parachuting and bungee jumping

1. Laver L., Pengas I. P., Mei-Dan O. Injuries in Extreme Sports. *J Orthop Surg Res*. 2017;12(59).
2. Cevik A. A., Kaya F. B., Acar N., et al. Injury, Hospitalization, and Operation Rates are Low in Aerial Sports. *Turkish J Emerg Med*. 2017;17(3):81–84.
3. British Skydiving. How Safe? https://britishskydiving.org/how-safe/. Accessed February 5, 2020.
4. Soreide K., Ellingson C. L., Knutson V. How Dangerous is BASE Jumping? An Analysis of Adverse Events in 20,850 Jumps from the Kjerag Massif, Norway. *J Trauma*. 2007;62(5):1113–1117.
5. Parker F. Girl Fell to Death on Bungee Jump after Mishearing Spanish Instructor's English. *Metro*. June 26, 2017. https://metro.co.uk/2017/06/26/ girl-fell-to-death-on-bungee-jump-after-mishearing-spanish-instructors-english-6736813/. Accessed December 30, 2019.
6. Graham B. Investigators Looking into Mystery Bungee Death. News. com.au. January 15, 2018. https://www.news.com.au/travel/travel-updates/incidents/investigators-looking-into-mystery-bungee-death/ news-story/d65c7c9c946068c214a7bf53a9c48dcf. Accessed December 30, 2019.
7. Søreide K. The Epidemiology of Injury in Bungee Jumping, BASE Jumping, and Skydiving. *Med Sport Sci*. 2012;58:112–129.
8. Fitzgerald J. J., Bassi S., White B. D. A Subdural Haematoma following 'Reverse' Bungee Jumping. *Br J Neurosurg*. 2002;16(3):307–308.
9. Hsieh M. T., Sun I. T., Chen C. H. Ocular Injuries after Bungee Jumping: A Case Report and Literature Review. *Taiwan J Opthalmology*. 2018;8(1):52–54.
10. Malone K. Train Surfing: It's Like Bungee Jumping without a Rope. In: Gilbert K., ed. *Sport, Culture & Society Vol 6: Sexuality, Sport and the Culture of Risk*. Meyer & Meyer Sport; 2005.

11. Strauch H., Wirth I., Geserick G. Fatal Accidents due to Train Surfing in Berlin. *Forensic Sci Int*. 1998;94(1–2):119–127.

## Hunting

1. Loder R. T., Farren N. Injuries from Firearms in Hunting Activities. *Injury*. 2014;45(8):1207–1214.
2. Bestetti V., Fisher E. E., Srivastava D. S., et al. If Hunters End Up in the Emergency Room: A Retrospective Analysis of Hunting Injuries in a Swiss Emergency Department. *Emerg Med Int*. 2015;2015:284908.
3. BBC News. Italian Boar Hunt Ends in Son Shooting his own Father. September 23, 2019. https://www.bbc.co.uk/news/world-europe-49791223. Accessed November 5, 2019.
4. Hamilton K., Rocque B., Brooks N. Spine and Spinal Cord Injuries after Falls from Tree Stands during the Wisconsin Deer Hunting Season. *WMJ*. 2017;116(4):201–205.
5. Mele, C. Rhino Poacher Killed by Elephant and Eaten by Lions, Officials Say. *New York Times*. April 7, 2019. https://www.nytimes.com/2019/04/07/world/africa/south-africa-poacher-rhino-lions.html. Accessed November 3, 2019.
6. Barnes T. Big Game Hunter 'Gored to Death by Buffalo' Moments after Shooting Another Member of Herd. *Independent*. May 30, 2018. https://www.independent.co.uk/news/world/africa/hunter-dead-buffallo-south-africa-big-game-claude-kleynhans-gored-a8376351.html. Accessed November 3, 2019.
7. BBC News. Hunter Killed in Attack by Polar Bear in Canada. August 29, 2018. https://www.bbc.co.uk/news/world-us-canada-45324627. Accessed November 5, 2019.
8. Kasturiratne A., Wickremasinghe A. R., De Silva N., et al. The Global Burden of Snakebite: A Literature Analysis and Modelling Based on Regional Estimates of Envenoming and Deaths. *PLoS Med*. 2008;5(11):e218.
9. Wootson C. R. Jr. Kenyan Officials did Little when a Hippo Killed a Local, Critics Say. Then a Foreigner was Mauled. *Washington Post*. August 13, 2018. https://www.washingtonpost.com/news/animalia/wp/2018/08/13/kenyan-officials-did-little-when-a-hippo-killed-a-local-critics-say-then-a-foreigner-was-mauled/. Accessed November 3, 2019.
10. Lyons K. Australian Crocodiles Blamed for Spate of Deaths in Timor-Leste. *Guardian*. June 11, 2019. https://www.theguardian.com/world/2019/jun/11/australian-crocodiles-blamed-for-spate-of-deaths-in-timor-leste. Accessed November 3, 2019.
11. Riches K. J., Gillis D., James R. A. An Autopsy Approach to Bee Sting-Related Deaths. *Pathology*. 2002;34(3):257–262.

12. HSE. *Overview of Fatal Incidents Involving Cattle.* 2015. http://www.hse.gov. uk/aboutus/meetings/iacs/aiac/090615/aiac-paper-150601.pdf. Accessed November 3, 2019.
13. Medical Equestrian Association. Risks of Injury & Risk Management. https: //www.medequestrian.co.uk/rider-safety/benefits-and-risks-of-riding/risks-of -injury-risk-management/. Accessed February 5, 2020.

## Motor racing

1. Laughlin L. The Isle of Men: The World's Deadliest Race. *Time.* August 2014. https://time.com/3071064/deadliest-race/.
2. Matthews J. Rally Death Spectators 'Not Warned' by Organisers, Inquiry Finds. Sky News. November 21, 2017. https://news.sky.com/story/rally-death-spectators-not-warned-by-organisers-inquiry-finds-11137073. Accessed November 7, 2019.
3. Oliver M. Three Die in Isle of Man TT Race Crash. *Guardian.* June 8, 2007. https://www.theguardian.com/uk/2007/jun/08/markoliver. Accessed November 6, 2019.
4. Knight S., Cook L. J., Olson L. M. The Fast and the Fatal: Street Racing Fatal Crashes in the United States. *Inj Prev.* 2004;10(1):53–55.
5. Queally J., Santa Cruz N. Out of Control: 17 Years. 179 Victims. The Deadly Toll of Street Racing in Los Angeles. *Los Angeles Times.* March 16, 2018. https://www.latimes.com/projects/la-me-street-racing/. Accessed November 6, 2019.
6. Wickens C., Smart R., Vingilis E., et al. Street Racing among the Ontario Adult Population: Prevalence and Association with Collision Risk. *Accid Anal Prev.* 2017;103:85–91.
7. Neundorf M. Never Forget that Motor Racing can be Deadly. *Gear Patrol.* September 25, 2015. https://gearpatrol.com/2015/09/25/dangers-of-motor-racing/. Accessed November 6, 2019.
8. Formula One World Championship. History of F1 Safety. https://www. formula1.com/en/championship/inside-f1/safety/history-of-F1-safety.html. Accessed November 7, 2019.
9. Kaul A., Abbas A., Smith G., et al. A Revolution in Preventing Fatal Craniovertebral Junction Injuries: Lessons Learned from the Head and Neck Support Device in Professional Auto Racing. *J Neurosurg Spine.* 2016;25(6):756–761.

## Scuba diving

1. Buzzacott P., Moore J. P., Bennett C. M., et al. *DAN Annual Diving Report 2018 Edition: A Report on 2016 Diving Fatalities, Injuries, and Incidents.* Divers Alert Network; 2018.

2. Vann R., Lang M., eds. *Recreational Diving Fatalities Workshop Proceedings*. Divers Alert Network. April 8–10, 2010. https://www.diversalertnetwork.org /files/Fatalities_Proceedings.pdf.
3. RoSPA. Tombstoning – 'Don't Jump into the Unknown'. https://www.rospa. com/Leisure-Safety/Water/Advice/Tombstoning. Accessed October 25, 2019.
4. Keegan N. Dive Danger: What is Tombstoning, Why is the Craze so Dangerous and How Many People have Died From It so far in the UK? All You Need to Know. *Sun*. June 22, 2017. https://www.thesun.co.uk/living/ 2632545/what-is-tombstoning-deaths-dangerous-uk/. Accessed October 15, 2019.

## Contact sports

1. McCabe P. How Many More Young People Must Die before Mixed Martial Arts is Banned? *Guardian*. April 15, 2016. https://www.theguardian.com/ commentisfree/2016/apr/15/mixed-martial-arts-mma-banned-joao-carvalho -fighter. Accessed January 27, 2020.
2. Drewett Z. Female MMA Fighter, 26, Dies from Brain Injury during Fight. *Metro*. November 19, 2019. https://metro.co.uk/2019/11/19/female- mma-fighter-26-dies-brain-injury-fight-11178931/. Accessed January 27, 2020.
3. Cacciola S. After Two Deaths Days Apart, Boxing Examines its Risks. *New York Times*. August 7, 2019. https://www.nytimes.com/2019/08/07/sports/- boxing-deaths.html. Accessed January 27, 2020.
4. Graham B. A. Two Deaths a Chilling Reminder of the Perils that Lurk in the Ring. *Guardian*. July 27, 2019. https://www.theguardian.com/sport/blog/ 2019/jul/27/boxing-deaths-reform-perils-ring. Accessed January 27, 2020.
5. Jones J. RIP Cowboy: Dwight Ritchie Dead at 27: Australian Boxer Dies in Freak 'Body Shot' Accident in Training after Twice Overcoming Cancer. *Sun*. November 9, 2019. https://www.thesun.co.uk/sport/10310367/dwight- ritchie-dead-27-australian-boxer-overcame-cancer-freak-accident-body-shot- training/. Accessed January 27, 2020.
6. Sawauchi S., Murakami S., Tani S., et al. Acute Subdural Hematoma caused by Professional Boxing. *No Shinkei Geka*. 1996;24(10):905–911.
7. Svinth J. R. Death under the Spotlight: The Manuel Velazquez Boxing Fatality Collection. *J Combat Sport*. October 2011. https://ejmas.com/jcs/ velazquez/Death_Under_the_Spotlight_2011_Final.pdf.
8. Thomas R. E., Thomas B. C. Systematic Review of Injuries in Mixed Martial Arts. *Phys Sportsmed*. 2018;46(2):155–167.
9. Jayarao M., Chin L. S., Cantu R. C. Boxing-Related Head Injuries. *Phys Sportsmed*. 2010;38(3):18–26.

10. Blecher R., Elliott M. A., Yilmaz E., et al. Contact Sports as a Risk Factor for Amyotrophic Lateral Sclerosis: A Systematic Review. *Global Spine J.* 2019;9(1):104–118.

11. McGran K. Hockey Player Dies after Fight. *Star.* January 3, 2009. https://www.thestar.com/news/gta/2009/01/03/hockey_player_dies_after_fight.html. Accessed January 27, 2020.

12. Deady B., Innes G. Sudden Death of a Young Hockey Player: Case Report of Commotio Cordis. *J Emerg Med.* 1999;17(3):459–462.

13. CBC News. Teen Hockey Player Dies after Puck Hits Throat. November 13, 2011 https://www.cbc.ca/news/canada/edmonton/teen-hockey-player-dies-after-puck-hits-throat-1.1066488. Accessed January 27, 2020.

14. *Los Angeles Times.* On-Ice Accident Kills Hockey Player. October 17, 1995. https://www.latimes.com/archives/la-xpm-1995-10-17-sp-57816-story.html. Accessed January 27, 2020.

15. Bull A. France Facing Up to Clamour for Rugby to Change after Spate of Tragedies. *Guardian.* December 18, 2018. https://www.theguardian.com/global/2018/dec/18/france-rugby-union-deaths. Accessed January 27, 2020.

16. Fortington L. V., Bekker S., Finch C. F. Online News Media Reporting of Football-Related Fatalities in Australia: A Matter of Life *and* Death. *J Sci Med Sport.* 2018;21(3):245–249.

17. Willingham A. J. Deaths on College and High School Football Fields are a Rare – but Reliable – Tragedy. CNN Health. October 1, 2018. https://edition.cnn.com/2018/09/21/health/football-deaths-season-injuries-high-school-college-trnd/index.html. Accessed January 27, 2020.

18. Schad T. Indonesian Soccer Player Dies after Collision with Teammate. *USA Today.* December 14, 2019. https://eu.usatoday.com/story/sports/soccer/2017/10/16/indonesian-soccer-player-choirul-huda-dies-collision-teammate/768472001/. Accessed January 27, 2020.

19. Fuller C. W. Catastrophic Injury in Rugby Union: Is the Level of Risk Acceptable? *Sport Med.* 2008;38(12):975–986.

20. De Menezes J. Phil Hughes Dead: List of Players who have Tragically Died on the Cricket Pitch. *Independent.* November 17, 2014. https://www.independent.co.uk/sport/cricket/phil-hughes-dead-list-of-players-who-have-tragically-died-on-the-cricket-pitch-9886460.html. Accessed January 27, 2020.

21. Clarke-Billings L. Hockey Player Died after Being Hit with Stick in Freak Accident. *Telegraph.* December 11, 2015. https://www.telegraph.co.uk/news/uknews/12046979/Hockey-player-died-after-being-hit-with-stick-in-freak-accident.html. Accessed January 27, 2020.

22. Callow J. Brazilian Futsal Player Dies in Freak Accident. *Guardian.* March 8, 2010. https://www.theguardian.com/sport/2010/mar/08/futsal-player-dies. Accessed January 27, 2020.

## Part Thirteen: Other Hazards

*Carbon monoxide*
1. NHS. Carbon Monoxide Poisoning. https://www.nhs.uk/conditions/carbon-monoxide-poisoning/. Accessed July 13, 2019.
2. RoSPA. Carbon Monoxide – The Silent Killer. https://www.rospa.com/home-safety/advice/carbon-monoxide-safety/. Accessed July 13, 2019.
3. Haines D. Carbon Monoxide Poisoning. *Med Leg J*. 2016;84(2):59.
4. Berezow A. Carbon Monoxide Kills More Americans than Mass Shootings, Terrorism Combined. American Council on Science and Health. March 6, 2017. https://www.acsh.org/news/2017/03/06/carbon-monoxide-kills-more-americans-mass-shootings-terrorism-combined-10954. Accessed July 13, 2019.

*Drowning*
1. WHO. Drowning. https://www.who.int/news-room/fact-sheets/detail/drowning. Accessed June 27, 2019.
2. National Water Safety Forum. Reports and Data. https://www.nationalwater-safety.org.uk/waid/reports-and-data/. Accessed June 27, 2019.
3. RoSPA. *Delivering Accident Prevention at Local Level in the New Public Health System*. March 2013. https://www.rospa.com/rospaweb/docs/advice-services/public-health/delivering-accident-prevention-context.pdf. Accessed June 27, 2019.
4. Leavy J. E., Crawford G., Portsmouth L., et al. Recreational Drowning Prevention Interventions for Adults, 1990–2012: A Review. *J Community Health*. 2015;40(4):725–735.
5. RoSPA. *Assessing Inland Accidental Drowning Risk*. https://www.rospa.com/rospaweb/docs/advice-services/leisure-safety/inland-waters-risk-assessment.pdf. Accessed June 27, 2019.
6. Szpilman D., Orlowski J. P. Sports Related to Drowning. *Eur Respir Rev*. 2016;25:348–359.

*Choking*
1. Kramarow E., Warner M., Chen L. H. Food-Related Choking Deaths among the Elderly. *Inj Prev*. 2014;20(3):200–203.
2. ONS. Choking Related Deaths Registered in England and Wales, 2014 to 2017. November 26, 2018. https://www.ons.gov.uk/peoplepopulationand-community/birthsdeathsandmarriages/deaths/adhocs/009342chokingrelated-deathsregisteredinenglandandwales2014to2017. Accessed December 27, 2019.

3. Harvard Medical School. Choking Alert: Strategies for Safe Swallowing. September 2016. https://www.health.harvard.edu/staying-healthy/choking-alert-strategies-for-safe-swallowing. Accessed December 27, 2019.
4. Toblin R. L., Paulozzi L. J., Gilchrist J., et al. Unintentional Strangulation Deaths from the 'Choking Game' among Youths Aged 6–19 Years – United States, 1995–2007. *J Safety Res*. 2008;39(4):445–448.
5. Gowens P. A., Davenport R. J., Kerr J., et al. Survival from Accidental Strangulation from a Scarf Resulting in Laryngeal Rupture and Carotid Artery Stenosis: The 'Isadora Duncan Syndrome'. A Case Report and Review of Literature. *Emerg Med J*. 2003;20(4):391–393.
6. Gharbaoui M., Naceur Y., Hmandi O., et al. Accidental and Occupational Ligature Strangulation in Northern Tunisia: Four-Case Study. *Egypt J Forensic Sci*. 2018;8:51.

## Hazardous jobs

1. HSE. *Workplace Fatal Injuries in Great Britain, 2019*. July 3, 2019. http://www.hse.gov.uk/statistics/pdf/fatalinjuries.pdf.
2. Davis M. E. Perceptions of Occupational Risk by US Commercial Fishermen. *Mar Policy*. 2012;36(1):28–33.
3. Bureau of Labor Statistics. *National Census of Fatal Occupational Injuries in 2017*. 2018. https://www.bls.gov/news.release/pdf/cfoi.pdf. Accessed November 3, 2019.
4. Safe Work Australia. Fatality Statistics by Occupation. 2016. https://www.safeworkaustralia.gov.au/statistics-and-research/statistics/fatalities/fatality-statistics-occupation. Accessed November 3, 2019.
5. Buckley J. P., Hedge A., Yates T., et al. The Sedentary Office: An Expert Statement on the Growing Case for Change Towards Better Health and Productivity. *Br J Sports Med*. 2015;49:1357–1362.
6. Gardner B., Smith L., Mansfield L. How did the Public Respond to the 2015 Expert Consensus Public Health Guidance Statement on Workplace Sedentary Behaviour? A Qualitative Analysis. *BMC Public Health*. 2017;17(47).

## High blood pressure

1. NHS. What is Blood Pressure? https://www.nhs.uk/common-health-questions/lifestyle/what-is-blood-pressure/. Accessed June 23, 2019.
2. PHE. Health Matters: Combating High Blood Pressure. January 24, 2017. https://www.gov.uk/government/publications/health-matters-combating-high-blood-pressure/health-matters-combating-high-blood-pressure. Accessed June 23, 2019.
3. Bundy J. D., Li C., Stuchlik P., et al. Systolic Blood Pressure Reduction and Risk of Cardiovascular Disease and Mortality: A Systematic Review and Network Meta-Analysis. *JAMA Cardiol*. 2017;2(7):775–781.

4. Rico-Campà A., Martínez-González M. A., Alvarez-Alvarez I., et al. Association between Consumption of Ultra-Processed Foods and All Cause Mortality: SUN Prospective Cohort Study. *BMJ*. 2019;365:l1949.
5. Post Hospers G., Smulders Y. M., Maier A. B., et al. Relation between Blood Pressure and Mortality Risk in an Older Population: Role of Chronological and Biological Age. *J Intern Med*. 2015;277(4):488–497.

## Infectious diseases

1. WHO. Infectious Diseases. https://www.who.int/topics/infectious_diseases/en/. Accessed January 18, 2020.
2. MedlinePlus. Infectious Diseases. https://medlineplus.gov/infectiousdiseases.html. Accessed January 18, 2020.
3. WHO. Campylobacter. January 23, 2018. https://www.who.int/news-room/fact-sheets/detail/campylobacter. Accessed January 18, 2020.
4. Bok K., Green K. Y. Norovirus Gastroenteritis in Immunocompromised Patients. *N Engl J Med*. 2013;368(10):971.
5. WHO. What is a Pandemic? February 24, 2010. https://www.who.int/csr/disease/swineflu/frequently_asked_questions/pandemic/en/. Accessed January 18, 2020.
6. WHO. *A Brief Guide to Emerging Infectious Diseases and Zoonoses*. 2014. https://apps.who.int/iris/bitstream/handle/10665/204722/B5123.pdf.
7. Baylor College of Medicine. Emerging Infectious Diseases. https://www.bcm.edu/departments/molecular-virology-and-microbiology/emerging-infections-and-biodefense/emerging-infectious-diseases. Accessed January 18, 2020.
8. CDC. 2009 H1N1 Pandemic (H1N1pdm09 virus). https://www.cdc.gov/flu/pandemic-resources/2009-h1n1-pandemic.html. Accessed January 18, 2020.
9. WHO. FAQs: H5N1 Influenza. https://www.who.int/influenza/human_animal_interface/avian_influenza/h5n1_research/faqs/en/. Accessed January 18, 2020.
10. WHO. Antibiotic Resistance. February 5, 2018. https://www.who.int/news-room/fact-sheets/detail/antibiotic-resistance. Accessed January 18, 2020.
11. IHME. Global Burden of Disease. http://www.healthdata.org/gbd. Accessed November 7, 2019.

## Mobile phones

1. NHS. Mobile Phone Safety. https://www.nhs.uk/conditions/mobile-phone-safety/. Accessed November 8, 2019.
2. Grimes D. R. Mobile Phones and Cancer – The Full Picture. *Observer*. July 21, 2018. https://www.theguardian.com/technology/2018/jul/21/mobile-phones-are-not-a-health-hazard. Accessed November 8, 2019.

3. National Cancer Institute. Cell Phones and Cancer Risk. https://www.cancer. gov/about-cancer/causes-prevention/risk/radiation/cell-phones-fact-sheet. Accessed November 8, 2019.
4. PHE. Mobile Phone Base Stations: Radio Waves and Health. May 16, 2019. https://www.gov.uk/government/publications/mobile-phone-base-stations-radio-waves-and-health/mobile-phone-base-stations-radio-waves-and-health. Accessed November 8, 2019.
5. Di Ciaula A. Towards 5G Communication Systems: Are there Health Implications? *Int J Hyg Environ Health*. 2018;221(3):367–375.
6. BBC News. Does 5G Pose Health Risks? July 15, 2019. https://www.bbc. co.uk/news/world-europe-48616174. Accessed November 8, 2019.
7. PHE. 5G Technologies: Radio Waves and Health. October 3, 2019. https://www.gov.uk/government/publications/5g-technologies-radio-waves-and-health/5g-technologies-radio-waves-and-health#summary. Accessed November 8, 2019.
8. WHO. Electromagnetic Fields and Public Health: Base stations and Wireless Technologies. May 2006. https://www.who.int/peh-emf/publications/facts/fs304/en/. Accessed November 8, 2019.

## Fairground rides and amusement parks

1. HSE. *Fairgrounds and Amusement Parks: Guidance on Safe Practice.* 3rd ed. November 2017. https://www.hse.gov.uk/pubns/priced/hsg175.pdf
2. Woodcock K. Global Incidence of Theme Park and Amusement Ride Accidents. *Saf Sci.* 2019;113:171–179.
3. Barnes T. Designers of Water Slide that Decapitated Boy 'Had No Technical Qualifications'. *Independent.* March 24, 2018. https://www.independent. co.uk/news/world/americas/water-slide-boy-verr-ckt-child-death-decapitation-designers-no-qualifications-schlitterbahn-a8272036.html. Accessed January 18, 2020.
4. Newton S. Fairgrounds: Accidents: Written question – 213367. https://www. parliament.uk/business/publications/written-questions-answers-statements/written-question/Commons/2019-01-29/213367/. Accessed January 18, 2020.
5. CPSC. *NEISS Data Highlights – Calendar Year 2018.* 2018. https://www. cpsc.gov/s3fs-public/2018 Neiss data highlights.pdf.
6. HSE. Bouncy Castles and Other Play Inflatables: Safety Advice. https://www. hse.gov.uk/entertainment/fairgrounds/inflatables.htm. Accessed January 18, 2020.
7. Siddique H. Pair Held Over Death of Girl Thrown from Inflatable Trampoline. *Guardian.* July 12, 2018. https://www.theguardian.com/uk-news/2018/jul/12/pair-held-over-death-of-girl-thrown-from-inflatable-trampoline-arrest-norfolk. Accessed January 18, 2020.

8. Feng J., Truelove S. Girl, 8, Crushed to Death after Inflatable Water Slide Collapses at Holiday Resort. *Mirror.* July 22, 2019. https://www.mirror.co.uk /news/world-news/girl-8-crushed-death-after-18633528. Accessed January 18, 2020.

9. Woodcock K. Amusement Ride Injury Data in the United States. *Saf Sci.* 2014;62:466–474.

10. Szeszet-Fedorowicz W. *Estimated Number of Injuries and Reported Deaths Associated with Inflatable Amusements, 2003–2013.* US Consumer Product Safety Comission. February 2015. https://www.cpsc.gov/s3fs-public/ Inflatable_Amusements_Deaths_and_Injuries_2015.pdf.

## Part Fourteen: Stuff You Can't Do Anything About

### Genes

1. NIH. Is Longevity Determined by Genetics? https://ghr.nlm.nih.gov/primer /traits/longevity. Accessed December 30, 2019.

2. Donlon T. A., Morris B. J., Chen R., et al. Analysis of Polymorphisms in 59 Potential Candidate Genes for Association with Human Longevity. *Journals Gerontol Ser A Biol Sci Med Sci.* 2018;73(11):1459–1464.

3. Moskalev A. A., Aliper A. M., Smit-McBride Z., et al. Genetics and Epigenetics of Aging and Longevity. *Cell Cycle.* 2014;13(7):1063–1077.

4. Van Raamsdonk J. M. Mechanisms Underlying Longevity: A Genetic Switch Model of Aging. *Exp Gerontol.* 2018;107:136–139.

5. Rappaport S. M. Genetic Factors are not the Major Causes of Chronic Diseases. *PLoS One.* 2016;11(4):e0154387.

6. WHO. Human Genomics in Global Health: Genes and Human Diseases. https://www.who.int/genomics/public/geneticdiseases/en/index3.html. Accessed December 30, 2019.

### Height

1. Davey-Smith G., Hart C., Upton M., et al. Height and Risk of Death among Men and Women: Aetiological Implications of Associations with Cardiorespiratory Disease and Cancer Mortality. *J Epidemiol Community Health.* 2000;54(2):97–103.

2. Perkins J. M., Subramanian S. V., Davey-Smith G., et al. Adult Height, Nutrition, and Population Health. *Nutr Rev.* 2016;74(3):149–165.

3. Keeshan B. C., Rossano J. W., Beck N., et al. Lung Transplant Waitlist Mortality: Height as a Predictor of Poor Outcomes. *Pediatr Transplant.* 2015;19(3):294–300.

4. Rohrmann S., Haile S. R., Staub K., et al. Body Height and Mortality: Mortality Follow-Up of Four Swiss Surveys. *Prev Med.* 2017;101:67–71.

5. Davies N. M., Gaunt T. R., Lewis S. J., et al. The Effects of Height and BMI on Prostate Cancer Incidence and Mortality: A Mendelian Randomization Study in 20,848 Cases and 20,214 Controls from the PRACTICAL Consortium. *Cancer Cause Control.* 2015;26(11):1603–1616.

## Race, ethnicity and country of birth

1. Betancourt J. R., Green A. R., Carrillo J. E., et al. Defining Cultural Competence: A Practical Framework for Addressing Racial/Ethnic Disparities in Health and Health Care. *Public Health Rep.* 2003;118(4):293–302.
2. PHE. *Public Health Outcomes Framework: Health Equity Report Focus on Ethnicity.* July 2017. https://assets.publishing.service.gov.uk/government/uploads/system/uploads/attachment_data/file/733093/PHOF_Health_Equity_Report.pdf.
3. Wohland P., Rees P., Nazroo J., et al. Inequalities in Healthy Life Expectancy between Ethnic Groups in England and Wales in 2001. *Ethn Health.* 2015;20(4):341–353.
4. Gruer L., Cézard G., Clark E., et al. Life Expectancy of Different Ethnic Groups using Death Records Linked to Population Census Data for 4.62 Million People in Scotland. *J Epidemiol Community Health.* 2016;70(12):1251–1254.
5. Race Disparity Unit. Ethnicity Facts and Figures: Health. https://www.ethnicity-facts-figures.service.gov.uk/health. Accessed November 11, 2019.
6. Lortet-Tieulent J., Soerjomataram I., Lin C. C., et al. U.S. Burden of Cancer by Race and Ethnicity According to Disability-Adjusted Life Years. *Am J Prev Med.* 2016;51(5):673–681.
7. Turner R. J., Brown T. N., Hale W. B. Race, Socioeconomic Position, and Physical Health: A Descriptive Analysis. *J Health Soc Behav.* 2017;58(1):23–36.
8. Assari S. Life Expectancy Gain Due to Employment Status Depends on Race, Gender, Education, and their Intersections. *J Racial Ethn Heal Disparities.* 2018;5(2):375–386.
9. Wallace S., Nazroo J., Bécares L. Cumulative Effect of Racial Discrimination on the Mental Health of Ethnic Minorities in the United Kingdom. *Am J Public Health.* 2016;106(7):1294–1300.
10. Paradies Y., Ben J., Denson N., et al. Racism as a Determinant of Health: A Systematic Review and Meta-Analysis. *PLoS One.* 2015;10(9):e0138511.
11. Levine R. S., Foster J. E., Fullilove R. E., et al. Black-White Inequalities in Mortality and Life Expectancy, 1933–1999: Implications for Healthy People 2010. *Public Health Rep.* 2001;116(5):474–483.
12. Shiels M. S., Chernyavskiy P., Anderson W. F., et al. Trends in Premature Mortality in the USA by Sex, Race, and Ethnicity from 1999 to 2014: An Analysis of Death Certificate Data. *Lancet.* 2017;389(10073):1043–1054.

13. Khan S. Q., Berrington de Gonzalez A., Best A. F., et al. Infant and Youth Mortality Trends by Race/Ethnicity and Cause of Death in the United States. *JAMA Pediatr.* 2018;172(12):e183317.

## Biological sex

1. ONS. Most Affluent Man Outlives the Average Woman for the First Time. October 21, 2015. https://www.ons.gov.uk/peoplepopulationandcommunity /birthsdeathsandmarriages/lifeexpectancies/articles/mostaffluentmanoutlives theaveragewomanforthefirsttime/2015-10-21. Accessed December 28, 2019.
2. PHE. Mortality Profile. https://fingertips.phe.org.uk/profile/mortality-profile. Accessed December 28, 2019.
3. ONS. *Avoidable Mortality in the UK: 2016.* April 18, 2018. https://www.ons. gov.uk/releases/avoidablemortalityinenglandandwales2016.       Accessed December 28, 2019.
4. Men's Health Forum. Key Data: Alcohol and Smoking. December 2014; March 2017. https://www.menshealthforum.org.uk/key-data-alcohol-and-smoking. Accessed December 28, 2019.
5. Men's Health Forum. Key Data: Mental Health – Statistics on Mental Health and Men. June 2016; September 2017. https://www.menshealthforum.org. uk/key-data-mental-health. Accessed December 28, 2019.
6. Men's Health Forum. Key Data: Understanding of Health and Access to Services – Statistics on Men's Health Literacy and Use of Services. https:// www.menshealthforum.org.uk/key-data-understanding-health-and-access-services. Accessed December 28, 2019.
7. Mayhew L., Harper G., Villegas A. M. *Inequalities Matter: An Investigation into the Impact of Deprivation on Demographic Inequalities in Adults.* ILC-UK. March 2018. https://ilcuk.org.uk/wp-content/uploads/2018/10/Inequalities -matter-An-investigation-into-the-impact-of-deprivation.pdf.
8. ONS. Suicides in the UK: 2017 Registrations. September 4, 2018. https:// www.ons.gov.uk/peoplepopulationandcommunity/birthsdeathsandmarriages /deaths/bulletins/suicidesintheunitedkingdom/2017registrations.       Accessed December 28, 2019.

## Sexuality

1. Cochran S. D., Mays V. M. Sexual Orientation and Mortality Among US Men Aged 17 to 59 Years: Results from the National Health and Nutrition Examination Survey III. *Am J Public Health.* 2011;101(6):1133–1138.
2. Cochran S. D., Mays V. M. Mortality Risks among Persons Reporting Same-Sex Sexual Partners: Evidence from the 2008 General Social Survey – National Death Index Data Set. *Am J Public Health.* 2015;105(2):358–364.

3. Cochran S. D., Björkenstam C., Mays V. M. Sexual Orientation and All-Cause Mortality Among US Adults Aged 18 to 59 Years, 2001–2011. *Am J Public Health*. 2016;106(5):918–920.

4. ILC. *Raising the Equality Flag: Health Inequalities among Older LGBT People in the UK*. May 2019. https://ilcuk.org.uk/wp-content/uploads/2019/05/ILC-Raising-the-equality-flag.pdf.

5. Hudson-Sharp N., Metcalf H. *Inequality among Lesbian, Gay, Bisexual and Transgender Groups in the UK: A Review of Evidence*. National Institute of Economic and Social Research. July 2016. https://assets.publishing.service.gov.uk/government/uploads/system/uploads/attachment_data/file/539682/160719_REPORT_LGBT_evidence_review_NIESR_FINALPDF.pdf

6. BBC News. Brunei Stoning: Which Places have the Death Penalty for Gay Sex? April 3, 2019. https://www.bbc.co.uk/news/world-45434583. Accessed December 29, 2019.

7. BBC News. US Man Charged with Triple Murder Targeting LGBT Victims. June 7, 2019. https://www.bbc.co.uk/news/world-us-canada-48564480. Accessed December 29, 2019.

8. Hall J. Russia Homophobic Murder: Two Detained after Man is Beaten and Tortured to Death in Anti-Gay Attack in Volgograd. *Independent*. May 14, 2013. independent.co.uk/news/world/europe/russia-homophobic-murder-two-detained-after-man-is-beaten-and-tortured-to-death-in-anti-gay-attack-8614334.html. Accessed December 29, 2019.

9. BBC News. Pair Jailed for Trafalgar Square Homophobic Killing. January 26, 2011. https://www.bbc.co.uk/news/uk-england-london-12283937. Accessed December 29, 2019.

## Left-handedness

1. McManus I. C., Moore J., Freegard M., et al. Science in the Making: Right Hand, Left Hand. III: Estimating Historical Rates of Left-Handedness. *Laterality*. 2010;15(1–2):186–208.

2. Mandal M. K., Dutta T. Left Handedness: Facts and Figures Across Cultures. *Psychol Dev Soc J*. 2001;13(2):173–191.

3. Altundag K., Isik M., Sever A. R. Handedness and Breast Cancer Characteristics. *J BUON*. 2016;21(3):576–579.

4. Martin W. L., Freitas M. B. Mean Mortality among Brazilian Left- and Right-Handers: Modification or Selective Elimination? *Laterality*. 2002; 7(1):31–44.

5. Steenhuis R. E., Østbye T., Walton R. An Examination of the Hypothesis that Left-Handers Die Earlier: The Canadian Study of Health and Aging. *Laterality*. 2001;6(1):69–75.

6. Cancer Research UK. Breast Cancer Statistics. https://www.cancerresearchuk. org/health-professional/cancer-statistics/statistics-by-cancer-type/breast-cancer. Accessed February 5, 2020.
7. Christman S. D., Henning B. R., Geers A. L., et al. Mixed-Handed Persons are More Easily Persuaded and are More Gullible: Interhemispheric Interaction and Belief Updating. *Laterality*. 2008;13(5):403–426.
8. Price M. The Left Brain Knows what the Right Hand is Doing. *Monitor*. 2009;40(1):60.
9. Barnett K. J., Corballis M. C. Ambidexterity and Magical Ideation. *Laterality*. 2002;7(1):75–84.

## Adverse childhood experiences

1. CDC. *Preventing Adverse Childhood Experiences (ACEs): Leveraging the Best Available Evidence*. 2019. https://www.cdc.gov/violenceprevention/childabuseandneglect/aces/fastfact.html. Accessed January 7, 2020.
2. NHS. Adverse Childhood Experiences (ACEs). http://www.healthscotland. scot/population-groups/children/adverse-childhood-experiences-aces/overview-of-aces. Accessed January 7, 2020.
3. Hughes K., Bellis M. A., Hardcastle K. A., et al. The Effect of Multiple Adverse Childhood Experiences on Health: A Systematic Review and Meta-Analysis. *Lancet Public Heal*. 2017;2(8):PE356–E366.
4. Ford K., Butler N., Hughes K. E., et al. *Adverse Childhood Experiences (ACEs) in Hertfordshire, Luton and Northamptonshire*. Centre for Public Health, Liverpool John Moores University. May 2016.
5. Minnesota Department of Health. Resilience to ACEs. https://www.health. state.mn.us/communities/ace/resilience.html. Accessed January 7, 2020.

## Other people's actions

1. RoSPA. Drinking and Driving Factsheet. October 2018. https://www.rospa. com/rospaweb/docs/advice-services/road-safety/drivers/drinking-and-driving.pdf. Accessed January 22, 2020.
2. The Geneva Declaration. *Global Burden of Armed Violence 2015: Every Body Counts*. May 8, 2015. http://www.genevadeclaration.org/measurability/global-burden-of-armed-violence/global-burden-of-armed-violence-2015. html.
3. Institute for Economics & Peace. *Global Terrorism Index 2019: Measuring the Impact of Terrorism*. November 2019. http://visionofhumanity.org/app/uploads/2019/11/GTI-2019web.pdf.
4. Office of Disease Prevention and Health Promotion. Determinants of Health. https://www.healthypeople.gov/2020/about/foundation-health-measures/Determinants-of-Health. Accessed January 22, 2020.

# References

5. Naik Y., Baker P., Walker I., et al. The Macro-Economic Determinants of Health and Health Inequalities: Umbrella Review Protocol. *Syst Rev.* 2017;6(1):222.
6. Nazareth M., Richards J., Javalkar K., et al. Relating Health Locus of Control to Health Care Use, Adherence, and Transition Readiness Among Youths With Chronic Conditions, North Carolina, 2015. *Prev Chronic Dis.* 2016;13:E93.

## The ageing process

1. Liochev S. I. Which is the Most Significant Cause of Aging? *Antioxidants.* 2015;4(4):793–810.
2. Campisi J., Kapahi P., Lithgow G. J., et al. From Discoveries in Ageing Research to Therapeutics for Healthy Ageing. *Nature.* 2019;571:183–192.
3. Pérez L. M., Amaral M. A., Mundstock E., et al. Effects of Diet on Telomere Length: Systematic Review and Meta-Analysis. *Public Health Genomics.* 2017;20(5):286–292.
4. Aunan J. R., Watson M. M., Hagland H. R., et al. Molecular and Biological Hallmarks of Ageing. *Br J Surg.* 2016;103(2):e29–e46.
5. Guinness World Records. Oldest Person Ever. https://www.guinnessworld records.com/world-records/oldest-person/. Accessed February 5, 2020.
6. Guinness World Records. Oldest Person Ever (Male). https://www.guinness-worldrecords.com/world-records/oldest-person-(male). Accessed February 5, 2020.
7. Hitchcott P. K., Fastame M. C., Penna M. P. More to Blue Zones than Long Life: Positive Psychological Characteristics. *Health Risk Soc.* 2018;20(3–4):163–181.
8. Chrysohoou C., Pitsavos C., Lazaros G., et al. Determinants of All-Cause Mortality and Incidence of Cardiovascular Disease (2009 to 2013) in Older Adults: The Ikaria Study of the Blue Zones. *Angiology.* 2016;67(6):541–548.
9. Buettner D., Skemp S. Blue Zones Lessons from the World's Longest Lived. *Am J Lifestyle Med.* 2016;10(5):318–321.
10. WHO. What is Healthy Ageing? https://www.who.int/ageing/healthy-ageing /en/. Accessed January 30, 2020.
11. NHS. Physical Activity Guidelines for Older Adults. https://www.nhs.uk/live -well/exercise/physical-activity-guidelines-older-adults/. Accessed August 10, 2019.
12. Tieland M., Trouwborst I., Clark B. C. Skeletal Muscle Performance and Ageing. *J Cachexia Sarcopenia Muscle.* 2018;9(1):3–19.

# Acknowledgements

The authors would like to thank:
All at Little, Brown, especially:
- Andrew McAleer, our wonderful editor, for his continuing enthusiasm, support, calmness and professionalism,
- Rebecca Sheppard for our friendly chats and for whipping the book into shape,
- Clara Diaz and Aimee Kitson for their excellent efforts in getting the book out there,
- Duncan Proudfoot for his kindness,
- Charlotte Cole for her diligent copyediting.

Stephanie Thwaites and Isobel Gahan at Curtis Brown for all their support and great ideas.

Charlie Brooker for the perfect quote for the cover.

All the celebrities for generously giving their time for free.

Gerald Beales for kindly helping compile all the hundreds of references.

Ariane would also like to thank:

David Conrad for suggesting we write this book together, and for being excellent to work with. I'm really looking forward to working together on our next book, *Happier*.

Graham Nunn for contributing jokes, letting me make lots of gags at his expense, and being the best ex-husband and friend a girl can have.

John Fleming, a.k.a. John Bon Jovial, for being an amazing illegal grandad and always helping lug my suitcase along on book tours.

Kia Abdullah for the warm and cosy author chats over a cuppa, and for always putting a smile on my face.

Emily Hill for her friendship, solidarity and support.

Nick Harrop for all his brilliantly tactful and supportive feedback and for showing me how much fun Q&As can be to write.

Lucy Spencer for bringing sunshine into my world and making my life so much fun.

Simon Le Bon and Hema Patel for giving me the courage to follow my heart and realise my dreams.

Peter Weilgony, P. A. and Simon Bligh for their much-appreciated generosity.

Angelo Marcos and James Harris for all the much-needed flat whites and writer chats.

All my incredible Patreon supporters, who generously helped fund the writing process for this book: Rik Steer, Mark White, Mary and Tim Fowler, Matthew Sylvester, Oliver Vass, Mark Ormandy, Steve Richards, Alan Brookland, Brian Engler, Jack Scanlan, Dave Nattriss, MusicalComedyGuide.com, Klaas Jan Runia, Mark Bailey, Keith Bell, Shane Jarvis, Rebekah Bennetch, Dominic McGladdery, Marcus P. Knight, Glenn Harris, Charlie Brooker, Lucy Spencer, John Fleming, Emily Hill, Gina Goldspink, Marc Alexander, Peter Weilgony, Dave Cross, Aragorn Strider and Sammy and Jelly.

My beloved Nana Shirin, aged ninety-five – sweet by name and sweet by nature – who gives me hope that one day I'll reach my nineties.

Damian Eadie, my hilarious genius soulmate, who I fell in love with after it was too late to edit all the stuff about being single out of the book! Thanks for your kindness, honesty, loyalty and for always making me laugh even when I don't feel like it. Here's to us – let's Countdown to being a hundred together!

And, most of all, my beautiful cheeky funny Lily – the best reason I could ever have for wanting to live to a hundred.

# Index

# Index

motorbikes 274, 276, 299
mould 211–13
mountain hikers 284
mountaineering 290–2
muscular strength 87–90, 112, 206

National Health Service (NHS) 145
natural disasters 234, 243–4
nature 234–9
nervous system damage 141
new psychoactive substances (NPS) 176
nitrate 101–2
norovirus 325
*Now Show, The* (TV show) 343
nutritional deficiency 140
nutritional supplements 140–2

obesity 143–6, 381
   childhood 349–50
   and diet 132, 134, 137
   and drinks 161, 163
   and marriage 5
   prevalence 143
   and social class 68
   and your neighbourhood 200
   *see also* overweight; weight gain; weight loss
     programmes
obstructive sleep apnoea 46
oesophageal cancer 129, 150
oil (fossil fuel) 275–6
oils, dietary 116–19
Okinawa 338, 368
oldest people in the world 367–8
olive oil 118, 119
omega-3 fatty acids 108–10, 117, 126
omega-6 fatty acids 117
opioids 176
Osman, Richard 106–7, 344–6, 379–80, 391
other people, actions of 365–6
ovarian cancer 258, 339
overweight 143–6, 248, 381
   and marriage 5
   prevalence 143
   and soft drinks 161
   *see also* obesity; weight gain; weight loss
     programmes
oxidation 118
oxidative stress 129, 131
oxygen 208, 234, 310
oysters 110

parabens 255–6
parachuting 293–5
Parkinson's disease 232
pedestrians, accidents involving 365
personality traits 39

pescatarians 125–6, 381
pesticides 102, 231–3
pet ownership 202–4
physical exercise 81–94, 368–70, 381
aerobic exercise 83–6
   'green' exercise 235
   and obesity 144–6
   and pets 202
   standing 91–4
   strength exercise 87–90
   *see also* cycling; gardening; walking
physical health, and subjective age 69, 70, 71
pirates 280
pneumonia 219
podcasts 47–8
policy making 365
post-traumatic stress disorder (PTSD) 57
poverty 61, 64, 66–8, 199–201, 349–50
   fuel poverty 212–13
   and healthcare 180, 181, 193–5
pregnancy 85, 109, 193–4, 231
premature ageing 250
prescription drugs 176
probiotics 137–8
processed foods 322
prostate cancer 113, 150
'protection' theories 3–4
protein 104, 108, 112–13, 121, 125
PTSD *see* post-traumatic stress disorder
Public Health England 347
puzzles 73–5

quadriceps 88

race 347–52
racism 350
radiation 328–30
randomised controlled trials (RCTs) 136
reading 76–9
relationships 1–41
religion 38–41
respiratory disease
   and air pollution 240
   and asbestos 214
   and biological sex 353
   and cleaning products 220
   and damp cold 211
   and diet 128
   and height 341, 342
   infectious 327
   and smoking 172
   *see also* lung cancer; lung disease
rheumatoid arthritis 129
right-handedness 360–1
risk-taking behaviours 353–4
Rivers, Joan 247

464